Zika and Other Neglected and Emerging Flaviviruses

Zika and Other Neglected and Emerging Flaviviruses

The Continuing Threat to Human Health

LISA A. BELTZ

ELSEVIER

Elsevier
Radarweg 29, PO Box 211, 1000 AE Amsterdam, Netherlands
The Boulevard, Langford Lane, Kidlington, Oxford OX5 1GB, United Kingdom
50 Hampshire Street, 5th Floor, Cambridge, MA 02139, United States

Notices
Knowledge and best practice in this field are constantly changing. As new research and experience broaden
our understanding, changes in research methods, professional practices, or medical treatment may become
necessary.

Practitioners and researchers must always rely on their own experience and knowledge in evaluating and
using any information, methods, compounds, or experiments described herein. In using such information or
methods they should be mindful of their own safety and the safety of others, including parties for whom they
have a professional responsibility.

To the fullest extent of the law, neither the Publisher nor the authors, contributors, or editors, assume any
liability for any injury and/or damage to persons or property as a matter of products liability, negligence or
otherwise, or from any use or operation of any methods, products, instructions, or ideas contained in the
material herein.

Library of Congress Cataloging-in-Publication Data
A catalog record for this book is available from the Library of Congress

British Library Cataloguing-in-Publication Data
A catalogue record for this book is available from the British Library

ISBN: 978-0-323-82501-6

For information on all Elsevier publications
visit our website at https://www.elsevier.com/books-and-journals

Publisher: Dolores Meloni
Acquisitions Editor: Charlotta Kryhl
Editorial Project Manager: Mona Zahir
Production Project Manager: Niranjan Bhaskaran
Cover Designer: Alan Studholme

Typeset by SPi Global, India

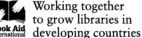

Working together
to grow libraries in
developing countries

www.elsevier.com • www.bookaid.org

I wish to dedicate this work to those children and adults affected by Zika virus diseases as well as their family members and support teams.

Contents

About the Author

Lisa A. Beltz began her career in infectious disease research in the Department of Microbiology and Public Health at Michigan State University, with a dissertation entitled "Suppression of Human T Lymphocyte Responses by *Trypanosoma cruzi*." She then spent 7 years conducting research as a post-doctoral fellow at the Johns Hopkins University Hospital System and at the University of Pittsburgh. Her research during this period focused on how simian and human immunodeficiency viruses (SIV and HIV), respectively, interact with simian and human bone marrow and blood.

Dr. Beltz then accepted a faculty position at the University of Northern Iowa, where she taught courses on biology while conducting research alongside the students she mentored. Dr. Beltz's research has investigated alterations in immune system function in response to exposure to green tea polyphenols, as well as the toxicological/immunotoxicological effects of environmental contaminants on human lymphocyte and monocyte viability and functioning. Afterward, she continued teaching while writing journal articles and books and giving conference presentations about infectious diseases of humans and bats. Dr. Beltz has previously written two books on this subject: *Emerging Infectious Diseases: A Guide to Diseases, Causative Agents, and Surveillance and Bats and Human Health*: Ebola, SARS, Rabies, and Beyond. She plans to continue writing about emerging and neglected diseases, particularly pathogenic human coronaviruses.

Acknowledgments

This book would not have been possible without the help and support of the editorial group at Elsevier Press, especially Mona Zahir, Charlotta Kryhl, and Priyadarshini Varadarajan. I also wish to acknowledge the support and help from my friends and colleagues at Malone University, especially Cindy Johnson, Gail Pigford, and Drs. Jeffery Goff and Christopher Payne, as well as Dr. Catherine Zeman at the University of Northern Iowa. Finally, I want to especially thank my family for supporting me when I virtually disappeared during the long hours of writing.

CHAPTER 1

Introduction to Flaviviruses

INTRODUCTION

The flaviviruses are the largest group of the Flaviviridae family that infects humans. Hepatitis C virus is also a member of the Flaviviridae family, but is not a flavivirus. Some flaviviruses cause severe pathology in both immunocompromised and immunocompetent people, while infection with other flaviviruses is typically asymptomatic or leads to only a mild, febrile disease. This book presents current and historical information about neglected and emerging/reemerging flaviviruses. The inclusion of historical data is important to understand the underpinnings of the current situation, especially since multiple flaviviruses are present or expanding into the same geographical area, complicating diagnoses due to the similarity of symptoms or to antigenic cross-reactivity. In some cases, including the overlapping ranges of different dengue virus (DENV) serotypes, the presence of two or more flaviviruses in a locale results in increased pathogenicity. A few of the most neglected viruses included in this book may only rarely infect humans and, even then, usually cause only febrile disease at this time, but have been known to result in serious, life-threatening disease in some people or have the potential to rise out of obscurity to do so. The ways in which specific viruses vary in these characteristics are the subject of subsequent chapters. These include viruses that may cause hemorrhagic fever (dengue, Omsk hemorrhagic fever, and Kyasanur Forest disease viruses), neurological disease (Zika, West Nile, tick-borne encephalitis, louping-ill, and Powassan encephalitis viruses), or both of these disease manifestations. Some of the mentioned viruses are transmitted by mosquitoes and others are transmitted by ticks. Some flaviviruses may also be transmitted to humans by drinking unpasteurized milk from infected animals. Other flaviviruses may also be transmitted by blood transfusion, organ transplantation, or sexually.

While not a flavivirus, the blood-borne hepatitis C virus is also a member of the Flaviviridae family and belongs to the *Hepacivirus* genus. It is very different from its flavivirus cousins in several ways. It only infects humans and chimpanzees, and it is transmitted via the exchange of bodily fluids, unlike flaviviruses. Hepatitis C virus also attacks the liver, causing either acute or chronic disease and, in addition to hepatitis, this virus is also responsible for many of the cases of liver cancer. It is unrelated to other hepatitis viruses and, unlike hepatitis A and hepatitis B viruses, there is currently no clinically approved effective vaccine. Due to the substantial differences between the hepatitis C virus and the flaviviruses, the hepatitis C virus is not a subject of this book.

DISEASES ASSOCIATED WITH FLAVIVIRUS INFECTION

Flavivirus-Induced Neurological Diseases

At least eight flaviviruses may cause mild-to-severe neurologic syndromes in humans. Different viruses cause different disease neurological manifestations, which will be described in separate chapters. Some of these manifestations are encephalitis; meningitis; acute flaccid myelitis; microencephaly; Guillain-Barré syndrome; and sensory and motor disorders. Some of the neurological disorders are found primarily in adults (Guillain-Barré syndrome), while others are present in fetuses or infants of mothers infected during pregnancy (microencephaly). Most of these viruses pass into the central nervous system (CNS) from the blood by crossing the blood–brain barrier (BBB) using several host- or virus-induced mechanisms.

Flaviviruses can replicate in brain microvascular endothelial cells (BMECs) in vitro and, in the process, decrease the effectiveness of the tight junction proteins that are found between the cells of the BBB, thus increasing the barriers' permeability.[1] Infected BMECs also permit the basolateral release of infectious virions in the absence of a cytopathic effect. Some of these viruses infect glial cells of the CNS, such as astrocytes and microglia (small, phagocytic immune system cells in the brain).[1] Activation of microglial triggers their production and secretion of inflammatory cytokines and chemokines that draw other leukocytes into the CNS. The infiltration of these inflammatory leukocytes can cause further disruption of the BBB as well as inducing neuropathology. Release and enzymatic activity of matrix metalloproteases by infected astrocytes damage the extracellular materials that hold the cells of the BBB tightly together. This allows for further flavivirus entry into the CNS.[1,2]

Zika and Other Neglected and Emerging Flaviviruses. https://doi.org/10.1016/B978-0-323-82501-6.00005-0

Flavivirus-Induced Hemorrhagic Fever Diseases

At least five flaviviruses are known to produce mild-to-fatal hemorrhagic disease in humans. While most people develop only fever with or without severe joint or muscle pain, other people develop the classic symptoms of potentially life-threatening hemorrhagic fever. In the midst of the current DENV pandemic, the incidence of dengue hemorrhagic fever (DHF) and dengue shock syndrome (DSS) is increasing as different DENV serotypes invade new geological regions. This leads to rising numbers of people who have been infected with one DENV serotype, followed by infection with a different serotype. In such cases, antibodies produced in response to the first DENV serotype may cause a pathogenic cross-reaction that leads to enhanced, rather than decreased, disease manifestations, in a process named antibody-dependent enhancement (ADE).

VIRAL STRUCTURE

General Information

Flaviviruses are spherical, enveloped viruses that are 40–50 nm in diameter (Fig. 1.1).[3]

Their genome consists of positive-sense, single-stranded RNA that is composed of approximately 11,000 nucleosides. This RNA lacks a poly-A tail, but contains 100 and 400–700 highly conserved nucleosides in its 5′ and 3′ untranslated regions (UTRs),

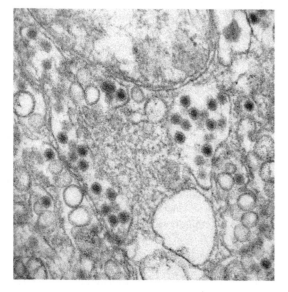

FIG. 1.1 Electron micrograph of Zika viruses inside cells. CDC/Cynthia Goldsmith, Dominique Rollin—content providers.

respectively. The 5′ terminal region, containing many AG dimers, is formed of two domains, both involved in the replication. The first domain is completely found within the 5′ UTR and has a branched stem-loop, a structure that serves as a promoter for flavivirus replication.[4,5] The second 5′ UTR domain extends in the genomes' single open-reading frame. Its contents include the nucleosides that are 5′ of the AUG region that folds into the second stem-loop structure, the AUC start site, the nucleosides downstream of AUG region, the capsid protein's coding region hairpin, the 5′ cyclization sequence, and a pseudoknot.[5]

Flavivirus' genomic RNA encodes a polyprotein that consists of 10 proteins, 7 of which are nonstructural (NS) genes. NS3 and its NS2B cofactor are found in the N-terminal serine protease domain. The NS3 C-terminal helicase domain performs three distinct activities, acting as an RNA helicase, a nucleoside triphosphatase, and a 5′ RNA triphosphatase.[6] In its membrane-bound form, NS5 is the largest and most conserved flaviviral NS protein, consisting of four dimers that undergo intermolecular interactions.[7] The N-terminal domain of NS5 contains a methyltransferase domain with three activities involved in RNA cap synthesis (guanylyltransferase, guanine-N7-ethyltransferase, and nucleoside-2′O-methyltransferase), while the NS5's C-terminal encodes the RNA-dependent RNA polymerase.[6]

The 3′ terminus of flavivirus' genome contains three domains within the 3′ UTR. Domain I is the most variable of the three. It contains two stem-loop structures in the form of pseudoknots and plays a role in the formation of subgenomic flavivirus RNAs (sfRNA1 and sfRNA2; RNA polymerase). The sfRNAs inhibit the host's innate immune response and aid in adaptation to different host species. Some of the components of the variable region differ substantially between the genomes of high and low pathogenic viral isolates, signifying that this region contains virulence factors.[5] Domain II of the 3′ UTR contains 1–2 conserved dumbbell-shaped structures required for replication and translation. Domain III is highly conserved among flaviviruses and contains sequences that interact with regions found at the 5′ end of the genomes that are necessary for genome circularization and genomic RNA replication. Domain III also contains a 3′ stem-loop structure that is flanked on its 5′ end by a short hairpin.[5]

The flaviviruses' single open-reading frame, after cleavage by cellular and viral proteases, also produces three structural proteins: the envelope (E) protein, membrane (M) protein, and capsid (C) protein.[4,8]

Flaviviruses' Structural Proteins

The E protein is the major structural glycoprotein, with 180 copies on the surface of each virion. It is highly conserved among the members of the genus and is the primary protein in the viral envelope. The E protein is multifunctional and is involved in receptor-mediated endocytosis and fusion with endosomal membranes. It additionally contains hemagglutination activity, which allows the virus to bind to the host cells' sialic acid moieties prior to membrane fusion.[9,10] Due to its abundance and location on the viral envelope, the E protein induces the host's immune system to produce protective hemagglutination-inhibiting (HI) and neutralizing antibodies.[4,5,11] E proteins are oriented parallel to the membrane and are organized 30 "rafts," each containing three E dimers. The dimers are situated in a head-to-tail manner and are transformed into active trimers after entering the target cell's acidified endosomes.

The E protein is composed of several domains.[12] Domain I (central domain) is approximately 120 amino acids long and can be N-glycosylated. Domain II is approximately 180 amino acids long and serves as the dimerization domain. It contains the fusion peptide as well as epitopes which cross-react with other flaviviruses and is important in diagnoses and vaccine development. The C-terminal region of Domain III has an immunoglobulin-like fold and is involved in binding to cellular receptors.[12] Naturally occurring mutations on the upper lateral surface of the E protein's Domain III are important determinants of neurovirulence and neuroinvasiveness. The presence or absence of a glycosylation site in this region plays a major role in whether or not the virus is able to escape neutralizing antibodies in mice.[10,13] Immediately downstream of Domain III is an area important for anchoring the virus to membranes, interacting with the precursor of the membrane protein (prM) and for acid-induced conformational changes. Its two transmembrane regions anchor the virus to host cells and allow signal translocation of the viral NS1 into the lumen of the cell's endoplasmic reticulum (ER).[4]

In addition to the E protein, the membrane (M) protein is found on the viral surface. It is derived from its prM precursor after its cleavage by the host cell's furin enzyme. prM prevents E protein from undergoing dimer-to-trimer transformation. The furin-induced cleavage allows activation of the E protein.[14]

Over 500 copies of the capsid protein form antiparallel dimers.[12] The capsid proteins act together with viral genomic RNA to form the electron-dense nucleocapsid. This provides an anchoring platform for prM and E proteins and viral assembly.[4]

Flaviviruses' NS Proteins

NS1 is multifunctional. It plays an important role in viral evasion of the host complement system of the immune response by decreasing the number of membrane attack complexes on its host cell's plasma membrane. This protects the virally infected cell from the production of complement-induced pores, which would normally result in cell lysis. The escape from complement destruction of the host cell allows the virus to continue its life cycle. NS1 also protects extracellular viruses.[12,15–17] Interactions between NS1 and NS4B regulate virus replication.[18] NS1 also acts in concert with NS3, NS2B, NS4A, and NS4B to extensively modify host cell's ER membranes.[19–21] These alterations in the lipid structure of the ER are important for viral RNA replication, translation, and assembly.

NS2A, NS2B, and NS4B are integral membrane proteins, but have different functions.[12] NS2A, NS3, and NS4B are involved in replication, viral assembly, and immunomodulation. The latter activity involves regulating the host cell's ER unfolded protein response as well as the interferon-β (IFN-β) signaling pathway, a key antiviral immune system agent.[22–27] NS2B also works in conjunction with NS3.

NS3 is the only known viral protein to serve as both a chymotrypsin-like serine protease in the N-terminal domain and a helicase/nucleotide triphosphatase (NTPase) that also includes ATPase activity.[12] This activity is regulated by cytoplasmic NS4A and releases energy from ATP for use by the viruses as well as the host cells.[28] The NS3 protease cleaves the newly transcribed viral polyprotein into its individual proteins, while the helicase is active during replication in strand unwinding prior to strand separation. It should be noted that flavivirus protease and helicase domains are arranged differently than those present in the other Flaviviridae member, hepatitis C virus, and are accordingly susceptible to different drugs.

NS5 has several functions. Its polymerase region incorporates ribonucleoside triphosphates into the nascent RNA during replication. Replication occurs in a close contact with the virally remodeled ER membrane.[12] NS5's capping functions include GTP binding and guanylyltransferase activity. The 5' cap is vital to Flaviviridae members since it directs viral polyprotein translation, protects the 5' end of the viral genome from cellular exonucleases, and is used by cells for self-nonself RNA discrimination.[29] The NS5 polymerase contains four potential protein kinase C (PKC) family members' phosphorylation sites. These sites are potential drug targets. Several antiviral NS5 drugs inhibit virus–cell membrane fusion during viral entry into host cells and dimer formation.

THE FLAVIVIRUS LIFE CYCLE

Viral envelope glycerophospholipids serve as ligands for cellular receptors.[30] Receptor binding promotes the entry of flaviviruses into the infected cell via pH-dependent, dynamin, and caveola-mediated endocytosis of the viruses.[14,31,32] The acidic pH conditions present in the endosomes induce conformational changes in the E protein that prompts fusion with the endosomal membrane[33] and the release of the nucleocapsid into the host cell's cytosol, where it subsequently uncoats.[14,34]

Flavivirus Assembly and Budding

The modified host ER is the site of translation and virion assembly.[35] Flavivirus genomic replication requires virally induced formation of replication complexes that are composed of 70–100-nm vesicles and are associated with invaginations of the ER membrane. Each invagination contains a pore that allows passage of materials between the ER lumen and the cytoplasm.[36–38] The replication complexes contain flavivirus replication components. Viral translation and proteolytic processing of the resulting polyprotein also appear to occur in paracrystalline arrays and convoluted membranes of the remodeled ER.[38–43]

The rearrangement of lipids is an important part of the ER membrane remodeling. The sphingolipids, primarily ceramide and sphingomyelin, are the primary lipid species to be altered. Both are involved in membrane curvature.[44,45] Cellular phospholipase A2 enzymes are vital to generating the phospholipids and lysophospholipids necessary for membrane remodeling in both mammalian and arthropod cells in vitro.[46] Fatty acids and sterol lipids, including cholesterol in some flaviviruses, are also used in membrane transformation.[47] The replication complexes also contain the double-stranded RNA produced during viral replication. By sequestering this viral intermediate RNA, the complexes avoid triggering the host innate immune response.

Viral particles composed of multiple capsid proteins and genomic RNA are assembled in the ER by the activity of NS2A, the transmembrane domains of NS2B, and NS3.[23,48,49] The highly basic viral capsid proteins travel to and associate with cytoplasmic, ER-derived lipid droplets via internal hydrophobic regions of the capsid protein. This association provides a scaffold for later viral genome encapsidation. Some capsid proteins enter the nucleus, particularly the nucleoli.[50] Immature viruses travel to the ER membranes for translation. Protein glycosylation occurred as $(Glc)_3(Man)_9(GlcNAc)$ is added to specific asparagine residues on the prM and E proteins where they are subsequently trimmed to produce high-mannose oligosaccharides. Afterward, the viral nucleocapsid is assembled and remodeled, producing vesicle-like structures in both vertebrate- and mosquito-derived cells that function as platforms for viral replication. It is there that double-stranded RNA and viral NS2B, NS3, NS4A, and NS4B are produced.[43,51] DENV genomic RNA associates with capsid proteins and the immature viral particles bud into the ER lumen, acquiring the part of the lipid bilayer containing viral E and prM proteins.[52]

Immature virus particles then travel to the Golgi apparatus. The acidic conditions in the trans-Golgi network transform trimeric prM/E spikes into prM/E dimers.[53–55] The prM protein is then cleaved by Golgi furin-like proteases to generate mature and immature virions that are then secreted from the host cell.[52] The now mature viral particles are then released from the host cell.[12,46,56] It should be noted that these processes may differ somewhat between different flaviviruses and differ further from the processes that occur in mammalian and vector host cells.

A BRIEF INTRODUCTION TO THE IMMUNE SYSTEM

The immune system is divided into several major categories: the innate and the adaptive immune systems. Both categories are composed of several types of leukocytes, their secreted molecules, and immune organs (bone marrow, spleen, thymus, tonsils, appendix, and nymph nodes) as well as small groupings of immune cells in the skin, intestine, and respiratory tract (Table 1.1).

Since flaviviruses are arboviruses, to a larger degree, their major means of entry is through the skin following the bite of a mosquito or tick. A specialized form of dendritic skin cells, the Langerhans cells, are found in that location and contribute to viral dissemination through the lymph nodes and into the circulatory system for further dispersal.

Introduction to the Innate Immune System

The innate immune system is inborn and rapidly responds to microbial threats, albeit with much weaker and shorter-lasting responses than those of the adaptive immune system. It is also nonspecific, since the same cell can respond to a wide variety of potential threats, including microbial infections. It does not produce immunological memory, so that it does not become faster or stronger upon further encounters with the same microbe. In order to function in an optimal manner, the cells of the innate immune system need to

TABLE 1.1
Types of Immune Cells and Their Functions

Cell Type	Type	Memory	Function
Neutrophil	Innate	No	Phagocytic Releases toxic enzymes and reactive O_2 species extracellularly
Monocyte Macrophage	Innate	No	Phagocytic Activates T helper cells Releases toxic enzymes and reactive O_2 species extracellularly
Natural killer cell	Innate	No	Releases molecules that create large pores in cells Releases molecules that cause cell to self-destruct Kills virally infected cells Releases antiviral cytokines
Dendritic cell	Innate	No	Prime activator of T helper cells Langerhans type protects against skin infection
B cell	Adaptive	Yes	Produces antibodies Activates T helper cells
T helper cells	Adaptive	Yes	Cornerstone of immune response Release many kinds of cytokines and chemokines
T killer cell	Adaptive	Yes	Releases molecules that produce large pores in cells Releases molecules that cause cell to self-destruct Kills virally infected cells

receive signals (cytokines) from some of the cells of the adaptive immune response, particularly from CD4$^+$ T helper lymphocytes. T helper cells themselves, however, require activation by some of the cells of the innate immune response, especially the dendritic cells and the monocyte/macrophages. Both innate and adaptive immune responses, therefore, depend upon each other in a complex, interactive manner that allows both major arms of the immune system to function optimally.

Some of the cell types that are important in producing either a protective or pathogenic innate immune response to viruses include neutrophils, monocytes and macrophages, natural killer (NK) cells, and dendritic cells. Neutrophils do not generally inactive viruses, but may be drawn to the site of infection and contribute to an immunopathologic inflammatory response.

NK cells eliminate microbes indirectly by killing infected cells rather than by killing the microbes themselves. By eliminating infected cells, microbes, especially viruses, are killed before they are able to replicate and infect new cells. The NK cells do so by releasing perforins, molecules that form pores in the infected cells, and granzymes, molecules that induce the infected cells to undergo apoptosis, a self-destruct process. NK cells and the CD8$^+$ T killer cells of the adaptive immune response are our best cellular defenses against

viral infections. One of the survival mechanisms used by flaviviruses is to prevent the death of their host cells by downregulating apoptosis and increasing prosurvival mechanisms. Decreasing the death of infected target cells is advantageous to the viruses, since it provides the viruses with more time to reproduce.

Monocytes and macrophages are two different stages in the life of the same cell type, with the newly produced immature monocytes staying in the blood for about 8 h before moving into various tissues where they mature, grow in size, and produce much stronger responses. The mature forms of the cells are the tissue-dwelling macrophages that differentiate in response to their location. Microglia are the form of macrophages that are found in the CNS. One of their functions of the different tissue types of macrophages is to phagocytize microbes, dead cells, and other debris. Macrophages bring these materials into the cells within membrane-enclosed vesicles (phagosomes) which fuse with lysosomes containing powerful digestive enzymes as well as toxic oxygen and nitrogen free radicals, resulting in the death and degradation of the viruses and other materials within the phagolysosomes.

Some viruses have developed methods of escaping degradation and leave the phagosome to enter into the cytosol or other organelles where they use viral and host compounds to complete their life cycle, including the production of viral genomic material, nucleocapsids, and sometimes other viral proteins. Multiple copies of the virus are then produced and assembled into complete progeny before exiting the host cell. Enveloped viruses, such as the flaviviruses, surround themselves with host cell membrane components that are studded with viral proteins, including the E protein that recognizes and binds to the appropriate host cell molecules before being brought into the new cell and beginning the process again. Such viruses not only replicate in the host phagocytic cells but use them as "Trojan horses" to spread throughout the body in search for the appropriate host cells bearing the viruses' receptor. The E protein is a major target for the adaptive immune response, especially antibodies.

Introduction to the Adaptive Immune System

The adaptive immune system is comprised of B and T lymphocytes and their products. B cells produce various types of antibodies with specific functions. They also help to stimulate T cell activity. There are several types of T cells, including $CD4^+$ T helper cells and $CD8^+$ T killer cells. There are also many types of T helper cells, which all release cytokines, immune messenger molecules that direct the other cells of the innate and adaptive immune systems, either increasing or decreasing their activity. They also produce chemokines, inflammatory molecules that attract other leukocytes into the infected area.

T killer cell activity in many ways resembles that of NK cells of the innate immune system. They also eliminate viruses indirectly, by killing virally infected cells. They also do so by producing and releasing perforins and granzymes. T killer cells differ from NK cells in that they are very specific, while NK cells are not. Unlike NK cells, T killer cells produce memory cells. $CD8^+$ killer cells, NK cells, and neutralizing antibodies are our best defenders against viral diseases, including those caused by flaviviruses. An overview of some types of immune system cells and some of their functions is found in Table 1.1.

The adaptive immune response starts to become functional in infants 6 months after birth. The components of the adaptive immune response produce a much more powerful response than is produced by the innate immune system. It requires 7–14 days, however, to respond to the threat the first time that one of these cells encounters its specific target. Adaptive immunity is extremely specific—an individual cell generally responds to one small section of one protein of one species of virus and not to other virus species of different

or the same genera. Cross-reactivity is an exception of this general rule and allows at least partial activity against a very similar structure on another microbe. An example of this cross-reactivity is seen in the case of the immune response to vaccinia virus, which cross-reacts with and provides protection against infection with the extremely virulent variola (smallpox) virus. In certain flaviviruses, cross-reactivity is protective. In this case, a vaccine against one flavivirus partially protects an immunized person against infection with another, similar flavivirus. However, weak cross-reactivity may instead result in the often-fatal ADE, especially if the weak cross-reaction is between different DENV serotypes.

One of the strengths of the adaptive immune response is that it produces immunological memory, in which the immune response is much more powerful and longer lasting the next time(s) that the same small region of the microbe is encountered. Vaccines are administered in order to stimulate the adaptive immune response to produce T and B memory cells that produce a much powerful protective response if the person is ever infected with that microbe in the future or, in the case of a previously infected person, protects against reinfection. Viruses that mutate rapidly, especially RNA viruses, may fail to trigger a T or B cell memory response if they alter the region of the virus that is recognized by these cells. Flaviviruses are RNA viruses and the viral enzyme that replicates their RNA is error-prone, leading to an increased rate of mutation in comparison with that seen when DNA is replicated.

Cytokines, Chemokines, and Inflammation

T helper cells are the primary source of cytokines and some of the chemokines, although other leukocytes and some other types of cells also produce them. Chemokines are chemoattractants that draw specific types of innate or adaptive immune system cells into an infected area, resulting in an inflammatory response. Neutrophils and monocyte/macrophages accumulate in infected areas and contribute to inflammation. Much of the immune system acts as a double-edged sword, protective in the correct amount, time, and location, but when excessive, leads to immune pathology. Under these circumstances, the inflammatory immune response may be necessary to eliminate the microbial threat, but if the response is prolonged, excessive, or in the wrong location, may kill the affected person.

Cytokines act as immune messenger molecules. Some cytokines contribute to inflammation, such as the T helper 1 cell (Th1) cytokines. The Th2 cytokines often act in opposition to the Th1 cytokines and may decrease inflammation in some cases. T regulatory cells (Tregs) are a type of CD4$^+$ T helper cell that regulates the production or activity of other T helper cell cytokines. When Tregs are overly active, they may downregulate the immune response to a large enough degree so as to prevent the other components of the immune response from clearing the microbial infection. This may result in large amounts of microbial-induced tissue damage and the death of the infected person.

The antimicrobial activity of some cytokines focuses on directing the killing of bacteria (Th2 cytokines), while others primarily direct the killing of viruses (Th1 cytokines and IFNs). The IFNs are a group of cytokines that are so named because they interfere with viral replication. Interferons are very active in the defense against viral diseases, including those caused by flaviviruses. Type I interferons (IFN-α and IFN-β) are produced by both immune and nonimmune cells. They have been used to treat a variety of viral infections, including infection by flaviviruses, either alone or in combination with other antiviral drug compounds. IFN-γ is an inflammatory type II IFN that is produced by Th1 and NK cells.

Antibodies

Five major classes of antibodies are produced by stimulated B cells. IgM is the first class of antibody that is produced and is present within 10–14 days after the initial infection with a given microbe. While relatively small amounts of antibodies are produced and are present for a relatively short period of time, the initial immune response triggers the production of immunological memory. As a result of B memory cells, antibodies are produced much sooner and to a larger titer during subsequent infections. These antibodies are also present for much longer periods of time. Later in the course of infection or during a subsequent infection, IgG antibodies are made. Testing for which classes of antibodies are being produced helps to determine whether a person is newly infected (making predominately IgM) or is late in the course of infection or recovered (primarily IgG).

Antibodies have several functions, some are more important during viral infections and others, during bacterial infections. Since viruses are obligate intracellular parasites, one of the most important functions of an antibody during a viral infection is to prevent the virus from binding to and entering its host's target cell. Neutralizing antibodies do just that. In the cause of flavivirus infection, these antibodies block the viral E protein from binding to its receptor on the host cell prior to being taken into the cell.

High levels of IgG antibodies generally remain in the blood for months after the person has recovered from a viral infection. Because of this long-lasting protection, one treatment option against flaviviruses is to administer either plasma or serum from a person who has recovered from the infection (convalescent plasma or serum) to an infected person. The antibodies in these fluids may help to decrease the severity of the recipient's disease or decrease the length of infection. Administration of convalescent serum has been used to treat many viral diseases, including those caused by flaviviruses.

THE IMMUNE RESPONSE TO FLAVIVIRUSES

Lipid metabolism shapes flaviviruses' interactions with the immune response. The cyclooxygenase-2 enzyme synthesizes prostaglandins from arachidonic acid, increasing inflammation and apoptosis in some flavivirus-infected cells, associating sphingolipid metabolism with the innate immune response.[30,57–60] Additionally, some flaviviruses alter cellular autophagy by modulating lipid droplet metabolism.[61] The lipid raft platforms produced by flaviviruses can also regulate the production of some cytokines and nitric oxide.[62,63] More importantly, the redistribution of intracellular cholesterol decreases the type I interferon Janus kinase/signal transducer and activator of transcription (JAK–STAT) antiviral pathway.[64] Compounds that target virus-induced changes in lipid metabolism may, therefore, help to restore the host immune response to flaviviruses.[30]

The two immune response effectors that are most effective in reducing or eliminating flavivirus titers and pathology are the type I IFNs IFN-α and IFN-β of the innate immune system, and neutralizing antibodies produced by the adaptive immune system in addition to the cytotoxic activity against infected cells. IFN-α is active against a wide range of flaviviruses in vitro and has a high selectivity index against cells growing in culture.[65] As discussed in later chapters, some flaviviruses have adapted to IFN-related antiviral protective responses by interfering with IFN-regulatory factor (IRF) activity, IFN interactions with their receptors, IFNs' downstream pathways, or cellular localization of IFN-stimulated gene (ISG) products. The JAK–STAT pathway is a common target for flavivirus defense systems. Flaviviruses and their components also "hide" in cells or in the lipid membranes of the remodeled ER to escape serum antibodies and the intracellular immune responses, respectively. Antibodies against the HI and neutralizing antibodies of the adaptive immune system are also very important in preventing flaviviral entry into host cells.

FLAVIVIRIDAE VACCINES AND TREATMENT

No licensed treatment or cure currently exists for flavivirus diseases, although there are effective vaccines against some human flaviviruses and others that are effective in horses, including a West Nile vaccine. Other flavivirus infections are preventable by cross-reactive vaccines against similar flaviviruses.

Many antiflavivirus drugs have been developed. It should be noted that the following drugs may only be active against specific viruses. These drugs may be placed into several categories, including previously developed antiviral compounds, such as ribavirin. Ribavirin is at least partially active against other virus families. It is active against flaviviruses in cell culture, but generally is not effective in vivo. Proposed mechanisms of action for ribavirin include the following: inhibition of inosine monophosphate dehydrogenase, viral RNA capping, or the viral RNA polymerase; mutagenesis; and promotion of an antiviral Th1 type of immune response.[65,66] Type I IFNs and ISGs can reduce flavivirus replication, but may be toxic to the vertebrate host. The combination of pegylated IFN-α, ribavirin, and a viral NS3/4A protease inhibitor may be more effective than any of these compounds alone.

A well-studied approach for broadly reactive antiflavivirus drugs attempts to induce chain termination of viral RNA and viral replication using nucleoside or nucleotide analogs.[67] This approach has also been largely ineffective, but several medicinal compounds that deplete guanosine triphosphate delay replication of some flaviviruses, including the four DENV serotypes and the relatively nonpathogenic Langat virus and Modoc viruses in vitro.[56] In vivo tests are needed to confirm the safety and usefulness of these compounds in infected animals and humans as well as their efficacy against other flaviviruses.

Nonnucleoside analogs can bind to and block the catalytic active site of the NS5 RNA polymerase, increasing and stabilizing viral capsid self-interaction and structural rigidity, thus allosterically interfering with both disassembly and assembly of nucleocapsids.[68] Other nonnucleoside analogs are allosteric inhibitors that bind to the entrance of the viral enzyme's RNA template tunnel. They also inhibit primer extension-based RNA elongation of the viral genome.[69] Other drugs inhibit NS5's RNA capping function by displacing GTP from the capping enzyme and blocking its viral guanylation activity.[29] By contrast, the antiviral drug viperin stimulates cellular proteasomal degradation of NS3,[70] while pyrrolones inhibit NS3's ATPase functions.[71] NS3 helicase activity is blocked by some compounds present in yellow and blue dyes.[72–74] Other

compounds also inhibit helicase activity by blocking helicase-catalyzed strand separation[75] and interfering with the binding of nucleic acids and ATP to the helicase.[76]

Several small-molecule viral inhibitors are effective against some flaviviruses both in vitro and in an in vivo mouse model.[77] Some of these inhibitors disrupt the organization of intracellular membrane-associated foci formed by NS4B as well as interactions between NS4B and lipid vesicles in vitro. These activities reduce viral replication in cell culture by causing the formation of elongated, snake-like NS4B assemblies.[78]

Other modes of action used by antiflavivirus drugs include the inhibition of host enzymatic activity. Some drugs act to disrupt lipogenesis and the lipid homeostasis that is critical to the remodeling of ER membranes during flavivirus replication, translation, and assembly. Several drugs inhibit the α-glucosidase activity necessary for the production of mature viral prM, E, and NS1 glycoproteins by blocking trimming of their N-linked glycans in the ER, leading to grossly misfolded glycoproteins that are targeted for degradation.[79] Other drugs target the ER-localized protein complexes, particularly oligosaccharyltransferase, which catalyzes N-linked protein glycosylation without decreasing cell proliferation.[80]

Other antiflavivirus drugs include those that target calcium-gated channels, blocking calcium ion release from the ER and mitochondria. Other drugs block the activity of atypical PKCs by decreasing the amount of ceramide lipids. PKCs normally regulate cellular lipid-dependent isoenzymes that help in the control of apoptosis, differentiation, proliferation, cellular transformation, motility, adhesion, and viability.[81] Still other drugs target host cells' CAMP-responsive element binding protein 1 (CREB1), cyclin-dependent kinases (CDKs), and purine catabolism, as well as the upregulation of the cellular prosurvival AKT pathway and antiapoptotic factor *bcl2* gene in neurons, regulate caspase activity, the release of heat shock protein 90; Na^+K^+-ATPase pump activity, and the Niemann–Pick C1-Like 1 (NPC1L1) cholesterol uptake receptor.[70,82–87]

A variety of other compounds have been found to have some antiflavivirus activity, including the following nutraceuticals: the green tea polyphenol epigallocatechin gallate, quercetin in red wine, curcumin from turmeric, several Chinese medicinal drugs, and essential oils.[88–93] Some drugs that were developed to kill other microbes have repurposed since they also have antiflavivirus activity, including several antimalarial compounds, such as chloroquine, and niclosamide, an antihelminth drug.[94–96]

TICK-BORNE VS MOSQUITO-BORNE FLAVIVIRUSES

Natural infection with flaviviruses almost exclusively occurs via mosquito or tick bites and often may be associated with hemorrhagic fever or neurological symptoms, including encephalitis or microcephaly in newborns. Other means of transmission include contact with infected animals or their by-products, including unpasteurized milk and cheese. Zika virus (ZIKV) may also be sexually transmitted and is viable in semen for months. The viruses and associated diseases that are covered in this book are the neglected or emerging/reemerging disease viruses that have the potential to become much more problematic in the future due to increased travel and migration of human populations, as well as increasing numbers of immunocompromised people. The latter include not just HIV⁺ people but also the very young and the elderly, those who are taking chemotherapy or antiinflammatory drugs, diabetics, the obese, malnourished people, and those who are infected with more than one microbe.[97]

Mosquito-Borne Flaviviruses

Mosquito-borne viral diseases may suddenly emerge and rapidly invade new regions and continents, sometimes leading to large epidemics or pandemics, while tick-borne viruses generally remain in stable foci.[98] The life cycle of mosquito-borne flaviviruses typically involves the transmission from mosquito vectors to vertebrate hosts and then back into mosquitoes. Humans may serve as amplifying hosts for mosquito-borne flaviviruses or act as dead-end hosts.[8,99,100] Birds and horses are hosts for many of these viruses and may remain asymptomatic or develop mild to life-threatening diseases. This is the case for West Nile virus (WNV) infection, which generally produces asymptomatic or mild disease in humans, but is often fatal to some species of birds and horses. Many of the pathogenic mosquito-borne flaviviruses are transmitted by either *Aedes* or *Culex* species mosquitoes, although other mosquito genera may also transmit these viruses.

All mosquito-borne flaviviruses are found in the Old World and many are now endemic in the Americas as well. They have been divided into the dengue, Japanese encephalitis, and yellow fever groups. The best studied mosquito-borne flaviviruses that cause moderate-to-severe human disease are the four serogroups of DENV; ZIKV; and WNV, emerging/reemerging viruses which are discussed in this book; and Japanese encephalitis virus (JEV); yellow fever virus (YFV); and St. Louis encephalitis virus (SLEV), not covered herein. DENV, ZIKV, and WNV are either expanding their range or

the diseases with which they are associated are becoming more pathogenic or increasingly common, as exemplified by the sudden emergence of ZIKV in South America in more pathogenic, neurological forms than the mild form with which it had initially been associated in parts of Africa, Asia, and the Pacific Islands. It is spreading northward at a rate of greater than 15,000 km per year.[101] After the initial wave of infection that appeared in Brazil, however, no similar ZIKV epidemic occurred in the subsequent 4 years.

The medical and public health systems were unprepared for both the emergence and increased pathology of ZIKV and WNV in the Americas.[102] Attempts at disease treatment or prevention only began after the viruses had gained a foothold in the region.[103] In an initial attempt to warn of a possible emergence of a microbe into a new geographical range, Evans[103] has developed a "watch list" for emerging mosquito-borne flavivirus diseases based on both viral and vector traits, including the species of the predicted mosquito vectors. Among the many traits considered in this watch list are mosquito abundance, likelihood of human exposure, and the host preference of the mosquito vectors. The watch list is meant to be the starting point for future predictive models for the emergence of zoonotic disease in the United States. This approach identified 37 mosquito species and 20 viruses of interest. The neglected Wesselsbron virus is among those flaviviruses that have the greatest number of predicted vector species.[103] In the case of DENV, however, several viral serotypes have been locally transmitted in Puerto Rico for decades. Despite the fact that DENV is only predicted to have three potential mosquito species endemic to the USA, as many as 2% of the residents along the Texas–Mexico border have evidence of recent infection, suggesting that it should also be on the watch list.[104]

DENV serogroups are spreading and overlapping in their ranges, resulting in growing numbers of cases of ADE, which may lead to the development of the life-threatening DHF or DSS, rather than the relatively mild, but extremely painful, dengue fever.[97] A possibility exists that ADE might also be seen in people infected first with one species of flavivirus and subsequently, infected by a different, but closely related, flavivirus (such as DENV and ZIKV) or by different members of a flavivirus species that are endemic in different regions of the world. A possible example of this would be infection with a WNV from the Americas or Africa, followed by infection with Kunjin virus (KUNV), an Australian subspecies of WNV. Exposure to viruses that are generally confined to very different areas of the world is made possible by the increased amount and speed of the human transportation systems, which not only rapidly transport humans to widespread regions of the world, but may also transport immature or mature mosquitoes as well. Mosquito larvae, for example, may be present in water accumulating in tires being transported between countries or continents.

Several other means exist by which immunologically naïve people are currently being brought into contact with flaviviruses that had typically only rarely infect humans and usually had caused, at their worst, mild disease. One such means of spreading these zoonotic infections is the increased level of urbanization and changes in ecosystems, such as forest removal or irrigation for the growth of crops. A second means is a human visitation to the remaining forested regions that bring both workers and travelers into contact with different species of mosquitoes, birds, and small mammals. A third means is living in close proximity to newly formed cropland, increasing exposure to rodents, bats, and nonhuman primates, which may adapt to the loss of their prior food sources and shelter by raiding or invading human cropland or food storage areas. Buildings may be used as alternative shelters for those animals that lost their previous habitat, especially rodents and bats. Other contributory factors in the spread of viruses into new human populations include adaptive genetic changes in the viruses, changes in host–vector relationships, bird and bat migration, changes in climate and wind patterns, and the planned or unplanned introduction of animals into new geographical regions. The accidental introduction of WNV-infected mosquitoes into New York harbors on freight ships is an example of the latter.[97]

Neglected Mosquito-Borne Flaviviruses

The neglected mosquito-borne flaviviruses that will be discussed in this book are the Usutu, Murray Valley encephalitis, Kunjin, Ilhéus, Kokobera, Stratford, Bussuquara, Rocio, and Wesselsbron viruses. Many of these viruses are found in different regions and ecosystems from around the world, use different mosquito vectors and reservoir hosts, and are associated with different diseases and habitats. In addition, Banzi, Edge Hill, Sepik, Spondweni, and T'Ho viruses might possibly cause mild, febrile disease in humans and, perhaps in the case of Edge Hill virus, fatigue, arthralgia, and myalgia,[103,105,106] but are not included in this book.

Usutu virus emerged in 1959 in Africa and in 2001 in Europe. It belongs to the JEV complex and occasionally causes severe neurological disease in humans, similar to that seen during WNV encephalitis. Usutu virus utilizes *Culex* mosquitoes as its vectors and several

species of birds as its reservoir hosts. The mosquito and bird host species differ in Europe and Africa.

Murray Valley encephalitis virus (MVEV) and KUNV are both found in Australia. They can cause encephalitis and some of the sequelae may be permanent, especially those associated with MVEV. Both viruses are members of the JEV complex. While MVEV was first detected in 1916, KUNV was not reported until 1960. KUNV is a subspecies of WNV. Both MVEV and KUNV utilize *Culex* mosquitoes as their primary vectors, but can also use *Aedes* mosquitoes. Both viral species use waterfowl, especially herons, as their reservoir host. While KUNV appears to be confined to Australia, MVEV is also found in Papua New Guinea.

Kokobera and Stratford viruses (KOKV and STRV, respectively) are found in Australia and Papua New Guinea. They are also members of the JEV complex, but are only distantly related to the other members of this group. Discovered in the early 1960s, infection with either virus may result in mild, febrile disease in humans. KOKV may also rarely cause acute polyarticular disease, myelitis, or encephalitis. KOKV has a *Culex* species mosquito vector, while STRV uses *Aedes* mosquitoes. The common reservoirs of KOKV are marsupials and, possibly, horses, while the reservoir host of STRV is unknown. Another regional virus that should be closely monitored is Fitzroy virus that was only isolated from *Aedes normanensis* mosquitoes in 2011 from Western Australia, due to rare, low titer, positive serological tests in humans. This virus is related to Wesselsbron virus from South Africa and Sepik virus in Papua New Guinea in the YFV group. While Fitzroy virus infects agricultural animals, such as cattle, goats, and sheep, it is not known to currently cause human or animal disease.[107] However, its association with domestic animals makes it a candidate for possible zoonotic transmission in the future.

Ilhéus (ILV), Bussuquara, and Rocio (ROCV) viruses are found in South America. ILV is also present in Central America, while Bussuquara virus and ROCV are restricted to Brazil. ILV and Bussuquara virus were first reported in the 1940s and 1950s, respectively, while ROCV was detected in the 1970s. While all three viruses may occasionally cause acute, severe febrile disease in humans, ILV and ROCV may also cause severe encephalitis. Bussuquara virus is only known to have caused disease in one person, although an asymptomatic person was found in Argentina. ILV and ROCV utilize *Psorophora ferox* mosquitoes as their vectors, but may use *Aedes* species as well. They both typically use birds as their reservoir hosts, but ILV may utilize horses and nonhuman primates as well. Rodents serve as reservoir hosts for the Bussuquara virus. Bussuquara virus, ILV, and ROCV are all the members of the JEV complex, but the latter two form their own subclades.

Wesselsbron virus is a significant cause of abortion in sheep, goats, and cattle in various regions of Africa. It was first reported in lambs in 1956. Even though the extent of seropositivity is high in certain regions, Wesselsbron virus infection rarely results in human disease. When disease does occur, it is generally a febrile, influenza-like illness. *Aedes* mosquitoes serve as the viral vector and black rats are the common reservoir host. Since up to 65% of the people in some regions of Nigeria are seropositive, Wesselsbron virus needs to be carefully monitored for changes in human pathogenicity.

Emerging/Reemerging Mosquito-Borne Flaviviruses

Emerging/reemerging infectious disease agents include not only newly detected microbes, but also those that are significantly increasing their geographical range or pathogenicity. Three of the mosquito-borne flaviviruses that are included in this book, WNV, the four serogroups of DENV, and ZIKV, are all increasing their range from the Eastern to Western Hemispheres and, at least in some groups of people, are transitioning from a relatively mild illness to severe and life-threatening diseases as they enter new regions of the world with immunologically naïve human populations.

For decades after its discovery in humans in Uganda in 1937 and its spread to Africa, the Middle East, Europe, South Asia, and Australia, infection by WNV was generally asymptomatic or only caused a mild, febrile infection. The situation began to change in the 1990s and, in a small number of people, began to cause severe neurological disorders, including encephalitis and meningitis as well as a polio-like syndrome and, in some cases, death. WNV first was detected in the Western Hemisphere in 1999 in New York City, where it killed a large number of birds, especially crows, blue jays, and related birds. Despite an extensive effort to control or eliminate the virus using insecticides, WNV spread across North America and into Central and South America in less than 10 years. Several species of *Culex* mosquitoes serve as WNV vectors, while birds, such as the house sparrow, are reservoir hosts.

First reported in humans in 1779, DENVs are typically responsible for a relatively mild, but extremely painful, febrile illness. DENV is divided into four serotypes that stimulate the production of antibodies that, rather than providing cross-protection among serotypes, often enhance pathogenicity to the

life-threatening manifestations of DHF and DSS. Although primarily found in tropical and subtropical regions in Africa and Asia, the geographical range of DENV serotypes is currently increasing in parts of the Western Hemisphere. This spread of multiple serotypes is increasing the numbers of people experiencing DHF and DSS. DENV is typically transmitted via the bite of infected *Aedes aegypti* mosquitoes, but *Aedes albopictus* is becoming increasingly important as a disease vector due to its ability to withstand cooler temperatures, thus allowing the spread of the disease into new regions. DENV disease is now characterized as a pandemic.

ZIKV was first reported in Africa in 1947, where it caused a relatively mild disease. As the virus spread to Asia, a more severe form of the disease was found in some people. In 2014–2016, the Asian strain spread to Brazil and was found to result in miscarriages or stillbirths and severe neurological disease in the surviving infants of women infected during pregnancy. The infants often had a developmental disease, microcephaly with skull deformities, and vision abnormalities. Some of the infected adults were found to have Guillain-Barré syndrome, another neurological disease with long-term sequelae. Humans are infected by the bite of the two species of *Aedes* mosquitoes that serve as DENV vectors and have overlapping ranges. They also may be transmitted sexually by infected men to women for long periods of time after ZIKV is no longer detectable in the blood.

Tick-Borne Flaviviruses

Tick-borne flaviviruses form a serogroup of the Flaviviridae family and are subdivided into mammalian and seabird groups.[108] A number of members of the former subdivision are known to be pathogenic to some humans, while others may cause human disease that is rare, mild, misdiagnosed, or unreported. Ticks generally take one blood meal between each of their developmental stages (larvae, nymph, and adult), so tick-borne viruses may be maintained in ticks for a very long time.[109,110] Accordingly, viral replication in ticks is generally slower than that in mosquitoes, which have a higher rate of viral turnover and a relatively rapid life cycle. This difference allows a high mutation rate in mosquito-borne flaviviruses when compared to the relatively stable genomes of tick-borne flaviviruses.[8,108,111] In nature, members of the mammalian subgroup of tick-borne flaviviruses use either rodents or insectivores as hosts. Humans typically have only a short viremic period and do not usually produce high enough levels of viremia to normally infect ticks. Humans, therefore, are generally considered to be dead-end hosts.[112,113]

Tick-borne flaviviruses are believed to have originated in Asia and then to have become widely dispersed, even reaching North America. Large numbers of human tick-borne encephalitis virus (TBEV) cases are reported in parts of Europe and Asia and cause many deaths. Other tick-borne flaviviruses are more geographically restricted, cause less disease in humans, and are less well studied. These include several of the viruses that are discussed in this book: louping-ill disease virus (LIV), Omsk hemorrhagic fever virus (OHFV), Kyasanur Forest disease virus (KFDV) and Alkhurma hemorrhagic fever virus (AHFV; a subspecies of KFDV); and Powassan encephalitis virus (POWV). Other tick-borne flaviviruses include Langat, Tyuleniy, Gadgets Gulley, Karshi, Royal Farm, Meaban, Kadam, and Saumarez Reef viruses.[108,114] While believed to be nonpathogenic to humans, this latter group of viruses should be monitored for possible zoonotic transmission and human disease. Also, Langat virus from Southeast Asia occasionally causes Siberia Fever and encephalitis when inoculated into humans, but does not appear to do so as a result of natural infection.[115]

Looping-ill virus is endemic almost exclusively in the United Kingdom and Ireland. It is a member of the TBEV complex. It was first detected in sheep in 1930 and was found in humans 4 years later. LIV-infected humans may experience severe neurological disease, leading to complete flaccid paralysis and death. The virus has several types of life cycles that involve complex interactions between the sheep tick vector (*Ixodes ricinus*) and sheep, red grouse, mountain hares, and roe and red deer. Humans are incidental hosts. Many of the widely distributed feral rabbits, an introduced invasive species, are also seropositive for LIV. While it is uncertain whether they play a role in the virus life cycle, the feral rabbits may be used, along with sentinel chickens, to monitor numbers of infected ticks in a region.

OHFV in humans is confined to some of the elevated regions of Western Siberia in Russia, although its common reservoir hosts, water voles and muskrats, are found throughout much of Eurasia. Another member of the TBEV complex, OHFV, was discovered in 1941 and has infected thousands of people, especially after the introduction of muskrats into the region. Infection may result in a biphasic, severe hemorrhagic fever disease. Many patients only experience the initial, febrile phase, while others develop a hemorrhagic disease that often also involves multiple organ systems. Despite the severity of the disease, its prognosis is favorable, with most people eventually recovering completely. The mortality rate is also low. Humans are usually infected by the bite of infected *Dermacentor reticulatus* or *Dermacentor mar-*

ginatus ticks, but may also become infected by drinking raw goat or sheep milk. Transmission may also occur by exposure to infected muskrat hides or bodily fluids.

KFDV was first reported in 1957 and is found in parts of India. AHFV, discovered in 1995, is a subspecies of KFDV that is found in Saudi Arabia and several other Mid-Eastern and African countries in the region. Both are members of the TBEV complex and may cause severe neurological disease, hemorrhagic fever, or both, even in a single patient. Humans may be infected with KFDV by the bite of *Haemaphysalis spinigera* or *Haemaphysalis turturis* ticks or by contact with infected rodents, most commonly, the Blanford rat, the striped forest squirrel, and the house shrew. Humans are infected with AHFV by the bite of *Hyalomma rufipes* or *Amblyomma lepidum* ticks or by contact with infected camel or sheep blood or milk. The common reservoir hosts for AHFV are camels, cattle, and birds.

POWV is the only tick-borne encephalitis flavivirus found in North America (Canada and the United States), where it was first detected in the late 1950s. In the late 1970s, POWV was also found in some parts of Russia. Another member of the tick-borne encephalitis complex, it is divided into two lineages. In the United States and Canada, members of POWV Lineage I are normally found in the Great Lakes region. Members of POWV Lineage II have recently been detected in the northeastern part of the United States. Although POWV infection may be asymptomatic, it typically results in disease. The neuroinvasive form may cause encephalitis, meningitis, and a poliomyelitis-like syndrome. While the mortality rate is approximately 10%, about half of the known patients with neurological disease develop chronic neurological sequelae. The seropositive rate is much higher than disease incidence would suggest. Humans become infected by the bite of an infected tick, usually *Ixodes cookei* or *Ixodes scapularis* in North America or *Haemaphysalis longicornis* in Russia. Rodents, particularly white-footed mice, woodchucks, and opossums as well as skunks are the common reservoir hosts. Viral range and disease incidence are increasing, and neuroinvasive and nonneuroinvasive diseases were added to the United States nationally notifiable disease list in the early 2000s.

Alongshan and Jingmen tick viruses were reported in 2020 in Inner Mongolia, China. They both may cause a mild, febrile illness in humans.[116,117] Interestingly, the genome of both viruses is segmented, containing four to five segments. They have been placed into the Jingmen virus group that is separate from the other members of the Flaviviridae family. This novel group is closely related to flaviviruses from humans, monkeys, and voles.[116]

PREVENTION

The best way to prevent infection by vector-borne microbes is to avoid contact with the vector and its secretions. This will not completely eliminate human infection since some flaviviruses have additional means of transmission, including consumption of unpasteurized milk, sexual contact, and mother-to-fetus or mother-to-child transmission. Also, many of the recommended methods of avoiding mosquitoes and ticks fail to totally protect against insect bites. Additionally, some preventive measures are not practical or affordable by people living in poverty. Also, apathy, misinformation about the diseases or their associated vaccines, and fear of Western-style health care are major factors that hinder prevention and treatment efforts. The methods described later are largely drawn from educational websites from the Centers for Disease Control and Prevention or the World Health Organization.

It is important to note that there is not a "one-size-fits-all" solution that is effective against infection by all insect-borne flaviviruses since different species of mosquitoes and ticks are found in very different environments and have different temperature and water tolerances; prefer to feed upon different host species or at different times of the day or night; and may prefer forested, grassland, rural, or urban areas. Even though people often assume that mosquito-borne illnesses are associated with warm, humid areas, hot spots for WNV in the United States are found in the Dakotas, Colorado, Texas, and California, but not in Louisiana or Mississippi (Beltz, unpublished data). West Nile viral disease incidence in humans does not correlate with precipitation and only weakly correlates with temperature. Additionally, the number of cases of West Nile viral disease in people living or working in a single county fluctuates greatly from year-to-year and in different seasons. Numbers of people who are clinically ill with WNV-associated disease correlate strongly with infection in mosquitoes in some, but not many, counties within a single state (Beltz, unpublished data).

Insect vectors adapt to expand into new geographical regions, as exemplified by the recent spread of *Ae. albopictus* mosquitoes into cooler climates. Arthropod vectors also adapt and gain resistance to insecticides. Reservoir host species, forced from their traditional areas by human activity or other factors, adapt and take residence in different niches of the region, as exemplified by the movement of rodents closer to human residences or fields as they search for new habitats and alternative food sources in response to deforestation and increased crop areas. All of these factors, and many more, make avoidance of vector and reservoir hosts very challenging.

Prevention of Infection by Flaviviruses

In order to prevent mosquito entry into homes, windows and doors need to be kept closed or covered with tight-fitting, intact screens. Mosquito netting may be used over infant carriers. During tick and mosquito season and while outdoors in areas with large numbers of these disease vectors, wearing light-colored, long-sleeved shirts and long pants reduces the amount of exposed skin and aids in detecting the ticks and mosquitoes that have landed on a person. It should be kept in mind, however, that people living and working outside in very hot areas typically do not wear clothing that covers their exposed skin, so alternative means of avoiding bites from vectors may be more practical. Also, even in some hotter regions of developed and affluent nations, some people choose to keep their doors open and do not use screens on windows.

When outdoors, especially at times during which mosquitoes are more prone to bite humans, such as dawn and dusk for many disease-bearing mosquitoes, the use of insect repellents reduces the numbers of mosquitoes landing and feeding on people. Repellents do not directly kill ticks or mosquitoes, but rather decrease the attractiveness of skin to these arthropods. Repellents containing one of the following two chemicals are believed to be most effective: DEET (*N*,*N*-diethyl-*m*-toluamide) or picaridin (KBR 3023 or Bayrepel). DEET may be applied to clothing and sparingly to exposed skin, but not to skin under clothing or that is broken or irritated. In order to apply DEET-containing repellents to the face or to the skin of children, the repellent should be sprayed onto an adult's hands and then rubbed on the child's skin. Since repellents may irritate the mouth and eyes, they should not be applied to children's hands. Repellents should be removed from the skin with soap and water after returning indoors. DEET has been shown to be safe for pregnant and breast-feeding women. These women are recommended to use insecticides since transovarian transmission may occur during pregnancy and breast-feeding may also transmit the virus to young children, even though infants rarely develop neuroinvasive diseases. DEET is not recommended for use in infants under the age of 2 months. It should also not be applied to dogs or cats since these animals lick their fur and would thus ingest the chemical. Insect repellents with DEET may be used at the same time as sunscreen.

The percentage of DEET that should be used depends upon the time to be spent outdoors. For example, 23.8% DEET provides protection for up to 5 h; 20% DEET protects for 4 h; 6.65%, for 2 h; and 4.75%, for 1.5 h. Oil of lemon eucalyptus (containing *p*-methane-3,

8-diol) is derived from a natural material and appears to provide the same degree of protection as repellents containing low concentrations of DEET, but should not be used on children under the age of 3 years. Another long-lasting repellent produced from natural materials is IR3535 (3-[N-butyl-N-acetyl]-aminopropionic acid, ethyl ester). If an individual sweats or becomes wet, the repellent may need to be reapplied.

Insecticides, like permethrin, kill adult insects. Permethrin may be used on clothing, footgear, bed nets, and camping gear, but not the skin. Permethrin kills mosquitoes and ticks and may continue to be active after repeated laundering.

Reducing Exposure to Ticks and Mosquitoes

Infection with tick-borne microbes is increasing in the United States as the number of natural predators of the reservoir or amplifying hosts, such as rodents and deer, is decreasing and, accordingly, the number of microbial hosts is increasing. Both rodents and deer have also been adapting to life in urban areas. Contact between humans and the microbial hosts is also increasing as more people are residing, working, and visiting parks and other remote or previously forested areas. The increased human presence is also significant in altering the ecology of these areas. Human presence alters food sources and natural habitats by decreasing woodlands, prairies, and wetlands. In parts of the western United States, people also suppress the fires that are necessary to maintain the natural ecosystem as they continue to build homes in remote, scenic areas. Fire suppression leads to the buildup of excessive flammable materials on the forest understudy, thus resulting in the production of ever larger and destructive fires.

One recommended means of decreasing viral transmission from mosquitoes to humans or their pets include the elimination of mosquito breeding grounds and areas of standing water, such as those found in flowerpots, buckets, wading pools, on swimming pool covers, or in clogged gutters. Holes may be drilled in tire swings to allow their drainage. Changing water in outdoor pet bowls and birdbaths twice a week kills the aquatic insect larvae. Communities may use chemical larvicides or insecticides to kill immature and adult mosquitoes, respectively. Larvicides are applied to the surface of the water. Insecticides (such as malathion, resmethrin, and sumithrin) may be sprayed by hand or trucks or from airplanes. These compounds, which are regulated by the United States Environmental Protection Agency, were used in New York City during the emergence of WNV in order to stop its geographical spread. Such compounds must be used repeatedly over

a large geographic area and, in the case of WNV, did not halt the march of the virus across much of the Western Hemisphere.

Tick-borne infections are becoming increasingly common as more people use tick habitats for recreational purposes, such as walking and hiking trails and parks, or building homes in forested regions. Some tick host species are undergoing population rises, including deer, and many other hosts are becoming adapted to humans and moving into suburban areas. There are many tick-borne infectious disease-causing organisms that infect humans: viruses, bacteria, and protozoans. These cause a wide variety of diseases, in addition to the flavivirus-associated diseases described in this book. Some of these found in the United States include Lyme disease, anaplasmosis, ehrlichiosis, Rocky Mountain spotted fever, babesiosis, tularemia, tick-borne relapsing fever, and Colorado tick fever.

If a tick does become imbedded in a person or animal, it should carefully be removed in a manner that removes the entire tick, including its head. Means of safely removing ticks are described in detail in the CDC's website. While transmission of most pathogens from ticks to their mammalian hosts usually takes one to several days, some microbes are transmitted rapidly, so ticks need to be removed as soon as possible. Early detection of ticks and their removal is thus important and involves close examination of the skin and scalp of humans or their pets after visiting tick habitats, especially in areas reporting large numbers of tick-borne diseases. Since the immature tick life stages that are more prone to attack humans are very small, this examination must be done carefully. Reducing human exposure to ticks may also include using antitick agents to dogs and outdoor cats. Removing underbrush immediately around homes also decreases contact between people and rodent reservoirs of ticks.

Precautionary Notes

One fact that is typically overlooked when recommending reducing areas of standing water or adding toxic chemicals to them is how these actions affect birds and other wild animals that rely on these areas as sources of their drinking water. Reducing the availability of water may seriously impact the ecosystem and environmental health of an area. In rural regions or wetlands, significant reduction of standing water, including that found in agricultural ditches and swamps, may not only be nearly impossible, but would damage the already threatened flora and fauna of the wetlands, resulting in potentially irreparable harm. Rice patties also require large amounts of standing water. Rice is not only a staple food for much of the world, but it also is a major economic crop. Significant decreases in rice production thus would endanger human health directly and indirectly.

Other means of protection are called for and need to take into consideration not only human health, but also our environment. Vaccines, if available, may be a more effective, practical way to protect humans and livestock from infection without harming the environment. Preventing or reducing the ill effects of infectious diseases requires a great degree of time, planning, and perhaps "thinking out of the box" in order to avoid unintended consequences, as we have seen too often in the past. Good intentions alone are often ineffective and may cause more harm than good. With careful planning, however, we may succeed in our attempts to keep people and our animals as well as wildlife and plants safe, in much of the same manner as we eliminated the natural transmission of smallpox. It may be well to include ecologists, infectious disease researchers, sociologists, and economists to the teams of public health and medical personnel before launching major campaigns to improve human health.

REFERENCES

1. Mustafá YM, Monteiro Meuren L, Coelho SVA, de Arruda LB. Pathways exploited by flaviviruses to counteract the blood-brain barrier and invade the central nervous system. *Front Microbiol.* 2019;10, 525.
2. Palus M, Bílý T, Elsterová J, et al. Infection and injury of human astrocytes by tick-borne encephalitis virus. *J Gen Virol.* 2014;95:2411–2426.
3. Füzik T, Formanová P, Rožek D, Yoshii K, Niedrig M, Plevka P. Structure of tick-borne encephalitis virus and its neutralization by a monoclonal antibody. *Nat Commun.* 2018;9:436.
4. Hurrelbrink RJ, McMinn PC. *The Flaviviruses: Pathogenesis and Immunity.* Academic Press; 2015.
5. Barrows NJ, Campos RK, Powell S, et al. A screen of FDA-approved drugs for inhibitors of Zika virus infection. *Cell Host Microbe.* 2016;20(2):259–270.
6. Bollati M, Alvarez K, Assenberg R, et al. Structure and functionality in flavivirus NS-proteins: perspectives for drug design. *Antiviral Res.* 2010;87:125–148.
7. Klema VJ, Ye M, Hindupur A, et al. Dengue virus nonstructural protein 5 (NS5) assembles into a dimer with a unique methyltransferase and polymerase interface. *PLoS Pathog.* 2016;12(2), e1005451.
8. Lindqvist R, Upadhyay A, Överby AK. Tick-borne flaviviruses and the type I interferon response. *Viruses.* 2018;10:340.
9. Heinz FX, Allison SL. The machinery for flavivirus fusion with host cell membranes. *Curr Opin Microbiol.* 2001;4:450–455.
10. Jiang WR, Lowe A, Higgs S, Reid H, Gould EA. Single amino acid codon changes detected in louping ill virus antibody-resistant mutants with reduced neurovirulence. *J Gen Virol.* 1993;74:931–935.
11. Heinz FX. Epitope mapping of flavivirus glycoproteins. *Adv Virus Res.* 1986;31:103–168.
12. Pulkkinen LA, Butcher SJ, Anastasina M. Tick-borne encephalitis virus: a structural view. *Viruses.* 2018;10:350.
13. Gao GF, Hussain MH, Reid HW, Gould EA. Identification of naturally occurring monoclonal antibody escape variants of louping ill virus. *J Gen Virol.* 1994;75:609–614.
14. Cruz-Oliveira C, Freire JM, Conceicao TM, Higa LM, Castanho MA, Da Poian AT. Receptors and routes of dengue virus entry into the host cells. *FEMS Microbiol Rev.* 2015;39:155–170.
15. Akey DL, Brown WC, Dutta S, et al. Flavivirus NS1 structures reveal surfaces for associations with membranes and the immune system. *Science.* 2014;343:881–885.
16. Rastogi M, Sharma N, Singh SK. Flavivirus NS1: a multifaceted enigmatic viral protein. *Virol J.* 2016;13:131.
17. Avirutnan P, Fuchs A, Hauhart RE, et al. Antagonism of the complement component C4 by flavivirus nonstructural protein NS1. *J Exp Med.* 2010;207:793–806.
18. Youn S, Li T, McCune BT, et al. Evidence for a genetic and physical interaction between nonstructural proteins NS1 and NS4B that modulates replication of West Nile virus. *J Virol.* 2012;86:7360–7371.
19. Miller S, Kastner S, Krijnse-Locker J, Buhler S, Bartenschlager R. Non-structural protein 4A of dengue virus is an integral membrane protein inducing membrane alterations in a 2K-regulated manner. *J Biol Chem.* 2007;282(12):8873–8882.
20. Roosendaal J, Westaway EG, Khromykh A, Mackenzie JM. Regulated cleavages at the West Nile virus NS4A-2K-NS4B junctions play a major role in rearranging cytoplasmic membranes and Golgi trafficking of the NS4A protein. *J Virol.* 2006;80(9):4623–4632.
21. Kaufusi H, Kelley JF, Yanagihara R, Nerurkar VR. Induction of endoplasmic reticulum-derived replication-competent membrane structures by West Nile virus non-structural protein 4B. *PLoS One.* 2014;9, e84040.
22. Li X-D, Deng C-L, Ye H-Q, et al. Transmembrane domains of NS2B contribute to both viral RNA replication and particle formation in Japanese encephalitis virus. *J Virol.* 2016;90:5735–5749.
23. Leung JY, Pijlman GP, Kondratieva N, Hyde J, Mackenzie JM, Khromykh AA. Role of nonstructural protein NS2A in flavivirus assembly. *J Virol.* 2008;82:4731–4741.
24. Ambrose RL, Mackenzie JM. West Nile virus differentially modulates the unfolded protein response to facilitate replication and immune evasion. *J Virol.* 2011;85(6):2723–2732.
25. Zmurko J, Neyts J, Dallmeier K. Flaviviral NS4b, chameleon and jack-in-the-box roles in viral replication and pathogenesis, and a molecular target for antiviral intervention. *Rev Med Virol.* 2015;25:205–223.

26. Liu WJ, Chen HB, Wang XJ, Huang H, Khromykh AA. Analysis of adaptive mutations in Kunjin virus replicon RNA reveals a novel role for the flavivirus nonstructural protein NS2A in inhibition of beta interferon promoter-driven transcription. *J Virol.* 2004;78:12225–12235.

27. Wang X, Liu WJ, Wang XJ, Mokhonov VV, Shi P. Inhibition of interferon signaling by the New York 99 strain and Kunjin subtype of West Nile virus involves blockage of STAT1 and STAT2 activation by nonstructural proteins. *J Virol.* 2005;79:1934–1942.

28. Shiryaev SA, Chernov AV, Aleshin AE, Shiryaeva TN, Strongin AY. NS4A regulates the ATPase activity of the NS3 helicase: a novel cofactor role of the non-structural protein NS4A from West Nile virus. *J Gen Virol.* 2009;90:2081–2085.

29. Stahla-Beek HJ, April DG, Saeedi BJ, Hannah AM, Keenan SM, Geiss BJ. Identification of a novel antiviral inhibitor of the flavivirus guanylyltransferase enzyme. *J Virol.* 2012;86:8730–8739.

30. Martín-Acebes MA, Gabandé-Rodríguez E, García-Cabrero AM, et al. Host sphingomyelin increases West Nile virus infection *in vivo. J Lipid Res.* 2016;57:422–432.

31. Peng T, Wang JL, Chen W, et al. Entry of dengue virus serotype 2 into ECV304 cells depends on clathrin-dependent endocytosis, but not on caveolae-dependent endocytosis. *Can J Microbiol.* 2009;55(2):139–145.

32. Zhu YZ, Xu QQ, Wu DG, et al. Japanese encephalitis virus enters rat neuroblastoma cells via a pH-dependent, dynamin and caveola-mediated endocytosis pathway. *J Virol.* 2012;86:13407–13422.

33. Stiasny K, Fritz R, Pangerl K, Heinz FX. Molecular mechanisms of flavivirus membrane fusion. *Amino Acids.* 2011;4(15):1159–1163.

34. Chao LH, Klein DE, Schmidt AG, Peña JM, Harrison SC. Sequential conformational rearrangements in flavivirus membrane fusion. *eLife.* 2014;3, e04389.

35. Mackenzie JM, Westaway EG. Assembly and maturation of the flavivirus Kunjin virus appear to occur in the rough endoplasmic reticulum and along the secretory pathway, respectively. *J Virol.* 2001;75(22):10787–10799.

36. Harak C, Lohmann V. Ultrastructure of the replication sites of positive-strand RNA viruses. *Virology.* 2015;479-480:418–433.

37. Apte-Sengupta S, Sirohi D, Kuhn RJ. Coupling of replication and assembly in flaviviruses. *Curr Opin Virol.* 2014;29:134–142.

38. Miorin L, Romero-Brey I, Maiuri P, et al. Three-dimensional architecture of tick-borne encephalitis virus replication sites and trafficking of the replicated RNA. *J Virol.* 2013;87(11):6469–6481.

39. Westaway EG, Mackenzie JM, Kenney MT, Jones MK, Khromykh AA. Ultrastructure of Kunjin virus-infected cells: colocalization of NS1 and NS3 with double-stranded RNA, and of NS2B with NS3, in virus-induced membrane structures. *J Virol.* 1997;71(9):6650–6661.

40. Mackenzie JM, Jones MK, Young PR. Immunolocalization of the dengue virus nonstructural glycoprotein NS1 suggests a role in viral RNA replication. *Virology.* 1996;220(1):232–240.

41. Welsch S, Miller S, Romero-Brey I, et al. Composition and three-dimensional architecture of the dengue virus replication and assembly sites. *Cell Host Microbe.* 2009;5(4):365–375.

42. Cortese M, Goellner S, Acosta EG, et al. Ultrastructural characterization of Zika virus replication factors. *Cell Rep.* 2017;18(9):2113–2123.

43. Gillespie LK, Hoenen A, Morgan G, Mackenzie JM. The endoplasmic reticulum provides the membrane platform for biogenesis of the flavivirus replication complex. *J Virol.* 2010;84(20):10438–10447.

44. Perera R, Riley C, Isaac G, et al. Dengue virus infection perturbs lipid homeostasis in infected mosquito cells. *PLoS Pathog.* 2012;8, e1002584.

45. Martín-Acebes MA, Merino-Ramos T, Blázquez A-B, et al. The composition of West Nile virus lipid envelope unveils a role of sphingolipid metabolism in flavivirus biogenesis. *J Virol.* 2014;88(20):12041–12054.

46. Liebscher S, Ambrose RL, Aktepe TE, et al. Phospholipase A2 activity during the replication cycle of the flavivirus West Nile virus. *PLoS Pathog.* 2018;14(4), e1007029.

47. Gollins SW, Porterfield JS. pH-dependent fusion between the flavivirus West Nile and liposomal model membranes. *J Gen Virol.* 1986;67(pt 1):157–166.

48. Voßmann S, Wieseler J, Kerber R, Kümmerer BM. A basic cluster in the N terminus of yellow fever virus NS2A contributes to infectious particle production. *J Virol.* 2015;89:4951–4965.

49. Patkar CG, Kuhn RJ. Yellow fever virus NS3 plays an essential role in virus assembly independent of its known enzymatic functions. *J Virol.* 2008;82:3342–3352.

50. Samsa MM, Mondotte JA, Iglesias NG, et al. Dengue virus capsid protein usurps lipid droplets for viral particle formation. *PLoS Pathol.* 2009;5, e1000632.

51. Villarea VA, Rodgers MA, Costello DA, Yang PL. Targeting host lipid synthesis and metabolism to inhibit dengue and hepatitis C viruses. *Antiviral Res.* 2015;124:110–121.

52. Byk LA, Iglesias NG, de Maio FA, Gebhard LG, Rossi M, Gamarnik AV. Dengue virus genome uncoating requires ubiquitination. *mBio.* 2016;7(3), e00804-16.

53. Li L, Lok SM, Yu IM, et al. The flavivirus precursor membrane-envelope protein complex: structure and maturation. *Science.* 2008;319:1830–1834.

54. Yu I-M, Zhang W, Holdaway HA, et al. Structure of the immature dengue virus at low pH primes proteolytic maturation. *Science.* 2008;319:1834–1837.

55. Kostyuchenko VA, Zhang Q, Tan JL, Ng T-S, Lok S-M. Immature and mature dengue serotype 1 virus structures provide insight into the maturation process. *J Virol.* 2013;87:7700–7707.

56. Mukhopadhyay S, Kuhn RJ, Rossmann MG. A structural perspective of the flavivirus life cycle. *Nat Rev Microbiol.* 2005;3:13–22.

57. Clarke JN, Davies LK, Calvert JK, et al. Reduction in sphingosine kinase 1 influences the susceptibility to dengue virus infection by altering antiviral responses. *J Gen Virol.* 2016;97:95–109.

58. Jan JT, Chen BH, Ma SH, et al. Potential dengue virus-triggered apoptotic pathway in human neuroblastoma cells: arachidonic acid, superoxide anion, and NF-kappaB are sequentially involved. *J Virol.* 2000;74:8680–8691.

59. Ghoshal A, Das S, Ghosh S, et al. Proinflammatory mediators released by activated microglia induces neuronal death in Japanese encephalitis. *Glia.* 2007;55:483–496.

60. Verma S, Kumar M, Nerurkar VR. Cyclooxygenase-2 inhibitor blocks the production of West Nile virus-induced neuroinflammatory markers in astrocytes. *J Gen Virol.* 2011;92:507–515.

61. Heaton NS, Randall G. Dengue virus-induced autophagy regulates lipid metabolism. *Cell Host Microbe.* 2010;8:422–432.

62. Chen CJ, Ou YC, Chang CY, et al. Src signaling involvement in Japanese encephalitis virus-induced cytokine production in microglia. *Neurochem Int.* 2011;58:924–933.

63. Chen CL, Lin CF, Wan SW, et al. Anti-dengue virus nonstructural protein 1 antibodies cause NO-mediated endothelial cell apoptosis via ceramide-regulated glycogen synthase kinase-3beta and NF-kappaB activation. *J Immunol.* 2013;191:1744–1752.

64. Mackenzie JM, Khromykh AA, Parton RG. Cholesterol manipulation by West Nile virus perturbs the cellular immune response. *Cell Host Microbe.* 2007;2:229–239.

65. Crance JM, Scaramozzino N, Jouan A, Garin D. Interferon, ribavirin, 6-azauridine and glycyrrhizin: antiviral compounds active against pathogenic flaviviruses. *Antiviral Res.* 2003;58:73–79.

66. McDowell M, Gonzales SR, Kumarapperuma SC, Jeselnik M, Arterburn JB, Hanley KA. A novel nucleoside analog, 1-β-D ribofuranosyl-3-ethynyl-[1,2,4] triazole (ETAR), exhibits efficacy against a broad range of flaviviruses *in vitro. Antiviral Res.* 2010;87(1):78–80.

67. Chen Y-L, Yin Z, Duraiswamy J, et al. Inhibition of dengue virus RNA synthesis by an adenosine nucleoside. *Antimicrob Agents Chemother.* 2010;54(7):2932–2939.

68. Pattnaik A, Palermo N, Sahoo BR, et al. Discovery of a non-nucleoside RNA polymerase inhibitor for blocking Zika virus replication through *in silico* screening. *Antiviral Res.* 2018;151:78–86.

69. Niyomrattanakit P, Chen YL, Dong H, et al. Inhibition of dengue virus polymerase by blocking of the RNA tunnel. *J Virol.* 2010;84:5678–5686.

70. Panayiotou C, Lindqvist R, Kurhade C, et al. Viperin restricts ZIKV and tick-borne encephalitis virus replication by targeting NS3 for proteasomal degradation. *J Virol.* 2018;92(7):e02054-17.

71. Belon CA, High YD, Lin TI, Pauwels F, Frick DN. Mechanism and specificity of a symmetrical benzimidazole-phenyl-carboxamide helicase inhibitor. *Biochemistry.* 2010;49:1822–1832.

72. Li K, Frankowski KJ, Belon CA, et al. Optimization of potent hepatitis C virus NS3 helicase inhibitors isolated from the yellow dyes thioflavine S and primuline. *J Med Chem.* 2012;55:3319–3330.

73. Ndjomou J, Kolli R, Mukherjee S, et al. Fluorescent primuline derivatives inhibit hepatitis C virus NS3-catalyzed RNA unwinding, peptide hydrolysis and viral replicase formation. *Antiviral Res.* 2012;96(2):245–255.

74. Chen C-S, Chiou C-T, Chen GS, et al. Structure-based discovery of triphenylmethane derivatives as inhibitors of hepatitis C virus helicase. *J Med Chem.* 2009;52:2716–2723.

75. Mukherjee S, Weiner WS, Schroeder CE, et al. Ebselen inhibits hepatitis C virus NS3 helicase binding to nucleic acid and prevents viral replication. *ACS Chem Biol.* 2014;9:2393–2403.

76. Shadrick WR, Mukherjee S, Hanson AM, Sweeney NL, Frick DN. Aurintricarboxylic acid modulates the affinity of hepatitis C virus NS3 helicase for both nucleic acid and ATP. *Biochemistry.* 2013;52(36):6151–6159.

77. Byrd CM, Dai D, Grosenbach DW, et al. A novel inhibitor of dengue virus replication that targets the capsid protein. *Antimicrob Agents Chemother.* 2013;57:15–25.

78. Bryson PD, Cho NJ, Einav S, et al. A small molecule inhibits HCV replication and alters NS4B's subcellular distribution. *Antiviral Res.* 2010;87(1):1–8.

79. Wu SF, Lee C-J, Liao C-L, Dwek RA, Zitzmann N, Lin Y-L. Antiviral effects of an iminosugar derivative on flavivirus infections. *J Virol.* 2002;76(8):3596–3604.

80. Puschnik AS, Marceau CD, Ooi YS, et al. A small molecule oligosaccharyltransferase inhibitor with panflaviviral activity. *Cell Rep.* 2017;21(11):3032–3039.

81. Blázquez AB, Vázquez-Calvo A, Martín-Acebes MA, Saiz J-C. Pharmacological inhibition of protein kinase C reduces West Nile virus replication. *Viruses.* 2018;10:91.

82. Xu M, Lee EM, Wen Z, et al. Identification of small molecule inhibitors of Zika virus infection and induced neural cell death via a drug repurposing screen. *Nat Med.* 2016;22(10):1101–1107.

83. Kim J-A, Seong R-K, Kumar M, Shin OS. Favipiravir and ribavirin inhibit replication of Asian and African strains of Zika in different cell models. *Viruses.* 2018;10:72.

84. Chen Y, Wang S, Yi Z, et al. Interferon-inducible cholesterol-25-hydroxylase inhibits hepatitis C virus replication via distinct mechanisms. *Sci Rep.* 2014;4:7242.

85. Nakagawa S-i, Umehara T, Matsuda C, Kuge S, Sudoh M, Kohara M. Hsp90 inhibitors suppress HCV replication in replicon cells and humanized liver mice. *Biochem Biophys Res Commun.* 2007;353:882–888.

86. Cheung YY, Chen KC, Chen H, Seng EK, Chu JJH. Antiviral activity of lanatoside C against dengue virus infection. *Antiviral Res.* 2014;111:93–99.

87. Sainz Jr B, Barretto N, Martin DN, et al. Identification of the Niemann-Pick C1-like 1 cholesterol absorption receptor as a new hepatitis C virus entry factor. *Nat Med.* 2012;18:281–285.

88. Carneiro BM, Batista MN, Braga ACS, Nogueira ML, Rahal P. The green tea molecule EGCG inhibits ZIKV entry. *Virology.* 2016;496:215–218.

89. Wong G, He S, Siragam V, et al. Antiviral activity of quercetin-3-β-O-D-glucoside against ZIKV infection. *Virol Sin.* 2017;32(6):545–547.

90. Mounce BC, Cesaro T, Carrau L, Vallet T, Vignuzzi M. Curcumin inhibits Zika and Chikungunya virus infection by inhibiting cell binding. *Antiviral Res.* 2017;142:148–157.

91. Behrendt P, Perin P, Menzel N, et al. Pentagalloylglucose, a highly bioavailable polyphenolic compound present in *Cortex moutan*, efficiently blocks hepatitis C virus entry. *Antiviral Res.* 2017;147:19–28.

92. Roy S, Chaurvedi P, Chowdhary A. Evaluation of antiviral activity of essential oil of *Trachyspermum ammi* against Japanese encephalitis virus. *Pharm Res.* 2015;3:263–267.

93. Lixia H, Jun C, Song H, FaHu Y, Jinwen T. Neuroprotective effect of (-)-tetrahydropalmatine in Japanese encephalitis virus strain GP-78 infected mouse model. *Microb Pathog.* 2018;114:197–203.

94. Shiryaev SA, Mesci P, Pinto A, et al. Repurposing of the anti-malaria drug chloroquine for ZIKV treatment and prophylaxis. *Sci Rep.* 2017;7:15771.

95. Han Y, Mesplède T, Xu H, Quan Y, Wainberg MA. The antimalarial drug amodiaquine possesses anti-Zika activities. *J Med Virol.* 2018;90(5):796–802.

96. Cairn DM, Boorgu DSSK, Levin M, Kaplan DL. Niclosamide rescues microcephaly in a humanized *in vivo* model of Zika infection using human induced neural stem cells. *Biol Open.* 2018;7, bio031807.

97. Beltz LA. *Bats and Human Health: Ebola, SARS, Rabies, and Beyond.* John Wiley and Sons; 2018.

98. Brackney DE, Nofchissey RA, Fitzpatrick KA, Brown IK, Ebel GD. Stable prevalence of Powassan virus in *Ixodes scapularis* in a northern Wisconsin focus. *Am J Trop Med Hyg.* 2008;79:971–973.

99. Gubler DJ. The changing epidemiology of yellow fever and dengue, 1900 to 2003: full circle? *Comp Immunol Microbiol Infect Dis.* 2004;27:319–330.

100. Gregory CJ, Oduyebo T, Brault AC, et al. Modes of transmission of Zika virus. *J Infect Dis.* 2017;216:S875–S883.

101. Zinszer K, Morrison K, Brownstein JS, Marinho F, Santos AF, Nsoesie EO. Reconstruction of Zika virus introduction in Brazil. *Emerg Infect Dis.* 2017;23:91–94.

102. Weaver SC, Forrester NL. Chikungunya: evolutionary history and recent epidemic spread. *Antiviral Res.* 2015;120:32–39.

103. Evans MV, Murdock CC, Drake JM. Anticipating emerging mosquito-borne flaviviruses in the USA: what comes after Zika? *Trends Parasitol.* 2018;34(7):544–547.

104. Hotez PJ. Neglected infections of poverty in the United States of America. *PLoS Negl Trop Dis.* 2008;2:256–311.

105. Briese T, Loroño-Pino MA, Garcia-Rejon JE, et al. Complete genome sequence of T'Ho virus, a novel putative flavivirus from the Yucatan Peninsula of Mexico. *Virol J.* 2017;14:110.

106. Mackenzie JS, Williams DT. The zoonotic flaviviruses of southern, south-eastern and eastern Asia, and Australasia: the potential for emergent viruses. *Zoonoses Public Health.* 2009;56:338–356.

107. Johansen CA, Williams SH, Melville LF, et al. Characterization of Fitzroy River virus and serologic evidence of human and animal infection. *Emerg Infect Dis.* 2017;23(8):1289–1299.

108. Dobler G. Zoonotic tick-borne flaviviruses. *Vet Microbiol.* 2010;140:221–228.

109. Parola P, Raoult D. Ticks and tick-borne bacterial diseases in humans: an emerging infectious threat. *Clin Infect Dis.* 2001;32:897–928.

110. Ebel GD, Kramer LD. Short report: duration of tick attachment required for transmission of Powassan virus by deer ticks. *Am J Trop Med Hyg.* 2004;71:268–271.

111. Nuttall PA. Molecular characterization of tick-virus interactions. *Front Biosci.* 2009;14:2466–2483.

112. Nuttall PA, Labuda M. Dynamics of infection in tick vectors and at the tick-host interface. *Adv Virus Res.* 2003;60:233–272.

113. Labuda M, Nuttall PA, Kozuch O, et al. Non-viraemic transmission of tick-borne encephalitis virus: a mechanism for arbovirus survival in nature. *Experientia.* 1993;49:802–805.

114. Grard G, Moureau G, Charrel RN, et al. Genetic characterization of tick-borne flaviviruses: new insights into evolution, pathogenetic determinants and taxonomy. *Virology.* 2007;361:80–92.

115. Webb HE, Wetherley-Mein G, Smith CEG, MacMahon D. Leukaemia and neoplastic processes treated with Langat and Kyasanur Forest disease viruses: a clinical and laboratory study of 28 patients. *Br Med J.* 1966;1:258–266.

116. Zhang X, Wang N, Wang Z, Liu Q. The discovery of segmented flaviviruses: implications for viral emergence. *Curr Opin Virol.* 2020;40:11–18.

117. Wang Z-D, Wang B, Wei F, et al. A new segmented virus associated with human febrile illness in China. *N Engl J Med.* 2019;380:2116–2125.

CHAPTER 2

Dengue Virus

INTRODUCTION

Dengue fever (DF) and the more serious forms of DENV infection, dengue hemorrhagic fever (DHF) and dengue shock syndrome (DSS), are currently found throughout much of the world. DF causes extreme bone pain. DHF and DSS are life-threatening, primarily in individuals who have been infected with one, and then another, of the four DENV serotypes. Dengue-related diseases are the most common vector-borne infections of humans, with 50–100 million cases of DF reported per year, primarily in tropical regions.[1] Several hundred thousand cases of DHF occur as well, with a fatality rate of 5% in treated individuals. This severe condition is most common in children and young adults. A very severe epidemic of DF and DHF occurred in 1958, involving 1.2 million people in 56 countries.[2] Over time, the epidemics have become larger and more frequent and, during the last 50 years, dengue-related diseases have risen almost 30-fold. This increase is due, at least in part, to increased human populations in urban centers and rapid transit of infected people via air travel, allowing the virus to become endemic in previously uninfected, local mosquito vectors' populations.[3,4]

The Pan American Health Organization[5] reported 3.1 million cases of dengue-related diseases in the Americas in 2019, 28,000 of which were severe and led to over 1500 deaths. These diseases are increasing rapidly in the Americas: the number of cumulative cases in the 1980s was 1.5 million, while 16.2 million cases were reported from 2010 to 2019. In addition to South and Central America, DENV diseases are found in North America. The Centers for Disease Control and Prevention (CDC)[6] reported 20 locally transmitted cases in the mainland of the United States in 2019. As to be suspected, the majority of these cases occurred in Florida, but Texas, North Carolina, and Washington, DC, also reported locally transmitted cases. DENV is also endemic in Puerto Rica and Guam. The World Health Organization[7] reported many endemic cases throughout Latin America in 2019, including over 2 million in Brazil, over 100,000 in Mexico, and over 140,000 in Nicaragua. DENV-1, DENV-2, DENV-3, and DENV-4 are found in Brazil and Mexico, putting the population in those countries at high risk for DHF and DSS. Only DENV-2 was found in Nicaragua.

DENV is usually transmitted to humans by two species of *Aedes* mosquitoes (Figs. 2.1 and 2.2).

Aedes aegypti is the primary vector for DENV and two other flaviviruses, yellow fever virus (YFV) and Zika virus (ZIKV), as well as for chikungunya virus. *Ae. aegypti* prefers to use humans as its primary host and, accordingly, lives in urban areas, especially near people's residences. This anthrophonic behavior may be due to vector domestication.[8] When humans move into an area and alter its fauna and flora, local life forms, including insects, must adapt or face possible removal from the area. Some blood-sucking insects evolve and adapt to the new ecosystem by changing from their preferred, former host animal species to preferring humans, who serve as a readily available, constant source of blood. During this process, the insect vector introduces microbes formerly associated with animals into human populations.[8]

Different strains of *Ae. aegypti* have a great degree of genetic variation that sometimes leads to large differences in their ability to successfully transmit DENV and YFV to humans. Genetic variations among mosquito strains may give some mosquitoes an adaptive advantage over other strains. Once a mosquito species has gained the ability to utilize humans as its host, it is likely to be introduced over large distances into new geographical regions due to the great mobility of their human hosts.[8] Vector domestication, resulting from human entry into and alteration of ecosystems, thus may contribute to the emergence of new microbial diseases. As humans continue to enter or increase their presence in new regions, this type of indirect zoonotic infection will, most likely, also continue. Additionally, just as *Ae. aegypti* evolved to use humans as their primary hosts, DENVs may be evolving in a manner that allows them to better utilize either *Ae. aegypti* or *Aedes albopictus* as their vector. Some DENV serotypes or strains within a serotype may thus become better adapted to a particular mosquito host and gain a survival advantage over other DENV strains.

Ae. albopictus has less of a biting affinity for humans, but is becoming more important as a DENV vector since it is adapting to life in cooler environments, thus expanding the range of DENV and the number of potential human hosts. This cold-adaptation may allow *Ae. albopictus* to exploit a new niche where it does not need

Zika and Other Neglected and Emerging Flaviviruses. https://doi.org/10.1016/B978-0-323-82501-6.00002-5

Aedes aegypti mosquito

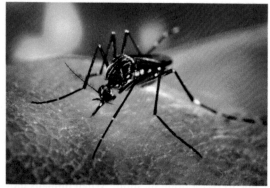

FIG. 2.1 *Aedes aegypti* mosquito. (Credit: CDC/Prof. Frank Hadley Collins, Dir., Cntr. for Global Health and Infectious Diseases, University of Notre Dame—Photo content provider; James Gathany—Photo credit.)

Aedes albopictus mosquito

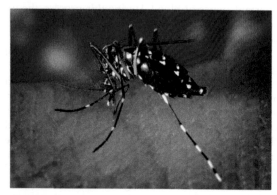

FIG. 2.2 *Aedes albopictus* mosquito. (Credit: CDC—Content provider; James Gathany—Photo credit.)

to compete with *Ae. aegypti*. It is likely that the mosquito species that are native to this more temperate environment will now also ingest DENV during their blood meals. Over time, these local mosquito species may also become able to serve as vectors that transmit DENV to the local human population. As was discussed earlier, some of the DENV serotypes or strains may become better adapted to *Ae. albopictus* and may become the predominant type of DENV in more temperate regions.

HISTORY

DF has been occurred in humans for at least several millennia. During the Chin Dynasty of China (265–420 AD), a disease with DENV-like symptoms was re-

corded. This disease was called "water poison" and was linked to exposure to flying insects. The description of a dengue-like illness is also found in a Chinese medical encyclopedia from 992 AD. Similar reports were recorded between 1635 and 1699 in the West Indies and Central America.[9] By the end of the 1700s, periodic epidemics of a disease whose symptoms are very similar to DF were reported in Asia and the Americas. Early reports of epidemics of DF in Asia and North Africa appeared in 1770.[10] Philadelphia, a large population center in the northeastern United States, experienced a large outbreak of DF in 1780.[9] These epidemics were periodic and infrequent. Often intervals of 10–40 years occurred between epidemics due, in large part, to its slow spread by sailing vessels. *Ae. aegypti* appear to have originated in Africa and then entered and become endemic in tropical or subtropical regions through trading ships carrying freshwater storage containers that could harbor and maintain mosquito breeding colonies.[11]

DF was first reported in Queensland, Australia, in 1873, and the first known dengue-associated death in this continent occurred in 1885. At least 13 major dengue outbreaks have occurred in Queensland since then. DENV subsequently spread into other regions of the continent. However, the last known cases in Western Australia were in the 1940s, and the last epidemic in the Northern Territory, in 1955.[4]

The seeds of the DF pandemic were planted in SE Asia during the Second World War as a result of the movement of military equipment that trapped rainwater containing *Ae. aegypti* eggs and larvae. This led to the spread of the mosquito vector to previously uninfected regions of the world.[12] During the war, due to the destruction of many water systems, the numbers of water storage facilities increased, providing new niches for mosquito larvae to exploit, especially if the water storage facilities were not adequately covered. The dengue outbreak in Southeast Asia was additionally spurred by the transit of hundreds of thousands of uninfected Japanese and Allied soldiers into the DENV-infected areas.[1,12] The mosquito vector hosts moved into most of the Central and South Pacific Islands that, due to their isolation and small human populations, could not support dengue epidemics for long periods of time.[1] People living in larger Pacific islands were also infected and, between 1953 and 1954, an epidemic of DHF occurred in Manila in the Philippines, following its appearance in Bangkok in 1950.[13]

Several decades later, DHF stuck Asia in Sri Lanka, India, Pakistan, Taiwan, China, and Singapore as the ranges of the mosquito vector and virus increased. Urbanization was becoming increasingly common.

This process moved the human hosts into a more compact mosquito feeding ground. The entry of infected people into these urban centers helped to spread the virus throughout these large populations of immunologically naïve human hosts.[1] Multiple DENV serotypes, predominately DENV-3, were present during an epidemic in the region. The DENV-3 strain associated with the epidemic differed from previous DENV-3 isolates. By 1975, DHF was the leading cause of hospitalization and death in children in the affected regions.[1] Some cases of DENV infection in other Pacific islands also manifested symptoms of DHF. Additionally, about 900,000 cases of either DHF or DSS occurred in Thailand between the years of 1958 and 1990, with a fatality rate of 1.6%.[14] The largest single epidemic in the region occurred in Vietnam in 1987 and resulted in 370,000 cases of DENV-related diseases. In the years since 1990, epidemics in SE Asia have continued to increase in intensity as the presence of multiple viral serotypes in a given region continues to become more frequent. Four times as many cases of DHF were reported in the last 15 years than had been detected during the previous 30 years. Recent modeling suggests as many as 390 million people are infected by DENV worldwide each year.[15]

In several areas of Africa and the Middle East, dengue-related diseases are also increasing. While the surveillance systems in the region are imperfect, the incidence of DF epidemics has been rising since 1980, most notably in East Africa (Kenya, Mozambique, Sudan, Djibouti, and Somalia) and in Saudi Arabia. All four DENV serotypes are active in these regions.[1] While sporadic cases of DHF have been reported in several countries, no epidemic of severe disease has yet been reported in this part of Africa. In addition to humans in western Africa and parts of SE Asia, DENV also circulates in local monkey populations. Also, in addition to *Ae. aegypti* and *Ae. albopictus*, *Aedes africanus* and *Aedes luteocephalus* are common DENV vectors in some parts of Africa.[4]

In the early 1980s, dengue-related diseases reached pandemic levels and have remained so ever since. The rapid expansion of dengue-related diseases was fueled by the corresponding expansion of the geographical range of the mosquito vectors along with all four virus serotypes.[16,17] It should be noted that in the late 1980s, more cost-effective and less laborious serotype-specific diagnostic tests were available that allowed the number of people infected with each serotype to be more accurately determined.[3] Even excluding more accurate testing protocols, hyperendemicity is continuing to grow as multiple DENV serotypes are occupying the same

region, resulting in the emergence of DHF and DSS.[1] This may not be the first time that DHF and DSS have emerged, since previous clinical reports of illness similar to DHF and DSS are present in medical records from northeastern Australia in 1897 and Greece in 1928. Since these reports are based upon symptoms rather than modern diagnostic techniques, it is possible that these earlier disease reports were produced by other, similar flaviviruses that are no longer circulating in the human population.

Dengue was unknown in the Western Hemisphere until the advent of European colonization and the introduction of the African slave trade into the Americas.[18] DENV's primary vector, *Ae. aegypti*, whose ancestor is believed to have originated in Africa, entered the Americas soon after the arrival of African slaves.[8] Programs directed by the Pan American Health Organization greatly reduced the numbers of *Ae. aegypti*. This mosquito species was eradicated in 18 regional countries and the number of DENV cases and the number of related YFV flavivirus plummeted. At that time, only sporadic cases of DF were found in some of the Atlantic islands that had failed to eradicate the mosquito vectors.[19] *Ae. aegypti* was reestablished in the Americas in the 1970s due to the failure or abandonment of mosquito control measures, including banning the use of DDT. As the numbers of mosquitoes increased, mosquito-borne diseases in humans also increased. By 1995, the incidence of DF was greater than that reported before the vector control program began.[9,10] Between 2011 and 2017, another series of DENV outbreaks occurred due to a large influx of tourists to see the 2011 Pan American Games in Mexico, the 2013 Confederations Cup, the 2014 World Cup, and the 2016 Olympics in Brazil.[10]

In 1970, DENV-2 and DENV-3 serotypes were detected in the Americas. DENV-3 caused several epidemics in Puerto Rico and Columbia in the mid-1970s. DENV-1 was introduced into the area in 1977, resulting in epidemics of DF in Jamaica, Cuba, Puerto Rico, and Venezuela in 1977–78 before spreading throughout the Caribbean, northward into Mexico and Texas, and southward into Central America and northern South America. DENV-4 was imported into the eastern Caribbean in 1981 and caused major epidemics throughout the surrounding areas.[1] The same year, a new and more virulent strain of DENV-2 that had originated in SE Asia (most likely from Vietnam) was imported into Cuba, leading to the first major epidemic of DHF in the Americas. Over 10,000 cases of DHF occurred during this outbreak; however, large-scale hospitalization and effective fluid replacement therapy limited the number of deaths to 158 people.[1]

The next major epidemic of DHF in the Americas began soon afterward in Venezuela, in 1989–90, resulting in over 6000 cases of disease and 73 deaths. Between 1990 and 1995, the Pan American Health Organization reported that DENV-2 led to a series of smaller epidemics in Columbia, Brazil, Puerto Rico, and Mexico. By 1997, 18 countries in the region had reported DHF cases. The CDC reported that a novel strain of DENV-3 from Sri Lanka had entered the Western Hemisphere in 1994 and led to an outbreak of DF in Costa Rica and Panama and an outbreak of DHF in Nicaragua.[20] Yellow fever incidence increased in tropical areas of the Americas as well.

The United States reported a small number of imported cases of DF in Texas in 1980, 1986, 1995, and 1997. While the virus has not yet become endemic in most of the continental United States, it is a major public health concern in Puerto Rica and other American-controlled islands in both the Atlantic and Pacific Oceans, including the US Virgin Islands, Samoa, and Guam.[6] The southern part of the United States is home to two species of appropriate mosquito vectors, most notably, *Ae. aegypti*, which is found along the Gulf Coast states from Texas to Florida. The virus's secondary vector, *Ae. albopictus*, entered the United States in the early 1980s and spread to over 25 states since then.

Several factors have contributed to the spread of DENV. RNA viruses, including DENV, have a high mutation rate that allows them to evolve in response to environmental changes and further expand into and exploit new niches. Additionally, the numbers of regional mosquito vectors rise as urbanization increases and adequate access to sewage treatment facilities decreases.[21] Pools of stagnating standing water also fuel the growth of mosquito populations. As stated previously, aggressive vector control programs greatly reduced the numbers of DENV vectors from most of Latin America during the 1940s and 1950s; however, increasing urbanization led to the reinfestation of many areas during the 1970s. Globalization, air travel, and commercial trade rapidly spread microbes, including DENV, into new locations with naïve, susceptible human hosts.[22] Between 1983 and 1995, the number of international travelers leaving the United States increased from 20 to 40 million people, half of which were bound for tropical regions.

THE DISEASES

The name "dengue" is derived from the Swahili "ki denga pepo" or seizure caused by an evil spirit.[18] Most DENV infections are asymptomatic and the virus is usually cleared from a person in approximately a week. In those people who are symptomatic, the illness may manifest itself as different forms: DF, DHF, and DSS, as well as causing neurological disease in some patients. All forms of the disease are associated with generalized vascular damage. Diffuse hemorrhage, edema, and congestion of organs occur in DHF and DSS, but not in DF.[2] In these two serious disease manifestations, antibodies produced during a prior infection with one DENV serotype, followed by infection with a different serotype, may lead to the formation of large immune complexes in the blood. These complexes contain large numbers of antibodies bound to microbial components. Due to their size, immune complexes may partially occlude blood vessels, resulting in the production of disseminated intravascular coagulation. The widespread coagulation depletes the blood of platelets and clotting factors. This decreases the ability of blood to clot and allows for the formation of hemorrhagic lesions. The mortality rate is 1%–10%, depending on the quality of the available health care. Additionally, DENV infection is associated with neurological disease in both children and adults with an incidence rate of 0.5%–20%.[23] DENV RNA is present in the brain and cerebrospinal fluid of patients with acute neurological disease.[24]

Dengue Fever

DF or "breakbone fever" is generally found in older children and adults. Infection may be asymptomatic or result in extremely painful, but short-term and self-resolving, illness. After an incubation period typically lasting from 4 to 6 days,[1] an infected person may develop fever of sudden onset, severe frontal headache, myalgia, and anorexia. This is followed by decreased numbers of neutrophils and platelets; severe eye, bone, and muscle pain; change in taste perception; nausea and vomiting; rapid heartbeat; and anxiety and depression. The extreme pain has been equated to that resulting from multiple broken bones. Later during the course of infection, petechial rashes may be found on the extremities, underarms, and mucous membranes due to hemorrhaging of small blood vessels in the skin, which may result from the host antibody response. The acute illness persists 8–10 days. While very painful, DF is seldom fatal, in contrast to the sometime high mortality rates associated with DHF and DSS. Following a long convalescent period, recovery is usually complete and without sequelae,[1] with the exception of some postinfection fatigue and depression. In rare cases, DF progresses to DHF or DSS.

Dengue Hemorrhagic Fever and Dengue Shock Syndrome

DHF and DSS are severe manifestations of DENV infection. Greater than 500,000 cases of DHF or DSS occur annually, with fatality rates ranging from 1% to 10%. Without appropriate supportive care, this rate may approach 30%.[18] DHF and DSS are generally found only in children under the age of 15 years.[2] Early disease manifestations include fever, anorexia, vomiting, and facial flush. Disease progression is accompanied by weakness, severe restlessness, cold extremities, facial pallor, profound abdominal pain, cyanosis (bluish hue to the skin), enlargement of and damage to the liver, petechial rash, and bleeding from the gums. Serious pathology is linked to hemorrhaging for 2–6 days after the onset of fever. Leukocyte and platelet numbers decrease as vascular permeability and fluid loss from the circulatory system increase, resulting in hypotension. In DHF, this may lead to capillary leak syndrome, with greater than 20% elevation in the hematocrit, hemoconcentration, pleural effusion, hypoproteinemia, and ascites.[2,25] In addition to hemorrhaging, the decrease in platelet levels may contribute to respiratory distress. The large drop in blood pressure may result in hypovolemic shock. Death may rapidly occur if the low blood plasma level is not quickly counteracted by fluid replacement.[25] Spontaneous hemorrhaging may also be fatal if it occurs in the gastrointestinal tract or within the cerebral medulla of the brain. Recently, increasingly greater numbers of DENV-infected people are developing the disease in additional organs, including myocarditis, hepatitis, and acute renal failure in the heart, liver, and kidneys, respectively. The involvement of more organ systems is accompanied by higher fatality rates.[26]

DSS may also occur as a result of severe decreases in blood pressure and hemoconcentration due to the loss of plasma from the circulatory system into the tissues. This disease manifestation may be suspected in DENV-infected people having a weak, rapid pulse; narrow pulse pressure (the difference in systolic and diastolic blood pressures); hypotension; cold, clammy skin; and restlessness.[2] DSS occurs in one-third of severe dengue cases and is most commonly seen in children. The low numbers of platelets increase coagulation time. Major bleeding may occur from multiple sites of the body with or without the presence of shock. Supporting treatments include the administration of intravenous fluids to raise blood volume and blood pressure to more homeostatic levels.[2]

Factors Influencing the Development of DF vs DHF or DSS

Several factors combine to determine whether a given individual infected with one of the DENV serotypes or strains develops the relatively mild DF or the more severe DHF or DSS.[27] The increase in DENV virulence may be linked to some trait that varies among different populations of infected people, including the strength and type of an individual's immune response. Numbers and proportions of immunocompromised individuals have been increasing in developed areas due to many factors, including increased survival of premature or ill newborns and infants, lengthening of human life spans and increased numbers of elderly people, the use of immunosuppressive drugs in people with autoimmune diseases or cancer, and infection with HIV. Diabetics, those on dialysis, and the obese are also at higher risk for developing severe forms of multiple infectious diseases. People also differ in their tendency to produce a primarily proinflammatory and antiviral Th1 cell response or an antiinflammatory and antiviral Th2 response.

Increased DENV virulence could also correlate with genetic factors that differ among populations. As DENVs expand their geographical range, they encounter diverse groups of people with different genetic traits. The adaptive immune response requires interactions with certain specific recognition molecules that vary among individuals. These molecules include the major histocompatibility complex class I or class II molecules (MHC I and MCH II). Different individuals express different alleles of these immune-recognition molecules on the surface of their cells. Some types of MHC molecules are associated with greater susceptibility to diseases of the immune system, while other MHC types are associated with greater disease resistance. The differential expression of MHC molecules among individuals has also been linked to differential susceptibility to microbial diseases, including those of viral origin. On a larger scale, different human populations have a tendency to express more or less of certain MHC molecule alleles than other populations. This could affect how different human populations respond to different disease agents, such as DENV, and whether they are more or less prone to develop DF, DHF, or DSS.

The development of severe disease is also dependent upon the virulence of the infecting viral serotype. Some viruses belonging to the DENV-2 serotype are more virulent than those of other serotypes.[27] Differing degrees of virulence also exist within a serotype: the disease associated with the DENV-2 strain present in Puerto Rico in 1969 was mild; however, the DENV-2 strain introduced into Cuba during the early 1980s was associated with a higher incidence of DHF and DSS. The latter strain was more closely related to virulent DENV-2 strains from SE Asia than to the older, Puerto Rico strain. If the second DENV infection involves viruses of Southeast Asian origin, there is often a greater risk of developing severe disease.

Gender and racial characteristics also affect disease severity.[27] Female children are more susceptible to developing lethal DSS than are males. Caucasians and Asians are at greater risk for severe infection than people of African descent. These racial differences may be related to differing MHC molecule expression, which is genetically determined and varies among different racial groups, as previously discussed. The decreased virulence among people of African origin as well as the relative rarity of DHF and DSS in Africa has led to a proposed "dengue resistance gene" that is present in some African populations. Whether such a resistance gene exists or is linked to the expression of certain MHC complex molecules is currently unknown.

Other host factors may also affect disease severity. Nearly 95% of DHF or DSS cases are present in children younger than 15 years. Surprisingly, infants with moderate to severe protein malnutrition are less likely to develop DHF or DSS, even if they produce levels of cytokines and anti-DENV antibodies that are similar to DENV-infected infants who are not malnourished.[28] Perhaps placing DENV-infected infants on a low-protein diet may improve disease outcome. Children with peptic ulcers are at increased risk of severe hemorrhaging, as are menstruating females. Ulcers are typically due to infection with *Helicobacter pylori* bacteria in the stomach. Infection with *H. pylori* is often associated with poverty.

THE VIRUSES

DENVs belong to the mosquito-borne group of the *Flavivirus* genus and are structurally related to other mosquito-borne flaviviruses, such as ZIKV, YFV, and Japanese encephalitis virus. Both mammalian and mosquito protein kinase G, a cGMP-dependent protein kinase, phosphorylate the DENV-2 NS5 protein, a nonstructural viral protein that replicates flavivirus RNA. Correct protein phosphorylation greatly enhances DENV production in both mammals and mosquito hosts. Additionally, phosphorylation increases flight activity in *Ae. aegypti* mosquitoes.[29]

DENV exists in four serotypes (DENV-1, DENV-2, DENV-3, and DENV-4), which are believed to have emerged approximately 2000 years ago. The existence

of a fifth DENV serotype has also been suggested.[30] The nucleoside sequences of the different serotypes' genomes vary by as much as 40% in the envelope genes whose protein products are the major targets for both antibody- and T cell-mediated immune responses. DENV-1 and DENV-3 are the most closely related members of the group, while DENV-4 has the greatest extent of genetic diversity. Some of DENV-2 and DENV-3 strains found in the Americas appear to be less virulent than the corresponding Asian strains.[9] No immunologic cross-reactivity exists among the different dengue serotypes, thus allowing hyperendemicity (simultaneous infection with more than one DENV serotype) to arise. The four serotypes have undergone an explosion in genetic diversity over the past 200 years, in some ways similar to the more recent explosion of HIV strains. This is likely due to the increased availability of new groups of susceptible human hosts who had not previously been exposed to the virus, perhaps reflecting increases in and interactions among human populations. Rapid movement, such as air travel, and intermingling of human groups who had formerly been separated geographically and culturally may have facilitated this process.[27]

Several mammalian cell types are infected by DENV, including dendritic cells (DCs) and Langerhans cells (immature DCs of the skin's epidermis), monocytes/macrophages, B lymphocytes, endothelial cells, mast cells, and hepatocytes. Interestingly, many of these target cells are part of the immune system. Their infection induces the expression of tumor necrosis factor-related apoptosis-inducing ligand (TRAIL) in primary DCs, monocytes/macrophages, and B lymphocytes. TRAIL is protective, regulating DENV replication in infected monocytes in a nonapoptotic manner. Interferons (IFNs), cytokines that serve as one of our primary antiviral defense systems, enhance TRAIL expression, and, in a positive feedback manner, TRAIL then enhances the expression of IFN-β and IFN-inducible antiviral genes.[31]

Early during the course of infection, mosquito-derived DENVs attach to Langerhans cells in a process that relies heavily upon the binding of the viral envelope glycoprotein (E protein) to a DC surface molecule, the mannose-specific lectin, DC-specific ICAM3-grabbing nonintegrin (DC-SIGN) in the presence or absence of a co-receptor.[32] Interestingly, hepatitis C virus, a non-flavivirus member of the Flaviviridae family, also uses DC-SIGN early during the cellular infection process. Langerhans cells are believed to serve as the primary mammalian host cells soon after DENV transmission from its mosquito vectors.[33] Although Langerhans cells typically have antiviral activity, in the case of DENV, when infected, these cells serve as hosts for viral replication and as the primary means of travel through the lymphatic system to lymph nodes at distant sites, as is also the case in other flaviviruses. Langerhans cells are approximately 10 times more susceptible to infection than blood or tissue monocytes or macrophages, respectively.

Other mammalian cell surface molecules serve as receptors for the binding of viral E protein in types of target cells that lack DC-SIGN. DENV binds to L-SIGN in liver endothelial cells and the mannose receptor in macrophages. A highly sulfated type of the heparin sulfate glycosaminoglycan acts as a receptor in epithelial cells.[34–36] In cells that bear both heparin sulfate and DC-SIGN, heparin sulfate does not alter interactions between DENV and DC-SIGN. The removal of the heparin sulfate from DC-SIGN-bearing cells does not decrease DENV infection.[32] Infectious DENV-2, however, is not able to bind to cultured kidney cells after the removal of heparin sulfate or its desulfuration.[37] Dermatan sulfate, but not chondroitin sulfate A, also plays a role in the infection of DCs.[38] Still, other cells bind to members of the cell surface receptor families TIM and TAM. These receptors normally function in the phosphatidylserine-dependent removal of cells undergoing apoptosis.[39]

DENV gains entry into its various target cells via clathrin-mediated endocytosis, during which the viruses are engulfed by clathrin-coated pits in the plasma membrane of the host cell. The pits then invaginate, carrying the bound DENV into the cell in clathrin-coated vesicles. Experimental inhibition of clathrin-mediated uptake blocks viral entry. The viruses are then taken to Rab5-positive early endosomes, which then mature into late endosomes that lose Rab5 expression while gaining that of Rab7. The acidic environment of the endosomes stimulates an irreversible trimerization of viral E proteins. Next, the DENV and endosomal membranes fuse, allowing the release of genomic RNA from the endosomes into the cytosol. This process requires acidic conditions as well as bis(monoacylglycero)phosphate.[34] Raising the endosomal pH blocks viral escape and inhibits the continuation of the DENV life cycle.

As is the case with other flaviviruses, DENV capsid proteins associate with both nuclear and cytoplasmic endoplasmic reticulum (ER)-derived subcellular compartments and with lipid droplets on the ER surface in both the virus's mammalian and mosquito hosts. These droplets provide a scaffold for viral genome encapsulation during the production of infectious viral particles.[40] During DENV infection, the number of lipid droplets increases. Inhibition of lipid droplet formation reduces DENV replication. In the ER membranes, translation and glycosylation also occur. The E protein of mosquito-derived DENV contains one to two N-linked high-mannose glycosylation sites. All DENV genotypes contain a possible glycosylation site at Asn 67, a trait that is unique among flaviviruses, as well as a glycosylation site at Asn 153 in DENV-1 and DENV-3.[32]

The nucleocapsid is assembled and remodeled in the ER, producing vesicle-like structures where double-stranded RNA and the viral nonstructural proteins NS2B, NS3, NS4A, and NS4B are produced.[41,42] Prior to budding from the ER, the DENV genomic RNA associates with viral capsid proteins and then surrounds itself with part of ER lipid bilayer that contains viral E and premembrane proteins (prM).[43] It is estimated that the DENV envelope contains approximately 8000 lipid molecules, making lipids the most abundant component of the flavivirus particle.[44] The virus particles then are passed along to the Golgi apparatus where the prM is cleaved to generate mature and immature virions that are then secreted from the host cell.[43]

DENV and Lipids—Fatty Acids and Phospholipids

Lipid metabolism plays an essential role in the DENV life cycle and the virus subverts the relevant host enzymes in order to increase its own replication. The virus-induced changes begin and end at specific times during the DENV life cycle.[45,46] The glycerophospholipids, phosphatidylserine and phosphatidylethanolamine, are required for viral entry into its target cells. Infection by DENV activates the host enzyme fatty acid synthetase and de novo lipid synthesis. This alters the lipid content of specific cellular membranes, including the amounts of unsaturated phosphatidylcholine and glycophospholipids as well as sphingolipids (ceramide, sphingosines, and sphingomyelin).[47,48] In addition to their roles in membranes, sphingolipids are also bioactive messengers that regulate apoptosis and autophagy.

Studies of the lipidome of DENV-infected cells reveal that 15% of the lipid metabolites differ significantly from those found in uninfected vertebrate and mosquito cells. These alterations in lipid content destabilize and change the curvature of cellular membranes, increasing their permeability to DENV as well as effecting the recruiting and assembly of membrane protein complexes. Intracellular trafficking is also affected by DENV-induced sphingolipids.[47] Additionally, the membrane-bound lipids help to control the synthesis and elongation of the palmitic, stearic, and oleic acids that serve as building blocks for the production of more complex lipids.

Fatty acid synthesis is connected to viral replication. The DENV NS3 protein recruits fatty acid synthase in order to increase fatty acid production.[49] People infected with DENV-3 have higher levels of lipid peroxidation in their plasma than uninfected people as determined by higher levels of malondialdehyde (MDA) around the time of defervescence. These levels are also greater in DHF and DSS than in DF cases, indicating that infection induces oxidative stress.[50] For a more comprehensive review of changes in lipid metabolism, see Martín-Acebes et al.[46]

The phospholipid receptors play a major role in the DENV life cycle. The normal function of the TAM (Tyro3, Axl, and Mertk) and TIM (T cell immunoglobulin domain and mucin domain) phosphatidylserine receptor families is to facilitate the phagocytic removal of apoptotic cells in a phosphatidylserine-dependent manner. DENV's membranes also contain this phospholipid, and the TAM and TIM receptor families indirectly or directly, respectively, recognize the virus and act as DENV entry factors. Ectopic expression of TAM or TIM receptors allows DENV to infect cells that are normally resistant to infection. Accordingly, DENV infection of susceptible cells is blocked by antibodies directed against the members of either of these receptor families.[34] In addition to phospholipids and their receptors, DENV infection also increases cellular uptake of low-density lipoproteins and the cell surface expression of their receptors.[51]

DENV and Lipids—Autophagy and Sphingolipids

DENVs alter host cell autophagy, a process that normally utilizes toxic lysosomal contents to block viral replication.[45,46] During autophagy, lipids are sequestered in double-membrane vesicles, the autophagosomes, which engulf some components of the cytoplasmic material, including viral genomes.[52] DENV and many other positive single-stranded RNA viruses, such as hepatitis C virus (HCV) and several Picornaviridae family members, induce autophagy. In these cases, however, autophagy does not harm the viruses, but rather is required for their replication. Viral RNA is present within autophagosomes and blocking autophagy also blocks DENV replication.[53,54] DENV-2 and DENV-3 escape destruction by inhibiting fusion between the autophagosomes and lysosomes, thereby preventing viral exposure to digestive enzymes and other toxic molecules sequestered within the lysosomes.

DENV also triggers autophagy-dependent processing of lipid droplets and triglycerides and releases free fatty acids. This process uses glycerolipids containing one to three fatty acids covalently attached to their glycerol backbone by an ester bond, including phosphatidylcholine, phosphatidylethanolamine, phosphatidylserine, and phosphatidylinositol. Hydrolysis of the ester bonds releases free fatty acids, which increases cellular β-oxidation in the mitochondria and generates greater amounts of ATP, enhancing viral replication.[42,49]

The DEV life cycle also requires sphingolipids and sterols, particularly cholesterol. Sphingolipids are fatty acids linked to a sphingoid by an amide bond and include ceramide and its products, the sphingosines and sphingomyelins. Viral replication complexes are enriched in sphingolipids and cholesterol when compared to the host ER. In addition to acting as a precursor for sphingosines and sphingomyelins, ceramide helps to regulate apoptosis. Following DENV RNA replication in the cytoplasm, sphingosines are involved in cellular signaling and adherence to matrices required for DENV assembly. Sphingomyelins interact with cholesterol to help control the lipid bilayer fluidity needed to form the cholesterol-rich rafts used during DENV polyprotein processing.[42] Cholesterol levels increase early during DENV infection.[55]

TRANSMISSION

DENV is transmitted to humans primarily by the bite of female *Ae. aegypti* or *Ae. albopictus* mosquitoes.[56] The outbreaks of dengue correlate to the size of the vectors' population in a given area. They usually occur during the wet season and following heavy rain since these events increase the number of potential mosquito breeding sites. *Ae. aegypti* are black-and-white mosquitoes that are generally aggressive, domestic, day-biting insects that prefer to use humans for their blood meals. Their biting activity begins in the 2 h after sunrise and ends prior to sunset. They adapt well to urban settings and lay their eggs in small stagnant pools of water or in water that has collected in vessels used to trap and store rainwater, flower vases, pet water bowls, and urban castoffs, such as nonbiodegradable plastic containers, cellophane, and discarded tires. *Ae. aegypti* are found south of 35 °N latitude.

Ae. albopictus, by contrast, is a rural mosquito originating in Asia that has been adapting to urban settings.[56] It is believed to have been introduced into the United States in the 1980s in Asian truck tires brought into the country to be retreaded. *Ae. albopictus* are much more cold-tolerant than *Ae. aegypti*, allowing them to extend their range by 7 °N latitude. The increased tolerance to cold results from the process of diapause, a suspension of egg hatching during winter months, and is similar to hibernation. *Ae. albopictus* is currently found throughout much of the eastern United States. Humans are less targeted by these mosquitoes than by *Ae. aegypti*. Several other mosquito species may also serve as DENV vectors: *Ae. scutellaris* in Polynesia, *Ae. niveus* in Malaysia, and *Ae. furcifer–taylori* in West Africa help to maintain the mosquito–monkey cycle.

Once a mosquito has ingested blood containing DENV from an infected person, it remains infective to humans for the remainder of its life without itself suffering any ill effects from its viral passenger.[6] In addition to acquiring DENV during blood meals from infected human hosts, female mosquitoes may pass DENV to their offspring through their eggs or to their mates through sexual transmission.

Other than mosquito-to-human transmission, several other relatively rare instances of human-to-human transmission have been reported.[6] Several cases of vertical transmission from infected mothers to newborns have been reported and are most likely due to the presence of DENV in breast milk.[57] Nosocomial transmission is also possible via needlesticks contaminated by the virus from an infected patient's blood. Rare instances of infection have been reported following renal or bone marrow transplantation. A small number of instances of transmission via blood transfusion are known to have occurred as well. Many countries require a deferral period from blood donation following DENV infection.[6]

THE IMMUNE RESPONSE
DENV and Innate Immune Response—Nitric Oxide

Normally after entering a person, DENV binds to the host heat-shock proteins 70 and 90 and CD14, which may serve as viral receptors during the infection of blood monocytes and tissue macrophages.[58,59] Infection stimulates interleukin (IL)-12 and IFN-γ production, activating the interferon response factor (IRF)-1 and the Janus kinase/signal transducer and activator of transcription-1 (JAK/STAT-1) pathways, which rely on the binding of phosphorylated STAT-1 to STAT-2. These pathways not only are important in the activation of type I IFNs (IFN-α and IFN-β), but they also increase the expression of the inducible nitric oxide synthesis (iNOS) gene transcription, resulting in the production of toxic nitric oxide (NO) radicals. NO is involved in a wide range of activities in their mammalian hosts, some of which are vital to normal cellular activity as well as other, harmful actions. The positive actions of NO include the relaxation of smooth muscles and increasing

blood flow to several areas, including the heart during a heart attack; decreasing blood pressure; inhibiting platelet activation; and affecting both neurotransmission and immune system responses. NO also is a potent antimicrobial agent that modifies thiol and metal centers via the formation of S–NO and S–S bonds in microbial proteins that are involved in critical catalytic and regulatory functions. IFN-γ induces NO production by iNOS in monocytes/macrophages and DCs. These closely related cells serve as hosts to many different viruses, DENV among them.[33] In monocyte/macrophage and kidney cell lines, NO reduces DENV replication. The NO donor, S-nitroso-N-acetylpenicillamine, inhibits de novo RNA synthesis by suppressing DENV-2's NS5 RNA-dependent RNA-polymerase activity. Exogenous NO also suppresses RNA synthesis in 60% of the primary isolates of DENV-2 ($n=40$).[60]

DENV and Innate Immune Response—Intracellular Signaling Pathways

DENV binds to the N-terminal caspase activation and recruitment domain (CARD)-like and the C-terminal transmembrane domains of the host adaptor protein mitochondrial antiviral signaling protein (MAVS). This binding then activates the retinoic acid-inducible gene-I (RIG-I)-like receptor (RLR). RLR binding to double-stranded RNA (dsRNA) triggers conformational changes that expose CARD domains, allowing for subsequent signaling through CARD–CARD domain interactions.[61] MAVS then interacts with TANK-binding kinase 1 (TBK1) and IκB kinase ε (IKKε), which phosphorylates IRF3 at several serine/threonine residues, permitting its translocation from the cytoplasm to the nucleus. In the nucleus, IRF3 activates the transcription factor nuclear factor-kappa B (NF-κB) and induces secretion of IFN-β by the mitochondrion-associated endoplasmic reticulum membrane RIG-I/MDA5 signaling pathway of cellular helicases.[62]

In addition to the RLR system, Toll-like receptor 3 (TLR3) recognizes viral dsRNA, but instead of using the MAVS adaptor protein, TLR3 works with Toll interleukin-1 receptor domain-containing adaptor inducing IFN-β (TRIF). As described earlier, this pathway also interacts with TBK1 and IKKε to eventually induce IFN-β secretion. The combination of IFN-β, NO, and other anti-DENV compounds is usually followed by patient recovery and resistance to reinfection by the same DENV serotype via the activity of memory T and B lymphocytes.

In order to evade threats posed by the innate immune system, DENV's NS4A interacts with MAVS, blocking the binding of MAVS to RIG-I and repressing

RIG-I-induced IRF3 activation and, consequently, abrogating IFN production.[61] DENVs' NS2B/NS3 also inhibits the phosphorylation and nuclear translocation of IRF3. DENV-4's NS2A and NS4B inhibit RIG-I-, MDA5-, MAVS-, and TBK1/IKKε-mediated IFN-β transcription pathways by greater than 80%.

Stimulator of interferon genes (STING) is part of a separate intracellular signaling pathway that induces IFN-α and IFN-β expression. STING is cleaved and inactivated by NS2B/NS3 in human DCs.[45,63] NS2A/NS4B from DENV-1, DENV-2, and DENV-4 blocks the phosphorylation of TBK1 and IRF3, decreasing IFN-β induction. DENV-1's NS4A also inhibits TBK1 activity.[64] This is in keeping with the fact that DENV-1 infection is associated with increased disease severity.

An additional mechanism by which DENV-2 avoids the IFN system is via viral dsRNA activation of protein kinase regulated by double-stranded RNA (PKR). While PKR promotes innate immune activity against several viruses, including WNV, this is not always the case. In the DENV-2-infected A459 epithelial cell line, PKR appears to downregulate IFN-β activity since abrogating activity of this kinase increases IFN-β expression, activates two mitogen-activated protein kinases (p38 and JNK) and IRF-3, and allows nuclear translocation of NF-κB.[65] Viral inhibition of IFN activity uses the RIG-I pathway and PKR's dsRNA binding, rather than kinase, activity. Interestingly, DENV does not inhibit IFN signaling in HepG2 liver or THP-1 monocytic cell lines. These particular cell lines have a lower ratio of PKR:RIG-I than is found in A459 cells. It is thus possible that PKR and RIG-I are competing for the binding of DENV dsRNA and the PKR:RIG-I ratio present in a given cell determines whether the IFN-β pathway is stimulated or downregulated.[65]

DENV and the Adaptive Immune Response—Antibodies and ADE

Antibodies that develop during the primary DENV infection provide potentially lifelong reinfection by the same DENV serotype. These antibodies briefly (less than 3 months) also protect against infection with other DENV serotypes. As antibody concentrations decrease over this time period to subneutralizing levels, they begin to instead increase DENV replication by the process of ADE triggered by an infection with a different DENV serotype. ADE increases the likelihood of developing DHF and DSS, due in part to the activity of cytokines and chemokines, such as tumor necrosis factor-α (TNF-α) and migration inhibitory factor (MIF).[66,67] Large amounts of TNF-α cause fever, inflammation, and decreases in blood pressure that may lead to shock and

death. MIF keeps macrophages in the area of infection. DENV-infected young children are also at high risk of developing DHF or DSS during the first year of life due to the lingering, low-level presence of maternal IgG antibody acquired transplacentally. Eventually, the risk of ADE is minimized as antibody levels fall still further.

The risk of developing DHF or DSS due to ADE is influenced by both the individual's immune response and the serotype of DENV involved in the secondary infection.[68] The development of DHF is also associated with the reactivation of CD8+ memory T lymphocytes formed during infection with the first DENV serotypes that cross-react with and are reactivated by the serotype present during the secondary infection. These memory T cells secrete potentially inflammatory cytokines, such as TFN-α and IFN-γ.[68] The levels of the soluble TNF-α receptor and IL-8 are also increased. These compounds mediate the increase in vascular permeability that is present in DHF and DSS patients.[69,70]

Large immune complexes also play an important role in producing ADE. These complexes bind to FcγRIIa IgG antibody receptors on the cell surface of monocytes/macrophages and DCs. This leads to increased infection of these cells and augmentation of viral replication within them. Immature DCs are refractory to ADE due to their high levels DC-SIGN and equivalent levels of FcγRIIa and FcγRIIb. FcγRIIa is stimulatory, while FcγRIIb contains an inhibitory motif. During DC maturation, the expression of the stimulatory FcγRIIa increases and DC-SIGN expression levels decrease, permitting ADE to occur.[71] The infection of DCs is followed by cellular proliferation, hypertrophy of the ER, and swelling of mitochondria, together with delayed apoptosis. Infected DCs express the maturation markers B7-1, B7-2, HLA-DR, CD11b, and CD83.[38] B7-1 and B7-2 serve as important costimulatory molecules during the activation of T lymphocytes. DENV also induces and manipulates the unfolded protein response (UFR), which normally responds to increased ER stress.[72] Viral NS2B/NS3 protein induces X-box binding protein 1, resulting in expansion of the ER and greater viral replication, due to the reduction in the UPR response and decreased DENV-induced cytopathic effect.[45,73]

CD4+ T lymphocytes are also involved in ADE. CD4+ T helper cells are stimulated by the presentation of viral antigens by MHC II molecules. As discussed previously, the type of MHC class II molecules produced by an individual is genetically determined, varies by racial group, and is related to the severity of the infection. DENV-2 stimulates a powerful antiviral CD4+ Th1 response by human peripheral blood mononuclear cells. This induces the production of the protective cytokine IFN-γ, but not the antagonistic CD4$^+$ Th2 cytokine IL-4. By contrast, the addition of subneutralizing titers of DENV-1-specific, IgG-containing immune sera induces ADE upon subsequent infection of these cells by DENV-2. This is accompanied by an increased lymphocyte proliferation index and decreased IFN-γ production.[74] Exogenous IFN-γ significantly reduces ADE in these cells.

The risk of developing ADE is greater when viruses of the DENV-2 serotype initiate the secondary infection. During the 1977 epidemic of DENV-1 in Cuba, 4.5 million cases of DF were reported without any cases of DHF or DSS. After an epidemic of DENV-2 in 1981, however, over 10,000 people developed severe disease: 95% of these had previously been infected by a different DENV serotype. Disease severity in 1981 was minimal in young children since they had not been previously infected by DENV-1 in 1977 and, thus, did not develop ADE. As noted previously, women are more prone to develop severe disease manifestations than are men. This tendency may well be linked to gender-specific differences in the immune response since both T and B lymphocyte activities are influenced by estrogens (female sex hormones). Such differences between the genders heavily influence the increased prevalence of several autoimmune conditions in women, such as systemic lupus erythematosus (lupus).

DENV and the Adaptive Immune Response—Cytokines

DENV infects and replicates in immature human myeloid DCs, including epidermal DCs (Langerhans cells) as well as those in the dermis, and its extent varies among individuals. Viral infection of these cells leads to the maturation and activation of infected as well as neighboring, uninfected DCs. Infection of these cells induces the production of several Th1-related cytokines, such as TNF-α, IFN-α, and small amounts of IL-12, but not the production of the Th2 cytokine IL-6.[38] Exposure to the Th1 cytokine IFN-γ increases the infected DCs' activation state and production of IL-12, a powerful stimulator of Th1 responses. Levels of IFN-γ in the microenvironment surrounding virally infected DCs thus appear to be a major factor in regulating whether a Th1 or Th2 response predominates.[75] DENV-stimulated natural killer cells (NK cells) may be an important early source of IFN-γ early during infection. The percent of circulating activated NK cells is greater in children with DHF than in those with dengue fever.[76]

Soundravally et al.[50] found significantly greater levels of TNF-α and IFN-γ in the plasma of persons infected with DENV-3 around the time of defervescence than in the plasma of the uninfected controls. Levels of IFN-γ later decrease with increasing disease severity so that the ratio of TNF-α to IFN-γ is greater in those with DF than in those with DHF or DSS. Infection of a monocytic leukemia cell line in vitro, however, induces a Th2-type response in both the cell lines and in peripheral blood mononuclear cells ex vivo.[74] Monocyte infection decreases transcription and translation of IL-12, IFN-γ, and TNF-α.[77] FcγR ligation completely halts IL-12 transcription, while rapid and large increases are seen in the levels of IL-10 transcription. This is in accord with increased levels of the Th2 cytokines IL-6 and IL-10 during ADE and the corresponding decrease in the levels of IL-12 in patients with severe disease when compared to the levels found in people with mild secondary infections who were initially infected by DENV-1 and then were infected by DENV-2 20 years later.[77,78] IL-10 levels are also higher in patients with secondary vs primary DENV infection.[78] While IFN-γ and TNF-α are produced by all infected cell types during ADE, cell-type-specific cytokine production patterns are observed for IL-10 and type I IFNs.

During the acute stage of DENV infection, increased levels of soluble IL-2R, soluble CD4, IL-2, and IFN-γ are present in the blood of children with DF and DHF. These levels are higher in patients with DHF than in those with DF. In addition to these immune molecules, soluble CD8 levels are also increased during DHF. Increased levels of IL-2, IFN-γ, TNF-α, and soluble TNF receptors are present during DENV infection as well and are higher during DHF than during DF.[69,70]

In in vitro studies using a primary cell culture system, the FcγR arrays differ among the various DENV host cells, even among macrophages and monocyte-derived DCs obtained from the same donor, perhaps contributing to their differing cytokine responses to ADE. Only the monocytes secreted IL-10 and they did so only during ADE. Type I IFN release from macrophages is high in the presence of neutralizing levels of antibodies, but falls during subneutralizing levels of antibody during ADE.[71] Even though the numbers of infected monocytes differ only slightly, secretion of IL-10 differs greatly among individuals according to regulatory single nucleotide polymorphisms in their IL-10 promoter region. GCC-, ACC-, and ATA-containing haplotypes are associated with high, intermediate, and low levels of IL-10 production, respectively. The haplotypes vary among populations: Asians generally have relatively low frequencies of the GCC variant (3%), while Caucasians have a 20% frequency. Looking at other DENV host cells, macrophages produce both type I IFNs during ADE, while mature DCs primarily secrete IFN-β.[71]

TNF-α is involved in ADE-related disease pathology. The previously noted decrease in TNF-α production by monocytes occurs early after infection and is transient.[72,77] The increased production of IL-6 by infected cells plays a role in liver damage, while IL-10 may damage coagulation systems.[79] IL-10 also suppresses the expression of the monocyte iNOS-1 enzyme, thus decreasing the production of NO. In addition to its roles in normal host activities, NO is an important mediator of protective immunity, inhibiting viral polymerase and protease activity and reducing DENV replication in monocytes.[60,80]

DENV interferes with type I IFN pathways interact in several ways. During ADE, IRF1 levels are reduced. Viral NS2A, NS4A, and NS4B dephosphorylate and inactivate STAT-1, while NS5 inhibits the JAK–STAT pathway by inhibiting JAK phosphorylation, which is vital for nuclear localization of STAT1/STAT2.[81,82] DENV-2's NS5 and NF4 also promote proteasomal degradation of human STAT-2. Disruption of the STAT-1/STAT-2 reduces the efficacy of IFN signaling pathways,[45,72] since these molecules normally interact with IRF9 to form the interferon stimulating gene factor 3 (ISGF3) complex. The complex then translocates to the nucleus and binds to the IFN-stimulated response elements in the promoter regions of IFN-stimulated genes (ISGs). These genes induce the production of antiviral proteins and proinflammatory cytokines. DENV disruption of any step in these pathways helps it to escape type I IFN-mediated responses.

Virus activation of several alternative signaling cascades, such as the mitogen-activated protein kinase p38 and the phosphatidylinositol 3 kinase cascades, also induces the production of proinflammatory cytokines and chemokines.[45] Additionally, DENV infection of monocyte-derived primary human macrophages that are stimulated by granulocyte macrophage colony-stimulating factor release (GM-CSF), release L-1β and IL-18 from inflammasomes. These, in turn, stimulate the activation of the proinflammatory Th17 subset of CD4+ T helper cells, contributing to severe disease.[83] By contrast, DENV-infected primary blood monocytes stimulated by macrophage colony-stimulating factor do not produce IL-1β.

Infection of Langerhans cells, monocytes/macrophages, and lymphocytes often results in increased production of several interleukins and other cytokines, including TNF-α, IL-8, IL-10, IL-13, and IL-18. These cytokines may be involved in the development of DHF and increase its severity. IL-6 and perhaps IL-10 increase

vascular permeability and that may promote capillary leakage. In an in vitro model of ADE, exposing monocytic cells to ADE-causing antibodies and DENV led to the secretion of several of the cytokines previously described plus the proinflammatory hormone prostaglandin E_2.[84] The addition of supernatants containing cytokines from the monocytic cultures mentioned previously to an epithelial cell monolayer in vitro causes a rapid loss of transepithelial electrical resistance and disarrangement of several apical–junction complex proteins (occludin, ZO-2, and E-cadherin) which normally prevent excessive fluid loss from capillaries.[84] Such vascular leakage is present during DSS.[85] Moreover, the culture supernatants increase in vascular permeability in plasma and lung extracts in mice in vivo. However, direct DENV infection of these cells, mimicking a primary infection, did not have this effect in vitro or in vivo.[84]

IL-10 levels are higher in persons with DHF than in those with DF. IL-12 appears to moderate DHF severity. IL-12 levels decrease during infection as the CD4+ T helper cell-mediated immunity shifts from a Th1 to a Th2 response during the course of the disease. TNF-α may contribute to disease by stimulating IL-6 production and by inducing thrombocytopenia. At excessive levels, TNF-α also induces a dangerously high fever. People inheriting a gene that permits the production of higher than normal levels of TNF-α are at a greater risk of developing DHF. Treating mice with serum containing antibodies to this cytokine reduces mortality by 60%, further underscoring the importance of the role of TNF-α in the pathological process.

Levels of the type II IFN, IFN-γ, produced by Th1 cells are increased during infection. This cytokine functions in both protective processes and disease induction. On the one hand, this cytokine has antiviral activity while, and on the other hand, it boosts inflammatory IL-6 and IL-8 production. IFN-γ also increases the expression of the Fc antibody receptor of macrophages, allowing them to be infected by the virus. Interestingly, when CD4+ T helper cells were exposed to DENV of the same serotype as the original infecting strain, they produce large amounts of protective IFN-γ. By contrast, exposing the T helper cells to a differing DENV serotype leads to greater production of TNF-α instead. IFN-γ may thus be linked to long-lasting immunity against reinfection by viruses of the same serotype, while TNF-α may lead to the pathogenic response induced by secondary infection by viruses of a different serotype.

Mucosal-associated invariant T cells are innate T cells with potent antibacterial activity. During acute DENV infection, these cells elevate their expression of the activation markers CD38 and HLA-DR. As is the case for CD4[+] T helper cells, the activation of these T cells is dependent on IL-12 and, additionally, on IL-18. The role of these cells in DENV infection is as yet unknown, but they do produce IFN-γ following in vitro ZIKV infection of cells.[86]

DENV and the Adaptive Immune Response—Lymphocyte Responses

The type of lymphocyte response to infection may help to determine the severity of diseases. High-affinity CD8[+] T killer cells may aid in controlling viral expansion. Numbers of these cells, as well as B lymphocytes and NK cells, are lower in individuals who develop DHF than in those who do not develop severe disease. Additionally, DENV infection lessens the ability of T to divide when stimulated.

NK cells and CD8[+] T killer cells provide the best host defense against viral infections, including flaviviruses. DENV-specific CD8[+] T killer cells also provide cross-protective responses to infection by ZIKV in mice, while passive transfer of DENV-immune serum is not protective against subsequent ZIKV infection.[87] In the case of DENV infection, B lymphocytes produce neutralizing antibodies that provide life-long protection against a secondary infection with the same viral serotype.

Lymphocytes also may be involved in immuno-pathogenesis, the development of which is at least partially influenced by which human MHC alleles are expressed in a given individual and the strength of their anti-DENV T cell response. DENV features also affect the severity of DENV-related disease, including which viral epitopes are expressed and recognized by T cells.[87] Low-affinity T cells against DENV contribute to immune-mediated pathology by the secretion of inflammatory cytokines by serotype-specific, cross-reactive CD8[+] memory T killer cells. Pathogenic CD8[+] memory T killer cells are relatively refractory to DENV-induced cytolysis while retaining their ability to secrete the inflammatory TNF-α cytokine and the MIP-1β chemokine during secondary infection by another DENV serotype.[68] The production of subneutralizing antibodies during secondary infection is associated with disease severity via ADE. Other types of antibodies against DENV antigens appear to cross-reactive with human platelets, leading to platelet aggregation and destruction by the complement cascade. This is followed by their ingestion and removal by macrophages in a manner similar to that occurring in the autoimmune disease thrombocytopenic purpura. Other products of complement activation, the anaphylatoxins, may lead to shock and death during DSS.

IL-10-producing T regulatory cells (Tregs) help to block excessive immune responses by downregulating the activity of both CD4[+] T helper cells and CD8[+] T killer cells. Insufficient numbers or activity of Tregs could thus contribute to the overactive inflammatory response to DENV infection. During the acute phase of infection, however, Tregs undergo expansion and the Treg:effector T cell ratio significantly increases, especially in adult patients with mild, but not severe, disease. In children, absolute numbers of Tregs are similar during mild or severe disease.[69] Tregs activated by dengue antigens reduce the secretion of vasoactive cytokines by effector T cells, decreasing plasma leakage and improving disease outcome. While DENV-mediated stimulation of peripheral blood mononuclear cells from noninfected donors, it does not affect IFN-γ levels. The production of IFN-γ by patients' CD4[+]CD25[+] activated cells, however, decreases in the presence of Treg cells. Accordingly, the depletion of Tregs significantly increases IFN-γ release.[69,70] The proliferation of CD4[+]CD25[neg] T cells during acute dengue infection is similar to that found during convalescence (over 55%), but this proliferation is reduced by 85% in the presence of exogenesis Tregs. The levels of IL-10 are also comparable in cells from acutely infected and recovered subjects.[69]

The Mosquito Immune Response to DENV Infection

A wide variety of viruses, including DENV, require a functioning ubiquitin–proteasome system to replicate in human endothelial and mosquito cells. During the DENV life cycle, following their release from endosomes, the now-cytoplasmic nucleocapsids are tagged by ubiquitin E1 for processing by proteasomes. During this process, the capsid protein is degraded and the "naked" viral RNA is released back into the cytoplasm.[88,89] Inhibition of ubiquitin activity in DENV-infected cells lengthens viral RNA retention in the nucleocapsid, thus blocking viral maturation.[43] Ubiquitin E1 is upregulated in DENV-infected cells and treatment for these cells with a specific ubiquitin E1 inhibitor reduces viral protein synthesis.[87,89] Treatment for infected primary human monocytes with low nM concentrations of the proteasome inhibitor bortezomib prevents exocytosis and the egress of all four DENV serotypes from human cell lines and may do so for mosquito cells as well.[90]

In addition to marking proteins for proteasomal destruction, some insect ubiquitins also help to control innate immune responses. The mosquito ubiquitin Ub3881 interacts with and regulates immune signaling by immune deficiency (Imd), leading to the transcription of innate immune genes, including antimicrobial peptides.[91] In addition, overexpression of Ub3881 upregulates the levels of several AMP genes, including cecropin, attacin, defensin, and diptericin, in addition to increasing levels of cleaved caspase-3, a marker of apoptosis. Microarray analysis of the DENV-infected *Ae. aegypti* transcriptome revealed that Ub3881 is the only mosquito ubiquitin protein that is highly downregulated during all stages of infection in both mosquito midgut and salivary glands. In in vitro studies of an infected mosquito cell line, Ub3881 targets both the DENV-2 E protein and capsid for degradation and destruction, reducing viral replication. Similar events occur in mosquitoes in vivo.[92,93]

Activation of the complement cascade neutralizes DENV-infected mammalian and insect host cells. Soluble NS1 is found in the plasma of DENV-infected patients and, in small amounts, in the supernatants of an *Ae. albopictus* cell line. Large amounts of soluble NS1 and members of the complement membrane attack complex (C5b-9) in human plasma correlate with a higher risk of developing severe dengue manifestations. Soluble NS1 is also found in the saliva of infected *Ae. aegypti* mosquitoes and differs from the form found in human plasma. Mammalian soluble NS1 bears high-mannose and complex N-linked glycans, while the NS1 form in insects has only high-mannose glycans. During a blood meal, soluble NS1 and DENV in mosquito saliva are released into the mammalian host. In both mosquito and mammalian cell types, soluble NS1 binds to several components of the complement system: C1s, C4, and the C4 binding protein of the classical pathway of complement activation. This binding results in C4 degradation and inhibition of both the classical and lectin pathways of complement activation.

All four DENV serotypes bind to the mannose-binding lectin (MBL) of the lectin pathway of complement activation in a manner that inhibits DENV attachment to insect cells without activating a complement pathway. Soluble NS1, however, competitively binds to the MBL, allowing the virus to bind to and enter mosquito cells.[94] The hexameric form of soluble NS1 also binds to lipids, forming lipoprotein particles that activate TLR-2, TLR-4, and TLR-6 of the innate immune system. This, in turn, stimulates the production of inflammatory cytokines that weaken vascular endothelial cell junction integrity.[94]

DENV and RNA Interference of Protein Synthesis

Another host defensive measure is the action of RNAi (RNA interference), which regulates the production of proteins, including antiviral IL-1 and TLRs, at the transcriptional and translational levels.[45] During their formation, RNAi must be processed by several host proteins. The NS4B protein of all four DENV serotypes together with host siRNA (small interfering RNA) blocks the activity of several proteins involved in the processing of host miRNA (microRNA) during the formation of RNAi, including Dicer, Drosha, Ago1, and Ago2. The loss of antiviral RNAi permits increased viral replication. This NS4B inhibitory activity is independent of its IFN-inhibitory actions.[95] The inhibitory regions of viral NS4B are found in transmembrane domain-3 and domain-5, but not in the NS4B N-terminal region. The terminal region encodes the signal sequence and is part of the viral replication complex.[95] Of the known host cell miRNA ($n = 151$), the expression of 94.7% is also inhibited by DENV, while 1.9% is upregulated. WNV also interferes with host RNAi activity.

PREVENTION

Vector control programs have been very effective in the control of dengue and other insect-borne diseases, including yellow fever and malaria. Such programs, however, are currently almost nonexistent in countries with endemic dengue. Unfortunately, some of the species of mosquito vectors have developed resistance to commonly used insecticides. Some other, less expensive, insecticides, such as DDT, have been banned due to ecological concerns that arose when these insecticides were used excessively in agriculture. Development and implementation of vector control programs are vital to control not only the diseases spread by insects, such as mosquitoes, ticks, and fleas, but also rodents that serve as both vectors and disease reservoirs. In the absence of effective vector control, individuals may attempt to avoid being bitten by the use of screening, protective clothing, and insect repellents.

One of the ways currently employed to decrease the number of infected *Ae. aegypti* mosquitoes is peridomestic spraying, in which droplets of insecticide are sprayed in and around houses of dengue-positive cases.[96] Either thermal fogs or cold fogs are used and may be dispensed from vehicle-mounted or hand-held equipment. This method is an emergency procedure that is used to eliminate adult mosquitoes. It is politically attractive due to the high visibility of the process. Fogging, however, comes with several shortcomings that may lull the area residents into a false sense of security, including the need for people to open the doors and windows of their homes to permit the droplets to enter the dwelling and the need for periodic re-application.

The treatment for materials, such as window curtains, water container covers, and bed nets with insecticides is another preventative method that effectively reduces *Ae. aegypti* numbers in homes. This method may prove to be more useful for DENV prevention than residual spraying of the domiciles' interior walls, even though it has been effectively employed in the campaign against *Anopheles* species mosquitoes that transmit malaria. Unlike *Anopheles* mosquitoes that alight on walls, *Ae. aegypti* often rest on other materials, such as hanging clothes, for which spraying would be inappropriate. By modifying insect-control measures that have proven successful against other arboviruses, methods may be developed to again reduce DENV vector numbers or exposure to the relevant *Aedes* species and decrease the extent of the current dengue pandemic.

Vaccination is another powerful means of preventing infection by many pathogenic microbes. In the case of DENV, however, vaccine development is more complicated than it is for many other pathogenic viruses. Due to the risk of inducing ADE in which antibodies to one serotype of DENV may enhance the pathogenicity of other serotypes, the research community may need to design a vaccine that induces immunity to all four dengue serotypes simultaneously. Dengvaxia, a vaccine that targets the four serotypes of DENV, as well as YFV, is licensed for use in several Latin American countries. However, it is costly and associated with serious issues that call into question its effectiveness in disease prevention and, more problematically, raise the possibility that this vaccine may increase the risk for severe disease in dengue-naïve people.[10] By contrast, phase 1 clinical trials of a yellow fever-dengue 2 combination vaccine (ChimeriVax-DENV2) have shown it to be safe, unaffected by pre-existing immunity to YFV, and able to induce a long-lasting, cross-neutralizing antibody response to all dengue serotypes.

TREATMENT

The treatment for DENV-associated diseases is currently largely supportive. Prompt oral or intravenous isotonic fluid replacement therapy is recommended by the World Health Organization to counter the results of plasma leakage from capillaries, the resulting hemoconcentration, and the life-threatening drop in blood pressure during DHF and DSS. If untreated, the fatality rates are 40%–50%, while adequate fluid replacement lowers the death rate to 1%–2%. Blood transfusions should be used with extreme caution due to fluid overload. Platelet transfusions are also used in patients with severe bleeding.

Several types of therapeutic drugs are being used or are under development. These act by inhibiting viral binding and entry into target cells; decreasing nucleoside production or causing their depletion; suppressing ISG activity; and blocking the activity of the enzymes RNA polymerase, methyltransferase, helicase, serine protease, α-glucosidase I, and the kinases that are involved in cellular signaling events; preventing capsid and nucleocapsid assembly; and disrupting lipid metabolism.

Inhibition of Viral Binding and Entry

Polyanions, like heparin derivatives; hyaluronic acid; and some seed extracts block viral binding to and entry into target cells.[35] Additionally, some agents that block cellular adhesion of bacteria, algae, and fungal spores also inhibit DENVs' binding to their target cells.

The viral E protein contains a pocket that binds to the detergent *n*-octyl-β-D-glucoside. This pocket must undergo a conformational change prior to fusion with the host cell membrane.

Agents that bind to this pocket may potentially able to block the E protein's change in shape and prevent DENV from entering the cell.[97]

Reduction of Nucleoside Levels

Mycophenolic acid, 6-azauridine, and urea VX-497 have been used to block nucleoside production or lead to their depletion. Ribavirin and several other antiviral agents suppress purine synthesis by inhibiting the host cell enzyme IMP dehydrogenase, resulting in a depletion of guanine. Other nucleoside inhibitors, NITD 982 and Brequinar, block host cell dihydroorotate dehydrogenase, an enzyme required for pyrimidine biosynthesis.[98] While effective against DENV-2, NITD 982 is significantly less active against the other three DENV serotypes in cell culture in vitro and is not active in mice in vivo, perhaps due to the abundance of uridine in the animals' plasma.

Suppression of ISG Activity

The expression of Repressor of yield of DENV (RyDEN), a zinc-ribbon protein containing ISG, inhibits the replication of all DENV serotypes, as well as Kunjin virus and HCV. RyDEN forms a complex with the cellular mRNA binding proteins PABPC1 and LARP1, which are necessary for efficient replication and translation of DENV.[99] Some other human ISGs, including interferon-inducible transmembrane proteins, ISG15, ISG20, viperin, and BST2, suppress in vitro virus infection. RyDEN siRNA also acts against the viral cytoplasmic NS3 and viral mycophenolic acid to block DENV replication.[99]

Inhibition of NS5 Polymerase—Nucleoside Analogs

Nucleoside analogs, such as barbituric and thiobarbituric acids, inhibit the flaviviruses' NS5 RNA-dependent RNA polymerase viral polymerase. Such analogs are active both in vitro in cell cultures and in vivo in mice. Some are active against all four dengue serotypes as well as several other flaviviruses, including WNV, YFV, and Powassan virus, as well as HCV, another member of the Flaviviridae family. The adenosine analogs NITD008 and beta-D-2'-ethynyl-7-deaza-adenosine act as chain terminating, competitive inhibitors of the viral polymerase and are active against all DENV serotypes.[100,101] NITD008 is active both in vitro and in vivo, but can only be used short-term in rats and dogs without causing adverse effects. Another adenosine analog, 7-deaza-2'-C-methyl-adenosine, is selective and has good cell penetration in vitro and encouraging pharmacokinetics results in vivo in beagle dogs and rats as well as in macaques.[102]

Inhibition of NS5 Polymerase—Nonnucleoside Analogs

Several nonnucleoside compounds also inhibit DENV's polymerase. Podocarpusflavone and sotetsuflavone, extracts of the leaves of the New Caledonian gymnosperm *Dacrydium balansae*, strongly inhibit DENV-2's polymerase in vitro without being cytotoxic.[103] These extracts also inhibit the WNV, but not the HCV, RNA polymerase. *N*-Sulfonylanthranilic acid derivatives are another group of DENV polymerase inhibitors that block the enzyme's primer extension-based RNA elongation as well as the de novo synthesis of RNA by DENV-2 and DENV-4.[104] They are specific for DENV polymerase and are not effective against the WNV and HCV enzymes. Unfortunately, these inhibitors are not active in in vitro cell culture. Derivatives of 2,1-benzothiazine 2,2-dioxide act against the N pocket of the polymerase's thumb domain.[105,106] A new class of polymerase inhibitors chelates divalent ions from the enzyme's active site, blocking DENV polymerase activity due to its need for two divalent Mg^{2+} cofactors.[107] One of these metal ion chelators is a pyridoxine derivative that is effective against all DENV serotypes in the assays of purified enzyme activity as well as in a cultured kidney cell line.

Inhibition of DENV NS5 Methyltransferase

In addition to encoding the RNA polymerase, DENV NS5 also encodes an AdoMet-dependent methyltransferase domain which is responsible for capping the ends of viral mRNA. Since mammalian cells also contain methyltransferases that are critical to their mRNA maturation, great care must be taken to create inhibitors that are highly selective for the DENV methyltransferases. A fragment-based drug design has identified three ligands of this domain. Linking *N*-phenyl-[(phenylcarbamoyl)amino]benzene-1-sulfonamide and phenyl [(phenylcarbamoyl) amino]benzene-1-sulfonate derivatives results in a 10–100-fold stronger inhibition of the methyltransferase activity than the fragments alone.[108]

Inhibition of Viral NS3 Helicase

The DENV's NS3 protein has several functions, including helicase activity in which it unwinds dsRNA to produce the single-stranded RNA (ssRNA) used during replication by the NS5 polymerase. NS3 and NS5 are excellent drug targets since they are conserved in all DENV serotypes. Halim et al.[109] used computational tools to perform in silico screening of potential inhibitors of the NS3 helicase. Many of the active compounds interact with a groove between NS3's domains II and III.

Inhibition of Viral Serine Protease

DENV's NS2B-NS3 serine protease cleaves the inactive long viral precursor polyprotein into active, individual proteins. The protease is inhibited by peptides containing phenylalanine and phenylglycine derivatives, which act as arginine-mimicking groups.[110]

Inhibition of α-Glucosidase I

α-Glucosidase I is a cellular enzyme that is vital to correct folding of glycoproteins by removing sugar moieties during protein processing. Castanospermine is an alkaloid derived from black beans or the Moreton Bay chestnut trees. It prevents the host cell α-glucosidase I enzyme from trimming N-linked glycans, a process that is necessary for folding the viral structural proteins prM and E. Castanospermine is active against all four DENV serotypes, but is either partially or totally ineffective against the YFV and WNV members of the flavivirus genus, respectively. Additionally, castanospermine prevented death in an in vivo mouse model of DENV infection.[111] Deoxynojirimycin is related to castanospermine and also inhibits α-glucosidase, although with less efficiency.

Inhibition of Intracellular Signaling—Protein Kinases

Kinases are integral members of many of the intracellular signaling cascades that control quite a few cellular activities. These enzymes generally attach phosphate ions to either proteins or lipids, often stimulating the next component of the cascade in a domino-like fashion. One signaling pathway triggered by DENV infection stimulates the activity of the angiogenic factor vascular endothelial growth factor (VEGF) and TNF-α. This may result in life-threatening capillary leakage, severe hypotension, and shock during DHF and DSS. In a mouse model, serum levels of VEGF increase by the second day of infection, leading to about an 80% mortality rate.[112] Administration of sunitinib, a VEGF receptor tyrosine kinase inhibitor, decreased this rate to 50%–80% of that seen in untreated, infected mice. Sunitinib also reduces serum TNF-α and leukocyte and hematocrit levels, however, only slightly decrease tissue viral load. Combination therapy with sunitinib and an anti-TNF antibody reduces vascular leakage and synergistically protects against fatal DENV infection.[112] DENV kinases also play an important role in the evasion of host immune responses.

Inhibition of Intracellular Signaling—RIG-I

Administration of low, noncytotoxic doses of an optimized 5′ triphosphorylated RNA blocks DENV-induced RIG-I stimulation and infection of mice when given before or after challenge with virus. This RIG-I agonist blocked primary infection in primary human monocytes and monocyte-derived DCs as well as in human epithelial and fibroblastic cells, as well as insect cell lines. Importantly, it prevented the development of ADE. Protection depends on an intact RIG-I/MAVS/TBK1/IRF3 axis that is largely independent of STAT signaling.[113]

Rhodiola extracts decrease DENV levels in human peripheral blood mononuclear cells in a similar manner, by inducing ISG, RIG-I, and MDA5 gene expression and the IFN-β pathway.[114] *Rhodiola imbricate* is a plant present in the high-altitude, cold desert of the Indian trans-Himalayan region and is used medicinally in several countries in the region. *Rhodiola* extracts contain several active compounds, including phenylpropanoids, phenylethanol derivatives, flavonoids, terpenoids, and phenolic acids.

Inhibition of Capsid and Nucleocapsid Assembly

The viral capsid, which typically exists as a dimer or a trimer, is another target for anti-DENV drugs. One such drug is T-148, which acts by enhancing capsid self-interaction and tetramer formation in all DENV serotypes. This self-interaction interferes with entry into target cells as well as with assembly and disassembly of DENV nucleocapsids, probably by inducing structural rigidity and blocking the formation of higher-order capsid structures. It is active in vitro and also decreases viremia in mice.[115] DENV assembly typically occurs in the ER, so interfering with nucleocapsid assembly leads to the accumulation of immature viral components in the host ER.

Disruption of Lipid Metabolism

An increase in cellular cholesterol levels is required early after DENV infection since viral replication requires cholesterol. The increase in cholesterol levels occurs by enhancing exogenous cholesterol uptake through the low-density lipoprotein receptor and by increasing activity of the 3-hydroxy-3-methyl-glutaryl-CoA reductase, HMG-CoA, and squalene synthase activity.[42,51] Nordihydroguaiaretic acid (NDGA) is a polyphenol hypolipidemic agent derived from the creosote bush (chaparral). NDGA inhibits lipogenesis by altering the expression of genes whose products regulate fatty acid synthesis and degradation including adenosine monophosphate-activated protein kinase (AMPK), SREBP-1 and SRRBP-2, acetyl-CoA carboxylase, and fatty acid synthase. The addition of NDGA to DENV-4-infected hepatocarcinoma, monocytic leukemia, and kidney cell lines decreases viral replication, NS1 secretion, numbers of lipid droplets, and dissociation of the viral C protein.[51] Two other agents, cerulenin and C75, also inhibit fatty acid synthetase in cell lines and interact with DENV NS3 in a Rab18-dependent manner.[42]

SUMMARY OVERVIEW

Diseases: dengue fever, dengue hemorrhagic fever, dengue shock syndrome
Causative agent: dengue viruses, serotypes 1–4
Vectors: *Aedes aegypti* and *Aedes albopictus* mosquitoes
Common reservoirs: humans and monkeys
Mode of transmission: mosquito bite
Geographical distribution: tropical and subtropical regions throughout the world
Year of emergence: 1770 (dengue fever); 1953 (dengue hemorrhagic fever)

REFERENCES

1. Gubler DJ. Epidemic dengue and dengue hemorrhagic fever: a global public health problem in the 21th century. In: Scheld WM, Armstrong D, Hughes JM, eds. *Emerging Infections.* vol. 1. ASM Press; 1998.
2. Heymann DL. *Control of Communicable Diseases Manual.* 19th ed. American Public Health Association; 2008.
3. Messina JP, Brady OJ, Scott TW, et al. Global spread of dengue virus types: mapping the 70 year history. *Trends Microbiol.* 2014;22(3):138–146.

4. Gyawali N, Bradbury RS, Taylor-Robinson AW. The epidemiology of dengue infection: harnessing past experience and current knowledge to support implementation of future control strategies. *J Vector Borne Dis.* 2016;53:293–304.

5. Pan American Health Organization. Dengue. Accessed May 31, 2020. https://www.paho.org/en/topics/dengue.

6. Centers for Disease Control and Prevention. Dengue. Accessed May 31, 2020. https://www.cdc.gov/dengue/epidemiology/index.html.

7. World Health Organization. Dengue. Accessed May 31, 2020. http://www/who.int/denguecontrol.

8. Powell JR, Tabachnick WJ. History of domestication and spread of *Aedes aegypti*—a review. *Mem Inst Oswaldo Cruz.* 2013;108(suppl. I):11–17.

9. Murray NEA, Quam MB, Wilder-Smith A. Epidemiology of dengue: past, present and future prospects. *Clin Epidemiol.* 2013;5:299–309.

10. Salles TS, da Encarnação Sá-Guimarães T, de Alvarenga ESL, et al. History, epidemiology and diagnostics of dengue in the American and Brazilian contexts: a review. *Parasit Vectors.* 2018;11:264.

11. Jansen CC, Beebe NW. The dengue vector *Aedes aegypti*: what comes next? *Microbes Infect.* 2010;12:272–279.

12. Halstead SB. Emergence mechanisms in yellow fever and dengue. In: Scheld WM, Craig WA, Hughes JM, eds. *Emerging Infections 2.* ASM Press; 1998.

13. Hammon WM. Dengue hemorrhagic fever—do we know its cause? *Am J Trop Med Hyg.* 1973;22:82–91.

14. Monath TP, Heinz FX. Flaviviruses. In: Fields BN, Knipe DM, Howley PM, et al., eds. *Fields Virology.* Lippincott-Raven; 1996:961–1034.

15. Bhatt S, Gething PW, Brady OJ, et al. The global distribution and burden of dengue. *Nature.* 2013;496:504–507.

16. Kyle JL, Harris E. Global spread and persistence of dengue. *Annu Rev Microbiol.* 2008;62:71–92.

17. Kraemer MU, Sinka ME, Duda KA, et al. The global distribution of the arbovirus vectors *Aedes aegypti* and *Ae. albopictus.* *eLife.* 2015;4, e08347.

18. Holmes EC, Bartley LM, Garnett GP. The emergence of dengue: past, present, and future. In: Krause RM, ed. *Emerging Infections.* vol. 1. Academic Press; 1998:301–325.

19. Schliessman DJ, Calheiros LB. A review of the status of yellow fever and *Aedes aegypti* eradication programs in the Americas. *Mosq News.* 1974;34:1–9.

20. Centers for Disease Control and Prevention. Imported dengue: United States, 1993–1994. *MMWR.* 1995;44:353–356.

21. Gubler DJ. Epidemic dengue/dengue hemorrhagic fever as a public health, social and economic problem in the 21st century. *Trends Microbiol.* 2002;10:100–103.

22. Mackenzie JS, Gubler DJ, Petersen LR. Emerging flaviviruses: the spread and resurgence of Japanese encephalitis, West Nile and dengue viruses. *Nat Med.* 2004;10:S98–S109.

23. Li GH, Ning ZJ, Liu YM, Li XH. Neurological manifestations of dengue infection. *Front Cell Infect Microbiol.* 2017;7:1–13.

24. Ramos C, Sánchez G, Pando RH, et al. Dengue virus in the brain of a fatal case of hemorrhagic dengue fever. *J Neurovirol.* 1998;4:465–468.

25. Guzman MG, Gubler DJ, Izquierdo A, Martinez E, Halstead SB. Dengue infection. *Nat Rev Dis Primers.* 2016;2:16055.

26. Martins VCA, Bastos MS, Ramasawmy R, et al. Clinical and virological descriptive study in the 2011 outbreak of dengue in the Amazonas, Brazil. *PLoS One.* 2014;9(6), e100535.

27. Beltz LA. Dengue fever and dengue hemorrhagic fever. In: *Emerging infectious diseases: a guide to diseases, causative agents, and surveillance.* Jossey-Bass; 2011.

28. Hung NT, Lan NT, Lei H-Y. Association between sex, nutritional status, severity of dengue hemorrhagic fever, and immune status in infants with dengue hemorrhagic fever. *Am J Trop Med Hyg.* 2005;72(4):370–374.

29. Keating JABD, Rund SS, Hoover S, et al. Mosquito protein kinase G phosphorylates flavivirus NS5 and alters flight behavior in *Aedes aegypti* and *Anopheles gambiae.* *Vector Borne Zoonotic Dis.* 2013;3(8):590–600.

30. Normile D. Surprising new dengue virus throws a spanner in disease control efforts. *Science.* 2013;342:415.

31. Warke RV, Martin KJ, Giaya K, Shaw SK, Rothman AL, Bosch I. TRAIL is a novel antiviral protein against dengue virus. *J Virol.* 2008;82(1):555–564.

32. Navarro-Sanchez E, Altmeyer R, Amara A. Dendritic-cell-specific ICAM3-grabbing non-integrin is essential for the productive infection of human dendritic cells by mosquito-cell-derived dengue viruses. *EMBO Rep.* 2003;4(7):723–728.

33. Wu S-JL, Grouard-Vogel G, Sun Mascola JR, et al. Human skin Langerhans cells are targets of dengue virus infection. *Nat Med.* 2003;6:816–820.

34. van der Schaar HM, Rust MJ, Chen C, et al. Dissecting the cell entry pathway of dengue virus by single-particle tracking in living cells. *PLoS Pathol.* 2008;4, e1000244.

35. Chen Y, Maguire T, Hileman RE, et al. Dengue virus infectivity depends on envelope protein binding to target cell heparin sulfate. *Nat Med.* 1997;3(8):866–871.

36. Hung S-L, Lee P-L, Chen H-W, Chen L-K, Kao C-L, King C-C. Analysis of the steps in dengue virus entry into host cells. *Virology.* 1999;257:156–167.

37. Germi R, Crance J-M, Garin D, et al. Heparin sulfate-mediated binding of infectious dengue virus type-2 and yellow fever virus. *Virology.* 2002;292:162–168.

38. Ho L-J, Wang J-J, Shaio M-F. Infection of human dendritic cells by dengue virus causes cell maturation and cytokine production. *J Immunol.* 2001;166:1499–1506.

39. Meertens L, Carnec X, Lecoin MP, et al. The TIM and TAM families of phosphatidylserine receptors mediate dengue virus entry. *Cell Host Microbe.* 2012;12:544–557.

40. Samsa MM, Mondotte JA, Iglesias NG, et al. Dengue virus capsid protein usurps lipid droplets for viral particle formation. *PLoS Pathol.* 2009;5, e1000632.

41. Gillespie LK, Hoenen A, Morgan G, Mackenzie JM. The endoplasmic reticulum provides the membrane platform for biogenesis of the flavivirus replication complex. *J Virol.* 2010;84:10438–10447.

42. Villareal VA, Rodgers MA, Costello DA, Yang PL. Targeting host lipid synthesis and metabolism to inhibit dengue and hepatitis C viruses. *Antiviral Res.* 2015;124:110–121.

43. Byk LA, Iglesias NG, de Maio FA, Gebhard LG, Rossi M, Gamarnik AV. Dengue virus genome uncoating requires ubiquitination. *mBio.* 2016;7(3), e00804-16.

44. Reddy T, Sansom MS. The role of the membrane in the structure and biophysical robustness of the dengue virion envelope. *Structure.* 2016;24:375–382.

45. Green AM, Beatty PR, Hadjilaou A, Harris E. Innate immunity to dengue virus infection and subversion of antiviral responses. *J Mol Biol.* 2014;426(6):1148–1160.

46. Martín-Acebes MA, Vázquez-Calvo A, Saiz J-C. Lipids and flaviviruses, present and future perspectives for the control of dengue, Zika, and West Nile viruses. *Prog Lipid Res.* 2016;64:123–137.

47. Perera R, Riley C, Isaac G, et al. Dengue virus infection perturbs lipid homeostasis in infected mosquito cells. *PLoS Pathog.* 2012;8, e1002584.

48. Heaton NS, Perera R, Berger KL. Dengue virus nonstructural protein 3 redistributes fatty acid synthase to sites of viral replication and increases cellular fatty acid synthesis. *PNAS.* 2010;107:17345–17350.

49. Heaton NS, Randall G. Dengue virus-induced autophagy regulates lipid metabolism. *Cell Host Microbe.* 2010;8:422–432.

50. Soundravally R, Hoti SL, Patil SA, et al. Association between proinflammatory cytokines and lipid peroxidation in patients with severe dengue disease around defervescence. *Int J Infect Dis.* 2014;18:68–72.

51. Soto-Acosta R, Mosso C, Cervantes-Salazar M, et al. The increase in cholesterol levels at early stages after dengue virus infection correlates with an augment in LDL particle uptake and HMG-CoA reductase activity. *Virology.* 2013;442:132–147.

52. Rubinsztein DC, Shpilka T, Elazar Z. Mechanisms of autophagosome biogenesis. *Curr Biol.* 2012;22:29–34.

53. Panyasrivanit M, Khakpoor A, Wikan N, Smith DR. Co-localization of constituents of the dengue virus translation and replication machinery with amphisomes. *J Gen Virol.* 2009;90:448–456.

54. Mateo R, Nagamine CM, Spagnolo J, et al. Inhibition of cellular autophagy deranges dengue virion maturation. *J Virol.* 2013;87:1312–1321.

55. Rothwell C, Lebreton A, Ng CY, et al. Cholesterol biosynthesis modulation regulates dengue viral replication. *Virology.* 2009;389:8–19.

56. Ponlawat A, Harrington LC. Blood feeding patterns of *Aedes aegypti* and *Aedes albopictus* in Thailand. *J Med Entomol.* 2005;42:844–849.

57. Barthel A, Gourinat AC, Cazorla C, Joubert C, Dupont-Rouzeyrol M, Descloux E. Breast milk as a possible route of vertical transmission of dengue virus? *Clin Infect Dis.* 2013;57(3):415–417.

58. Chen YC, Wang SY, King CC. Bacterial lipopolysaccharide inhibits dengue virus infection of primary human monocytes/macrophages by blockade of virus entry via a CD14-dependent mechanism. *J Virol.* 1999;73:2650–2657.

59. Reyes-del Valle J, Chavez-Salinas S, Medina F, del Angel RM. Heat shock protein 90 and heat shock protein 70 are components of dengue virus receptor complex in human cells. *J Virol.* 2005;79:4557–4567.

60. Charnsilpa W, Takhampunya R, Endy TP, Mammen Jr MP, Libraty DH, Ubol S. Nitric oxide radical suppresses replication of wild-type dengue 2 viruses *in vitro. J Med Virol.* 2005;77:89–95.

61. He Z, Zhu X, Wen W. Dengue virus subverts host innate immunity by targeting adaptor protein MAVS. *J Virol.* 2016;90:7219–7230.

62. Hiscott J. Triggering the innate antiviral response through IRF-3 activation. *J Biol Chem.* 2007;282:15325–15329.

63. Aguirre S, Maestre AM, Pagni S, et al. DENV inhibits type I IFN production in infected cells by cleaving human STING. *PLoS Pathog.* 2012;8:1002934.

64. Dalrymple NA, Cimica V, Mackow ER. Dengue virus NS proteins inhibit RIG-1/MAVS signaling by blocking TBK1/IRF3 phosphorylation: dengue virus serotype 1 NS4A is a unique interferon-regulating virulence determinant. *mBio.* 2015;6(3). e00553-15.

65. Li Y, Xie J, Wu S, et al. Protein kinase regulated by dsRNA downregulates the interferon production in dengue virus- and dsRNA-stimulated human lung epithelial cells. *PLoS One.* 2013;8(1), e55108.

66. Atrasheuskaya A, Petzelbauer P, Fredeking TM, Ignatyev G. Anti-TNF antibody treatment reduces mortality in experimental dengue virus infection. *FEMS Immunol Med Microbiol.* 2003;35:33–42.

67. Chen LC, Lei HY, Liu CC, et al. Correlation of serum levels of macrophage migration inhibitory factor with disease severity and clinical outcome in dengue patients. *Am J Trop Med Hyg.* 2006;74:142–147.

68. Bashyam HS, Green S, Rothman AL. Dengue virus-reactive CD8[+] T cells display quantitative and qualitative differences in their response to variant epitopes of heterologous viral serotypes. *J Immunol.* 2006;176:2817–2824.

69. Kurane I, Innis BL, Nimmannitya S, et al. Activation of T lymphocytes in dengue virus infections. High levels of soluble interleukin 2 receptor, soluble CD4, soluble CD8, interleukin 2, and interferon-gamma in sera of children with dengue. *J Clin Invest.* 1991;88:1473.

70. Hober D, Delannoy AS, Benyoucef S, De Groote D, Wattre P. High levels of sTNFR p75 and TNF-α in dengue-infected patients. *Microbiol Immunol.* 1996;40:569–573.

71. Boonnak K, Slike BM, Burgess TH, et al. Role of dendritic cells in antibody-dependent enhancement of dengue virus infection. *J Virol.* 2008;82(8):3939–3951.

72. Pena J, Harris E. Dengue virus modulates the unfolded protein response in a time-dependent manner. *J Biol Chem.* 2011;286:14226–14236.

73. Yu CY, Hsu YW, Liao CL, Lin YL. Flavivirus infection activates the XBP1 pathway of the unfolded protein response to cope with endoplasmic reticulum stress. *J Virol.* 2006;80:11868–11880.

74. Yang KD, Yeh WT, Yang MY, Chen RF, Shaio MF. Antibody-dependent enhancement of heterotypic dengue infections involved in suppression of IFN-gamma production. *J Med Virol.* 2001;63(2):150–157.

75. Libraty DH, Pichyangkul S, Ajariyakhajorn C, Endy TP, Ennis FA. Human dendritic cells are activated by dengue virus infection: enhancement by gamma interferon and implications for disease pathogenesis. *J Virol.* 2001;75(8):3501–3508.

76. Green S, Pichyangkul S, Vaughn DW, et al. Early CD69 expression on peripheral blood lymphocytes from children with dengue hemorrhagic fever. *J Infect Dis.* 1999;180:1429–1435.

77. Chareonsirisuthigul T, Kalayanarooj S, Ubol S. Dengue virus (DENV) antibody-dependent enhancement of infection upregulates the production of anti-inflammatory cytokines, but suppresses anti-DENV free radical and pro-inflammatory cytokine production, in THP-1 cells. *J Gen Virol.* 2007;88:365–375.

78. Perez AB, García G, Sierra B, et al. IL-10 levels in dengue patients: some findings from the exceptional epidemiological conditions in Cuba. *J Med Virol.* 2004;73:230–234.

79. Nguyen TH, Lei HY, Nguyen TL, et al. Dengue hemorrhagic fever in infants: a study of clinical and cytokine profiles. *J Infect Dis.* 2004;189:221–232.

80. Takhampunya R, Padmanabhan R, Sukathida U. Antiviral action of nitric oxide on dengue virus type 2 replication. *J Gen Virol.* 2006;87:3003–3011.

81. Ho LJ, Hung LF, Weng CW. Dengue virus type 2 antagonizes IFN-alpha but not IFN-gamma antiviral effect via down-regulating Tyk2-STAT signaling in the human dendritic cell. *J Immunol.* 2005;174:8163–8172.

82. Laurent-Rolle M, Boer ERF, Lubick KJ, et al. The NS5 protein of the virulent West Nile virus NY99 strain is a potent antagonist of type I interferon-mediated JAK-STAT signaling. *J Virol.* 2010;84(7):3503–3515.

83. Wu MF, Chen ST, Hsieh SL. Distinct regulation of dengue virus-induced inflammasome activation in human macrophage subsets. *J Biomed Sci.* 2013;20:36.

84. Puerta-Guardo H, Raya-Sandino A, González-Mariscal L, et al. The cytokine response of U937-derived macrophages infected through antibody-dependent enhancement of dengue virus disrupts cell apical-junction complexes and increases vascular permeability. *J Virol.* 2013;87(13):7486–7501.

85. Kanlaya R, Pattanakitsakul SN, Sinchaikul S, Chen ST, Thongboonkerd V. Alterations in actin cytoskeletal assembly and junctional protein complexes in human endothelial cells induced by dengue virus infection and mimicry of leukocyte transendothelial migration. *J Proteome Res.* 2009;8:2551–2562.

86. Paquin-Proulx D, Avelino-Silva VI, Santos BAN, et al. MAIT cells are activated in acute dengue virus infection and after *in vitro* Zika virus infection. *PLoS Negl Trop Dis.* 2018;12(1), e0006154.

87. Wen J, Ngono AE, Regla-Nava JA, et al. Dengue virus-reactive CD8+ T cells mediate cross-protection against subsequent Zika virus challenge. *Nat Commun.* 2017;8:1459.

88. Kanlaya R, Pattanakitsakul SN, Sinchaikul S, Chen ST, Thongboonkerd V. The ubiquitin-proteasome pathway is important for dengue virus infection in primary human endothelial cells. *J Proteome Res.* 2010;9:4960–4971.

89. Choy MM, Sessions OM, Gubler DJ, Ooi EE. Production of infectious dengue virus in *Aedes aegypti* is dependent on the ubiquitin proteasome pathway. *PLoS Negl Trop Dis.* 2015;9(11), e0004227.

90. Choy MM, Zhang SL, Costa VV, Tan NC, Horrevorts S, Ooi EE. Proteasome inhibition suppresses dengue virus egress in antibody-dependent infection. *PLoS Negl Trop Dis.* 2015;9(11), e0004058.

91. Myllymaki H, Valanne S, Ramet M. The *Drosophila* imd signaling pathway. *J Immunol.* 2014;19:3455–3462.

92. Colpitts TM, Cox J, Vanlandingham DL, et al. Alterations in the *Aedes aegypti* transcriptome during infection with West Nile, dengue and yellow fever viruses. *PLoS Pathog.* 2011;7(9), e1002189.

93. Troupin A, Londono-Renteria B, Conway MJ, et al. A novel mosquito ubiquitin targets viral envelope protein for degradation and reduces virion production during dengue virus infection. *Biochem Biophys Acta.* 2016;1860(9):1898–1909.

94. Thiemmeca S, Tamdej C, Punyadee N, et al. Secreted NS1 protects dengue virus from mannose binding lectin-mediated neutralization. *J Immunol.* 2016;197(10):4053–4065.

95. Kakumani PK, Ponia SS, Rajgokul KS. Role of RNAi in dengue viral replication and identification of NS4B as a RNAi suppressor. *J Virol.* 2013;87(16):8870–8883.

96. Esu E, Lenhart A, Smith L, Horstick O. Effectiveness of peridomestic space spraying with insecticide on dengue transmission: systematic review. *Trop Med Int Health.* 2010;15:619–631.

97. Jadav SS, Kaptein S, Timiri A. Design, synthesis, optimization and antiviral activity of a class of hybrid dengue virus E protein inhibitors. *Bioorg Med Chem Lett.* 2015;25:1747–1752.

98. Wang Q-Y, Bushell S, Qing M, et al. Inhibition of dengue virus through suppression of host pyrimidine biosynthesis. *J Virol.* 2011;85(13):6548–6556.

99. Suzuki Y, Chin W-X, Han Q'E, et al. Characterization of RyDEN (C19orf66) as an interferon-stimulated cellular inhibitor against dengue virus replication. *PLoS Pathog.* 2016;12(1), e1005357.

100. Yin Z, Chen Y-L, Schul W, et al. An adenosine nucleoside inhibitor of dengue virus. *PNAS.* 2009;106(48):20435–20439.

101. Latour DR, Jekle A, Javanbakht H. Biochemical characterization of the inhibition of the dengue virus RNA polymerase by beta-D-2'-ethynyl-7-deaza-adenosine triphosphate. *Antiviral Res.* 2010;87:213–222.

102. Olsen DB, Eldrup AB, Bartholomew L, et al. A 7-deaza-adenosine analog is a potent and selective inhibitor of hepatitis C virus replication with excellent pharmacokinetic properties. *Antimicrob Agents Chemother.* 2004;48:3944–3953.

103. Coulerie P, Eydoux C, Hnawia E, et al. Biflavonoids of *Dacrydium balansae* with potent inhibitory activity on dengue 2 NS5 polymerase. *Planta Med.* 2012;78:672–677.

104. Niyomrattanakit P, Chen Y-P, Dong H, et al. Inhibition of dengue virus polymerase by blocking of the RNA tunnel. *J Virol.* 2010;84(11):5678–5686.

105. Lim SP, Noble CG, She CC, et al. Potent allosteric dengue virus NS5 polymerase inhibitors: mechanism of action and resistance profiling. *PLoS Pathog.* 2016;12(8), e1005737.

106. Cannalire R, Tarantino D, Astolfi A. Functionalized 2,1-benzothiazine 2,2-dioxides as new inhibitors of dengue NS5 RNA-dependent RNA polymerase. *Eur J Med Chem.* 2018;143:1667–1676.

107. Xu H-T, Colby-Germinario SP, Hassounah S, et al. Identification of a pyridoxine-derived small-molecule inhibitor targeting dengue virus RNA-dependent RNA polymerase. *Antimicrob Agents Chemother.* 2016;60:600–608.

108. Benmansour F, Trist I, Coutard B. Discovery of novel dengue virus NS5 methyltransferase non-nucleoside inhibitors by fragment-based drug design. *Eur J Med Chem.* 2017;125:865–880.

109. Halim SA, Khan S, Khan A, et al. Targeting dengue virus NS-3 helicase by ligand based pharmacophore modeling and structure based virtual screening. *Front Chem.* 2017;5, 88.

110. Weigel LF, Nitsche C, Graf D, Bartenschlager R, Klein CD. Phenylalanine and phenylglycine analogues as arginine mimetics in dengue protease inhibitors. *J Med Chem.* 2015;58(19):7719–7733.

111. Whitby K, Pierson TC, Geiss B, et al. Castanospermine, a potent inhibitor of dengue virus infection *in vitro* and *in vivo*. *J Virol.* 2005;79(14):8698–8706.

112. Branche E, Tang WW, Viramontes KM, et al. Synergism between the tyrosine kinase inhibitor sunitinib and anti-TNF antibody protects against lethal dengue infection. *Antiviral Res.* 2018;158:1–7.

113. Olagnier D, Scholte FEM, Chiang C, et al. Inhibition of dengue and chikungunya virus infections by RIG-I mediated type I interferon-independent stimulation of the innate antiviral response. *J Virol.* 2014;88(8):4180–4194.

114. Diwaker D, Mishra KP, Ganju L, Singh SB. Rhodiola inhibits dengue virus multiplication by inducing innate immune response genes RIG-I, MDA5 and ISG in human monocytes. *Arch Virol.* 2014;159:1975–1986.

115. Scaturro P, Trist IMT, Paul D, et al. Characterization of the mode of action of a potent dengue virus capsid inhibitor. *J Virol.* 2014;88(19):11540–11555.

CHAPTER 3

Zika Virus

INTRODUCTION

In 2014, a rare and mysterious disease began to be seen in newborns in Brazil. Babies afflicted with this disease had several distinctive features: severe microcephaly accompanied by neurological, developmental, and prominent skull abnormalities; decreased range of motion; and, in some cases, eye damage. The number of miscarriages and stillbirths also increased in the affected areas. The disorder spread rapidly throughout Latin America and to travelers to this region. The condition was named congenital Zika syndrome after the outbreak was found to be caused by Zika virus (ZIKV). This virus had previously been confined to eastern Africa, Southeast Asia, and some Pacific Ocean islands. The disease was originally self-resolving and typically associated with rash and painful joints, before it morphed to a severe, devastating disease of fetuses, newborns, and infants. ZIKV infection was later found also to be linked to Guillain–Barré syndrome (GBS), a rare neuromuscular condition in adults.

ZIKV is transmitted primarily by the bite of two species of mosquitoes, one of which prefers to live in close proximity to human habitations. It is also transmitted from mother to fetus and sexually long after infection. Brazil was preparing to host the Summer Olympics, and the fear of infection by attendees and their spouses overshadowed this long-anticipated event. Fortunately, the severe outbreak subsided almost as mysteriously as it had begun and concern about the infection soon disappeared from the media and from the attention of the general public, reduced again to obscurity. Since the precise factors that led to both the appearance and disappearance of this disease are unknown, the possibility of another outbreak continues to loom, especially given the wide range of the mosquito vectors in both eastern and western hemispheres and the similarity of ZIKV and dengue virus (DENV). The latter flavivirus is spread by the same mosquito vectors as ZIKV and is currently responsible for a pandemic in most parts of the world.

HISTORY

Zika virus was first reported in the Zika Forest of Uganda in 1947 among nonhuman primates, initially in a febrile sentinel rhesus macaque placed in the forest canopy. In the same year, it was also discovered in humans in Nigeria. A 1957 study detected neutralizing antibodies against ZIKV and another flavivirus, Wesselsbron virus, in 4.0% and 15.9%, respectively, of people who were tested in Mozambique.[1] ZIKV spread across Southeast Asia in the late 1960s and 1970s and was first detected in Malaysia in 1969 and in Indonesia in 1977. In 2007, the virus had reached Yap Island of Micronesia and then was reported in French Polynesia in 2013.[2,3] Although initially occurring sporadically or in small clusters, the outbreak in Yap Island was large and had a 73% infection rate for those older than 3 years, with 18% of those who were infected developing mild symptomatic illness.[2] Disease during the Yap Island and French Polynesia outbreaks was self-resolving, characterized primarily by rash and painful joints, although it was also responsible for 42 cases of GBS in adults in the French Polynesia outbreak.[3]

In 2014–15, ZIKV spread to the western hemisphere. Infections were then reported in Brazil, Chile, Colombia, Surinam, Guatemala, El Salvador, Mexico, Paraguay, Venezuela, and Panama, with most of the cases being in Brazil. ZIKV may have been introduced to that country during an international canoe-racing event, which included racers from the Pacific Islands. The virus also rapidly spread northward, reaching Mexico by November 2015.[3] ZIKV was determined to have a causal relationship with what was to be named "congenital Zika syndrome" in Brazil, as evidenced by the increased incidence of this form of ZIKV-associated disease soon after its introduction into the region. In Brazil, a combination of rare exposure and rare detective criteria was seen and corroborated by epidemiologic data, meeting many of Shepard's and Bradford Hill criteria for causality.[4]

Travel-associated cases were then reported in other parts of southern North America. In addition to many travel-related infections, autochthonous transmission of ZIKV from infected mosquitoes to humans was seen in Brownsville, Texas, and in Miami-Dade County, Florida, in late 2016.[5,6] In 2016, Florida had 1325 reported cases, more than 200 of which were reported in pregnant women. By far, most of the cases (1042) were travel related; however, 262 were due to local transmission. Nevertheless, by the end of November 2016, South

Zika and Other Neglected and Emerging Flaviviruses. https://doi.org/10.1016/B978-0-323-82501-6.00013-X

Florida appeared to have eliminated local transmission.[7] ZIKV in the western hemisphere peaked in 2016 and dropped substantially during the 2017–18 and 2018–19 seasons, despite its spread to many countries in South and Central America and Caribbean islands. Small, isolated outbreaks were also reported in other countries in Southeastern Asia and parts of Europe until 2019.[8] No large "second wave" has occurred.

THE DISEASES
Mild Disease
The majority of ZIKV infections either remain asymptomatic (80%) or result in only mild disease. In the latter, the most common symptoms of Zika infection are fever, maculopapular rash, headache, muscle and joint pain, conjunctivitis, and vertigo that lasts for several days to a week.[7]

Congenital Zika Syndrome and Other Disorders
Symptoms of congenital Zika syndrome in babies include severe microcephaly with partial collapse of the skull, intracranial calcifications, excessive and redundant scalp skin, clubfoot and other conditions related to limited range of motion of the joints and excessive muscle tone, or scarring or pigment changes in the back of the eye. These, and additional features, such as the brain overlapping the cranial sutures, a prominent occipital bone, and neurologic impairment, are consistent with fetal brain disruption sequence.[4] The diameter of the head of babies with microcephaly is much smaller than that found in normal babies of the same sex and age. Microcephaly also leads to smaller brain size and brain tissue and may be accompanied by improper nervous system development.[5] Babies who had been infected prior to birth may also experience damage to their eyes, including macular lesions and optic nerve abnormalities or damaged visual cortex, negatively impacting visual development, even in the absence of microcephaly. Some infected infants without signs of microcephaly at birth later develop postnatal microcephaly. Infection is additionally associated with miscarriage and stillbirth, hydranencephaly, and placental insufficiency, leading to intrauterine growth restriction. Arthrogryposis (joint contracture) is present in both arms and legs of 86% of infected children and may lead to limb paralysis.[9]

At autopsy, fetuses with microcephaly were found to have severely reduced brain size, no cerebral gyri, severe dilation of the cerebral lateral ventricles, dystrophic calcifications in the cerebral cortex, neuronophagy, gliosis, microglial nodules, and hypoplasia of the brain stem and spinal cord.[10,11] One study found that 5.8% of infants with microcephaly developed sensorineural hearing loss, mainly due to damage to the cochlea.[12] Some of these features may be due to the observed infiltration of mononuclear cells into the central nervous system (CNS), as discussed below. In an experimental model system, infection of mouse neural progenitor cells in vitro led to apoptosis, cell-cycle arrest, and decreased progenitor cell differentiation.[13] Astrocytes may also be heavily infected and may serve as one source of ZIKV that infects neurons.[11] It has been suggested that treatment with nerve growth factors may be useful in the repair of damaged brain cells.[14]

In a mouse model system, ZIKV was injected into amniotic fluid of embryonic animals in pregnant mice. A total of 86.4% ($n = 44$ pups) of the injected pups survived to birth, 76.3% of which reached adulthood. As these mice entered puberty, they displayed motor incoordination and visual dysfunctions due to anatomical defects in the cerebellar cortex. Numbers of Purkinje cells were decreased, retinas were thinner, and the optic nerves were diminished.[14] At 40 days postinfection, surviving mice had reduced body weight, brain volume, skull length, and cranial height compared to mock-injected mice. Thickness of motor, somatosensory, and visual areas was decreased, and the dentate gyrus of the hippocampus exhibited hypoplasia. The lamination of the cerebral cortex and subcortical structures, such as striatum, was not significantly affected, however, nor was the mice's anxiety level.[14] Arthrogryposis caused hind limb paralysis in two of the mice.

Guillain–Barré Syndrome and Neurological Disease
GBS is a rare nervous system disorder in which the immune system damages nerve cells and may result in weakness of arms and legs and paralysis that, in severe cases, affects the muscles that control breathing. These symptoms may persist for weeks to several months and, while most people fully recover, some appear to have permanent damage. The death rate is very low, however.[5] In 1976, some people vaccinated against the H1N1 "swine flu" developed GBS. Some regions with Zika outbreaks have also experienced increased incidence of GBS in adults. Research at the Centers for Disease Control and Prevention (CDC) indicates a strong association between GBS and Zika infection. Nevertheless, very few of those infected with ZIKV develop GBS, at least in the short term.[5] Other neurological disorders linked to ZIKV infection include myelitis, meningoencephalitis, and brain ischemia.[7]

Other Manifestations of ZIKV Infection

Other potential consequences of infection include retro-orbital and abdominal pain, diarrhea, thrombocytopenia with disseminated intravascular coagulation and hemorrhagic complications, hepatic dysfunction, acute respiratory distress syndrome, shock, and multiorgan dysfunction syndrome. Individuals with both CNS and hemorrhagic fever manifestations have been reported in other flavivirus infections as well. Hematospermia and orchitis have also been seen in humans and may lead to male infertility.[15]

THE VIRUS

ZIKV Serotypes

ZIKV is related to the four DENV serotypes, yellow fever virus (YFV), and West Nile virus (WNV). ZIKV has been split into three distinct groups: two African lineages and one Asian lineage.[3] A clinical Asian lineage isolate produced 10-fold more virus than the prototypic African strain, supporting the contention that the Asian group is more pathogenic than the African groups. The virus present in the Americas is more closely related to the Asian lineage. Puerto Rican isolates reveal significant variability in viral replication, but not in viral binding, to dendritic cells (DCs) from different donors. ZIKV infection of DCs in the Americas results in minimal cell activation. African ZIKV and Asian ZIKV differ in their replication kinetics, with the two African lineage virus groups having more rapid replication kinetics and infection magnitude and also inducing death of infected human DC.[16] DCs, especially the Langerhans form present in the skin, are responsible for carrying ZIKV into the bloodstream, allowing systemic infection. DC death may thus slow the dispersal of the virus, giving the immune system additional time to respond to the infection, leading to their decreased pathogenicity.

ZIKV and IFN Signaling Pathways

All studied ZIKV strains of either the African or Asian lineages block type I IFN (IFN-α and IFN-β) receptor signaling through the STAT1 and STAT2 pathways. The virus inhibits phosphorylation of these two molecules and induces STAT1 degradation in the proteasome. As is the case with other related flaviviruses, the 5′ and 3′ untranslated regions of the Zika polyprotein are involved in genome cyclization and replication. NS3 also acts together with NS2B to form the protease that cleaves the ZIKV polyprotein, a viral helicase, and nucleoside 5′-triphosphatase. Cleavage of the nucleoside triphosphates, especially ATP, provides energy for viral enzymatic activity.[17] ZIKV NS5 induces the destruction of human STAT2 through its interaction with the human E3 ubiquitin ligase seven in absentia homolog (SIAH). Acting together, NS5 and SIAH attach ubiquitin to human STAT2, thus tagging the protein for proteasomal degradation. Virus-induced removal of the STAT proteins disrupts IFN-stimulated signaling pathways, which play a major role in the ZIKV antiviral response.[18] Other flaviviruses, including DENV, also degrade STAT2, albeit using a somewhat different pathway.

The other major IFN signaling pathway utilizes RIG-1 and innate viral RNA sensors. This pathway is unaffected by the presence of ZIKV. Moreover, the administration of a RIG-I agonist restricts ZIKV replication in DC in vitro, demonstrating the importance of the RIG-1 pathway in anti-ZIKV defense.[16]

ZIKV Infection of Diverse Cell Types

ZIKV attachment to various types of vertebrate cells is mediated by several cellular attachment factors, including DC-specific ICAM3-grabbing nonintegrin (DC-SIGN) and members of phosphatidylserine kinase family TAM (Tyro3, AXL, and MERTK) and T cell/transmembrane, immunoglobulin, and mucin gene family-1 (TIM-1).[19] After entering skin cells, including Langerhans cells of the innate immune system, the virus travels to lymph nodes and, from there, into the bloodstream. In primates and humans, ZIKV targets placental and fetal tissue.[20] Importantly, ZIKV also infects Hofbauer cells (placental macrophages) as well as trophoblasts, and fetal endothelial cells.[21]

ZIKV is also neurotropic, infecting cortical neural progenitor cells and astrocytes of the CNS.[20] ZIKV RNA is also present in damaged brain mononuclear cells in newborns with microcephaly. Moreover, live virus has been cultured from the brain of a mouse fetus with severe brain abnormalities whose dam was experimentally infected early in pregnancy. The virus also productively infects human-induced pluripotent stem cell-derived cells from the neural lineage, such as cortical and motor neurons, as well as astrocytes, and dendrites. ZIKV causes cytopathic effect in these infected cells. ZIKV from the western hemisphere also infects neocortical and spinal neuroepithelial stem cells as well as their fetal homologs, the radial glial cells.[22] These cells express the viral AXL cell receptor, as do adult astrocytes, microglia, and endothelial cells, but not neurons. ZIKV decreases mitosis, depletes centrosomes, and causes mitochondrial sequestration of phospho-TANK-binding kinase 1 (TBK1). This leads to structural disorganization and death of these cells.[22]

Infection of mice with ZIKV has also been found to infect and kill peripheral nervous system neurons in vitro. It also infects neurons of peripheral nervous system in vivo as well as stem cell-derived human neural crest cells in vitro. Infection of these cells results in their death and transcriptional deregulation of greater magnitude than that seen in neurons from the CNS. Human stem cell-derived Schwann cells are also infected by ZIKV.[23] Infected mice exhibit behavioral changes, including motor incoordination and visual defects.[24]

ZIKV is neurotropic in its mosquito vectors and induces behavioral changes in these insects. ZIKV increases locomotor activity of captive Ae. aegypti and, perhaps, the geographical range of infected mosquitoes in the wild. Primary neurons obtained from the infected mosquitoes have greater spiking activity and numbers of synaptic connections, but the microtubule protein signals are reduced. Additionally, the expression of some components of the glutamate pathway is altered during ZIKV infection. Glutamate is the major excitatory neurotransmitter in normal vertebrates; thus, increases in its excitatory pathway may be at least partially responsible for increased neuron activity. The voltage-gated sodium channel is also upregulated in infected mosquito primary neuron cultures, triggering or maintaining the excitatory state of the CNS. Thus, unlike the case in vertebrates, viral infection in mosquitoes is benign and may actually be beneficial to ZIKV.[24]

Persistence of ZIKV in Selected Bodily Fluids and Anatomical Sites

Following experimental infection with ZIKV, several species of monkeys and mice exhibit a rapid decline in acute viremia and the type of early invasion of the CNS that is seen in humans, in addition to prolonged viral shedding and fetal pathology found in pregnant women and animals.[25] They are often used as animal models of human disease. ZIKV infects the CNS and lymph nodes of experimentally infected rhesus macaques, but remains in the cerebrospinal fluid (CSF) for up to 42 days and in the lymph nodes and colorectal biopsies for up to 72 days, weeks after viral clearance from the peripheral blood, urine, and mucosal secretions. ZIKV-specific neutralizing antibodies are detectable in peripheral blood within 7 days of infection and their presence correlates with the removal of virus from peripheral blood by day 10. Protective antibodies and cytokines, however, were undetectable in the CSF for at least 24 weeks, even in the face of ZIKV presence in this locale.[25]

The activity of several cellular signaling pathways correlates with persistent CSF and lymph node viral loads, including the mechanistic target of rapamycin

(mTOR), transforming growth factor-β (TGF-β), interferon (IFN)-α, and tumor necrosis factor-α (TNF-α) pathways. mTOR signaling and proinflammatory pathways appear to aid in the survival of ZIKV-infected cells and viral persistence, while extracellular matrix and platelet activation pathways, collagen formation, and many cell adherence molecules negatively correlate with viral loads. These include members of the MLLT (MLLT4), COL (COL14A, COL5A, COL6A), matrix-degrading metalloproteinase (MMP) (MMP1, MMP2, MMP3, MMP8, and MMP19), and SLC (SLC22A2, SLC6A13, SLC7A9, and SLC17A1) groups.[25] The extracellular matrix pathway is similarly affected by other flaviviruses, including DENV. Expression of the antiapoptotic genes BIK, BCL2A1, and BCL2L1 has a positive correlation with persistent viral load. The proapoptotic genes ASP8, CAV1, CLU, and LMNA have a negative correlation. In addition to its role in cell survival, mTOR signaling is involved in neurodevelopment, including proliferation of neural stem cells, neuronal circuit development, neural plasticity, and higher complex CNS functions. In transgenic mice, overexpression of mTOR during early embryonic development causes cortical atrophy and microcephaly, and, in adult mice, to neurodegeneration.[25]

ZIKV infection of the CNS and lymph nodes appears, therefore, to effectively create an atmosphere that encourages the survival of infected cells. In addition to parts of the central nervous and lymphoid systems, the gastrointestinal and genitourinary tracts are able to serve as "anatomical sanctuaries" for ZIKV, allowing the virus to remain protected and hidden for long periods of time after its clearance from the circulatory system.[25]

In addition to infecting and altering CNS and immune system functions, sporadic, low-level viral shedding also occurs in the urine, cervicovaginal secretions, saliva, and semen of infected monkeys. Infectious ZIKV is detectable in the semen of infected men as well. It persists for months after the virus is no longer detectable in the blood.[25] In an animal model system using mice with a transplanted human immune system, ZIKV infects human bone marrow monocytes and macrophages, B cells, and hematopoietic stem cells. These "humanized" mice produce human antibodies against ZIKV E and capsid proteins. Interestingly, ZIKV was not found to infect T cells anywhere in the mouse's body.[26]

ZIKV and Genomic Recombination

As is typically true for mosquito-borne flaviviruses, ZIKV alters its genome more rapidly than do tick-borne flaviviruses. In the case of ZIKV, genetic analysis reveals that numerous recombination events have occurred between different viral strains. Recombinant ZIKV strains have been found in several mosquito species, including *Ae. aegypti, Aedes dalzieli, Aedes africanus,* and *Aedes furcifer* and perhaps many other types of mosquitoes. The promiscuous feeding habits of the zoophilic mosquito, *Ae. dalzieli,* may play a role in the production of numerous recombinant strains since it feeds on animals, which are simultaneously infected by more than one ZIKV strain.[10] This allows for the exchange of parts of the genomic RNA between the different viral strains, producing recombinant viruses. Such recombinants may be either more or less virulent or able to infect humans better or worse than the original, parent viral strains. The ability of the immune response to recognize recombinant strains may also be altered.

TRANSMISSION

Mosquito Vectors and the Urban Transmission Cycle

ZIKV is primarily transmitted to humans in an urban cycle via the bite of select *Aedes* species mosquitoes, usually *Ae. aegypti* or *Ae. albopictus*. The former feed almost exclusively on humans and live in urban settings, while the latter is more typically found in suburban back yards and parks, feeding on other species of mammals, such as domestic pets, squirrels, and chipmunks.[27]

In the urban cycle, the virus is passed back and forth between humans and mosquitoes with no other amplifying host required. Once a mosquito acquires the virus during a blood meal from an infected human host, that mosquito is infected for the remainder of its life without being damaged itself. ZIKV is transmitted to its next human host during the mosquito's next blood meal. ZIKV has been isolated from many *Aedes* species mosquitoes plus a lesser number of other mosquito genera. Additionally, many species of mosquitoes are seropositive for ZIKV. Most of these mosquitoes, however, are not able to serve as vectors for the virus due to too low viral titers. Of the mosquitoes that are able to serve as ZIKV vectors, not many transmit the virus to humans, but may instead serve as vectors for other animal species. For example, at least 10 species of ZIKV-positive *Aedes,* including *Ae. africanus, Aedes apicoargenteus, Aedes luteocephalus, Ae. furcifer,* and *Aedes vittatus,* and one species of *Culex* mosquito are present in Africa.[27] Laboratory testing, however, indicates that only *Ae. luteocephalus* and *Ae. vittatus* are able to transmit ZIKV.[28] Several *Anopheles* and *Mansonia* species mosquitoes may also serve as ZIKV vectors in Africa.[10] For a comprehensive list of infected mosquito species, see Kauffman and Kramer.[27]

Ae. aegypti or *Ae. albopictus* mosquitoes serve as the major vectors of human infection in the Americas.[5] Both of these mosquito species also transmit other flaviviruses, including DENV, YFV, and chikungunya virus (not a flavivirus). Coinfection of these mosquitoes with ZIKV, DENV, and chikungunya virus occurs fairly often.[29] *Ae. aegypti,* the principal vector in the western hemisphere, is an aggressive mosquito, which typically lives in close proximity to people's residences, either indoors or outdoors. Humans are their preferred hosts.

While *Ae. aegypti* is the primary vector for ZIKV transmission to humans in many areas of the world, the secondary viral vector, *Ae. albopictus,* is becoming increasingly more of a threat for human transmission. In Central Africa, *Ae. albopictus* is found in Cameroon and in urban areas of Gabon. In Mozambique, Southeast Africa, it is beginning to replace *Ae. aegypti* as the primary vector.[10] *Ae. albopictus* is also an emerging ZIKV vector in temperate regions of North America and parts of Europe and Asia, due to its increasing ability to persist in regions with colder temperatures.

Since ZIKV is usually transmitted via the bite of infected mosquitoes, human infection is affected by the seasonal and geographical factors that influence mosquito vector abundance. Climatic conditions render most of the United States unsuitable for large numbers of *Ae. aegypti* during the winter months, except for southern Florida and south Texas, areas in which locally acquired cases of Zika have occurred. Poor socioeconomic conditions along the United States border with Mexico in Texas, as well as the mass entry of people from endemic regions of Latin America into the United States, also increase the number of infected people who can transmit the virus to these mosquitoes, and, subsequently, to people in the southern United States.[30]

Socioeconomic conditions are important factors in ZIKV infection of people. The large increase in the number of cases of neonatal microcephaly in 2015 occurred in a large, heavily populated urban area in Northeast Brazil. The spatial distribution of microcephaly revealed a strong association between disease incidence and living in areas with low socioeconomic levels. Only 2% of the microcephaly cases occurred in the wealthiest district of Brazil.[31] People living in poverty or in the large slums outside of Rio de Janeiro are much less likely to be able to afford air-conditioning than people of the other economic classes. They are more likely to lack intact screens for the doors and windows in their dwellings, if they even have a house or hut in which to live. Impoverished people also spend much more time outdoors. This increases their exposure to the mosquito vectors. Urban areas of subtropical or temperate North America with large, concentrated numbers of homeless people may also be at risk. This includes Mexico City, San Francisco, and large cities in California, where "tent cities" are increasingly springing up in the business areas of the cities.

Mosquito Vectors, the Sylvatic Transmission Cycle, and Vertebrate Hosts

In addition to an endemic, human-urban transmission cycle involving primarily two *Aedes* species mosquitoes, ZIKV is also maintained by sylvatic transmission between several species of monkey and ape hosts and many species of forest-dwelling mosquitoes. Few naturally or experimentally infected monkeys or apes are symptomatic and those who do become ill usually develop a mild, transient fever.[32] Old World monkeys that were naturally infected with ZIKV in the wild were reported in Uganda in the 1940s and, in 2016, in a region of Brazil undergoing a large outbreak in humans. Capuchin monkeys (*Sapajus flavius* and *Sapajus libidinosus*) produce neutralizing antibodies against not only ZIKV, but also many other species of flaviviruses, including all four serotypes of DENV, YFV, Ilhéus virus, and Saint Louis encephalitis virus.[32] This does not necessarily imply that the capuchin monkeys are infected with all of these viruses, since at least some of these antibodies could be cross-reacting with more than one flavivirus species.

ZIKV is found more often in forested regions than in areas with other types of land cover. Regional rainfall levels in West Africa are indicative of the potential of ZIKV to infect forest mosquitoes.[28] Interestingly, a pool of male *Ae. furcifer* mosquitoes was ZIKV positive, suggesting that vertical transmission of the virus from an infected female to offspring may occur in West Africa since male mosquitoes do not feed on blood.[2] Free-living populations of at least some Old World monkey species are also found in South America, including African green monkeys, which serve as Zika hosts in Africa. This indicates the potential for sylvatic transmission in South America as well as that which now occurs in Africa.[28]

A study of potential ZIKV primate hosts in Africa found no active ZIKV infection in wild Tanzanian baboons and Gambian African green monkeys. However, up to 16% of these animals were seropositive, indicating, at the least, that they had prior exposure to viral antigen or that they may have had previously undetected infection. The rate of seropositivity is higher in the northern portion of sub-Saharan Africa than in the more southern regions.[33]

In addition to primates, guinea pigs, rats, mice, rabbits, bats, gazelle, wildebeest, lions, African water buffalo, hippopotami, elephants, impalas, zebras, wild birds, and snakes can be infected by ZIKV either naturally or following experimental inoculation. Interestingly, most wild mammals naturally infected by ZIKV, including nonhuman primates, display few clinical signs.[34] While many of the above wild animal species have little contact with humans, anti-ZIKV antibodies are also found in domestic animals, such as sheep, goats, horses, cows, and ducks.[10]

When male marmosets, a form of New World monkey, are experimentally infected intramuscularly with an African ZIKV strain, they display characteristics similar to those seen early during human infection. Infection in these monkeys is generally asymptomatic, but infectious virus persists in their semen and saliva longer than in their serum or urine. Additionally, neutralizing antibodies are able to protect the monkeys against subsequent challenge with a ZIKV strain isolated in Brazil (Asian lineage).[35] The antiviral IFN signaling pathway was also upregulated when tested at 3, 7, and 9 days postinfection. While this animal model thus may be useful in studies of viral persistence and shedding, it remains to be determined whether experimental infection of pregnant marmosets will cause fetal abnormalities.

Human-to-Human Transmission

Since ZIKV is able to cross the placenta, pregnant women are able to infect their fetuses. Although the virus is present in breast milk and several babies are known to have been infected via this route, they have not yet developed health problems.[5] The long-term effects of infection of children by breastfeeding can only be answered over the course of time; however, studies using animal models may be informative.

ZIKV can be transmitted sexually from male-to-female, female-to-male, and male-to-male. ZIKV remains viable in both semen and the female reproductive tract for many months after infection is no longer detectable in blood. In fact, the percentage of sexual transmission of ZIKV from infected male mice to dams may reach 50% for up to 19 days postinfection, posing a serious risk to their offspring.[36]

THE IMMUNE RESPONSE

While detectable levels of viremia during ZIKV infection typically last for approximately a week in immunocompetent individuals, it is prolonged in pregnant women due to their partially suppressed immune systems. Both innate and adaptive immune responses appear to play a role in limiting viral replication, especially IFN activity.

IFN-induced transmembrane proteins 1 and 2, activated by ZIKV infection, decrease viral replication. Mice without type I IFN activity are more susceptible to disease.[20] A specific mutation arose in the NS1 gene of the Asian lineage of ZIKV. This mutation inhibits induction of the IFN-β gene by decreasing the phosphorylation of TBK1. When this mutation was genetically engineered into a ZIKV strain that possessed the wild-type NS1 sequence, the ability of the hybrid virus to induce IFN-β production was reduced. When neonatal mice were inoculated with mutated virus by the intracranial route, the mice developed higher virus loads in the brain and higher neurovirulence in comparison with mice with the wild-type gene.[37] Other viral nonstructural proteins, NS2A, NS2B, NS4A, NS4B, and NS5, also reduce production of either type I IFN or different components of the RIG-1 signaling pathway. NS2A, NS2B, and NS4B decrease TBK1 phosphorylation, NS4A alters interferon regulatory factor 3 (IRF3) phosphorylation, and NS5 acts at a time following IRF3 phosphorylation by interacting directly with IRF3.[37]

The importance of adaptive immunity is evidenced by the robust production of antibodies during ZIKV infection, including high-potency, virus-specific, neutralizing antibodies that target the E protein.[20] One such neutralizing antibody, ZIKV-117, blocks infection by both African and Asian-American lineage ZIKV strains, but not by any of the DENV serotypes. The antibody limits early viral replication, placenta and fetal pathology, and death in experimentally infected pregnant mice.[38]

As is often the case, at least some anti-ZIKV antibodies cross-react with other flaviviruses, particularly DENVs. Such cross-reactive neutralizing antibodies against both ZIKV and DENV have been found to increase ZIKV replication both in vitro and in vivo in mice. This raises concern that cross-reactive antibodies may lead to antibody-dependent enhancement of disease (ADE).[20] During DENV infection, ADE-related pathology results from cross-reactive antibodies produced when infection with one DENV serotype is followed by infection with a different DENV serotype (see Chapter 2). It is possible that antibodies produced against an African ZIKV strain may produce ADE during a subsequent infection with an Asian strain of the virus or with another, closely related flavivirus in areas where these viruses coexist or vice versa. Given this possibility, it is necessary to approach the therapeutic use of cross-reactive antibodies with caution. This is a matter

of concern since several DENV serotypes are endemic in many of the regions where ZIKV is now found or to which it is spreading. Additionally, the large number of ZIKV CD4[+] T helper cell epitopes may, in some cases, also respond to related epitopes from other flaviviruses, enhancing the production of the proinflammatory cytokine interleukin (IL)-17A, perhaps inducing immunopathology upon subsequent exposure to DENVs. Prolonged activity of cross-reactive T cells against the NS3 helicases of African ZIKV and DENVs is known to cause inflammatory immune responses, including robust IFN-γ and TNF-α production. No such specific T cell responses were found to be mounted against the ZIKV and DENVs NS3 proteases.[39,40] It should be noted that no increased ZIKV replication or adverse clinical outcome occurred in monkeys primed by exposure to either DENVs or YFV followed by subsequent challenge with ZIKV.[20] It is unknown whether this is also the case in humans. It may be relevant that cross-reactive IgM and IgG anti-ZIKV antibodies were detected against all four DENV serotypes in an American ZIKV-infected patient who had never been infected with DENV. These antibodies alone did not cause ADE,[41] but the possibility remains that ADE might develop if the patient were to be infected later with DENV.

T lymphocytes may play an important role during ZIKV infection since CD4[+] T helper cell and CD8[+] T killer cell responses to both structural (capsid and envelope) and nonstructural (NS1) proteins are produced in ZIKV-infected monkeys and humans. However, while IFN-γ is detectable in most monkeys within 5 weeks of infection and CD8[+] T killer cells aid in controlling ZIKV replication in mice, T lymphocyte activity and Th1 cytokines do not correlate with virologic control, at least in the nonhuman primates.[20,25] Mucosal-associated invariant T cells, however, are potentially relevant in controlling ZIKVs. They are innate immune system T cells with potent antibacterial activity. They also produce IFN-γ after exposure to ZIKV in vitro. IFN-γ production by these cells depends upon the presence of IL-12 and IL-18, but not the T cell receptor. These invariant cells are stimulated during acute DENV infection as well.[42]

Since both DENVs and ZIKV infections are present in some of the same geographical locations and are transmitted by the same mosquito species, DENV/ZIKV coinfections also occur. CD4[+] T helper cells and CD8[+] T killer cells from coinfected persons express several chemokine receptors, such as the CC-chemokine receptor 5 (CCR5) and two CXC receptors, CXCR1 and CXCR3, in vitro without stimulation. Coinfection also decreases the production of IFN-γ, TNF-α, and IL-2 by CD4[+] T helper cells when compared to cells from people infected by only one of these flaviviruses.[43] It will be important to determine how coinfection affects other immune parameters, especially when developing vaccines against either virus species.

Myeloid DCs isolated from adults during acute ZIKV infection have altered transcriptional signatures, including downregulated expression of interferon-stimulated genes (ISGs) and innate immune sensors. The transcription of at least 67 host molecules that support ZIKV infection is, however, strongly upregulated during infection with this virus. These include AXL, which serves as the primary receptor for ZIKV; SOCS3, which downregulates ISG expression; and IDO-1, which induces regulatory T cell responses. These findings indicate that ZIKV modifies the DC transcriptome in a manner that favors infection of these cells as well as avoids the antiviral immune response.[44] This is of importance since some types of DCs host ZIKV early during infection in vivo and are also vital to CD4$^+$ T helper cell activation. Moreover, in vitro work indicates that fetal or neonatal myeloid DCs have a higher susceptibility to ZIKV infection than do adult cells.[44]

In vivo, acute ZIKV infection upregulates the expression of the inflammasome components NOD2, NLRP3, CXCL10, BTG2, BST2, OSM, as well as expression of the proinflammatory cytokines and chemokines TNF-α, IL-1, IL-18, CCR7, CCL2, and CCL20, and the immunomodulatory agents IL-10 and TGF-β from T regulatory (Treg) cells. The mTOR signaling pathway is activated as well. This important pathway regulates both immune functions and neurologic development. Genes controlling monocyte, NK cell, and CD4$^+$ helper T cell pathways are upregulated, while genes stimulating components of CD8$^+$ T killer cell and B cell signaling pathways and major histocompatibility complex class I (MHC-I) pathways are downregulated, including CD40, GATA3, RHOH, PIK3CG, BANK1, and the B cell receptor. Thus, during acute ZIKV infection, proinflammatory, antiviral, and immunomodulatory pathways are upregulated, while some other immune system responses are downregulated.[25]

Type I IFN-α/β and type II IFN-γ play very important roles in controlling and eliminating most viral infections. The type I IFNs do not, however, play a major role in defense against ZIKVs due to the countermeasures employed by the virus to escape this aspect of the host innate immune response. These measures include reduced expression of IFN-α/β and their corresponding downstream ISG activity.[45] As discussed above, when ZIKV NS5 induces proteasomal degradation of STAT2, anti-ZIKV activation of type I ISGs is dampened.

NS1 and NS4A also decrease IFN-mediated activity. Nevertheless, expression of the ISGs OAS2, IFT1/2/3, ISG15, IRF7, IFI44, MX1, and MX2 does occur and peaks on day 6 post infection.[25] While activity of IFN-λ, a type III IFN, is also reduced, IFN-γ activity is less affected by ZIKV immune countermeasures.[45] Activity of the IFN-α and IFN-γ signaling pathways is correlated with acute viral loads. A similar correlation is seen between the NK cell and IL-10 signaling pathways as well as the oxidative phosphorylation and mTOR signaling pathways (mTORC1 and PI3K–AKT–mTOR). A negative correlation, however, exists between the extracellular matrix, epithelial–mesenchymal transition, myogenesis, and signal transduction and plasma membrane pathways.[25]

When inflammatory infiltrates from the autopsies of infected stillborn and neonatal infants are studied, a complex mixture of immune cells and cytokines emerges. The infiltrates contain antigen-presenting cells and astrocytes, NK cells, M1 and M2 macrophages and microglia, CD4$^+$ T helper cells (predominately Th2 cells), CD8$^+$ T killer cells, and Treg. Of the T helper cells, while Th2 cells predominate, increased levels of Th1, Treg, Th9, Th17, and Th22 cells are also present. The Th2 cytokines IL-4, IL-10, IL-33, IL-37, and TGF-β1 are present, as well as a large variety of proinflammatory cytokines, including type I IFNs, IFN-γ, IL-1β, IL-6, IL-12A, and TNF-α. The Th9 T cell subset increases the production of histamine and glutamate in cortical neurons, Th17 cells induce the production of reactive oxygen and nitrogen intermediates, and Th22 cells recruit inflammatory cells to the area. Expression of both the antagonistic enzymes, inducible nitric oxide synthase (iNOS) and arginase, is also increased. Along with a diverse number of inflammatory mediators, IL-33 expression is very intense in areas of neuronal necrosis. This cytokine is directly involved in necroptosis.[11] NK cells play only a minor role in anti-ZIKV defense since viral infection upregulates the expression of MHC class I proteins on host cells, which, in turn, inhibits NK cell activation.[46] Increased expression of MHC class I molecules involves the RIG-1 pathway, mediated by IFN-β and NF-κB.

Microglia are by far the most prominent type of leukocyte in the CNS under normal conditions and function as brain macrophages. When primary microglia are infected by ZIKV in vitro, they stimulate an inflammatory response similar to that seen in humans in vivo, producing high levels of the proinflammatory cytokines TNF-α, IL-6, and IL-1β, in addition to stimulating iNOS to produce nitric oxide, a nitrogen and oxygen free radical that is toxic to microbes. Conditional medium from infected microglia cultures inhibits the proliferation and neuronal differentiation of neural precursor cells from mice brains.[47] Inhibiting production of these cytokines decreases astrocytic differentiation of neural progenitor cells and increases neurogenesis, suggesting that microglia may play an important role in ZIKV immunopathology, including the production of new neurons.

Infection of a first-trimester trophoblast cell line by ZIKV causes levels of protective type I IFNs to decrease, while proinflammatory responses increase, suggesting that young fetuses may also be exposed to this pathogenic environment in utero. This is particularly important since placental inflammation is associated with a higher risk of brain damage in normal preterm newborns. Toll-like receptors 3 and 8 both are involved in this pathogenic response. While YFV and DENVs also replicate efficiently in placental trophoblasts, ZIKV stimulates a stronger proinflammatory and a weaker IFN response by these cells than that induced by the other two species of flaviviruses, neither of which are known to cause fetal disease.[48]

PREVENTION
Vaccines

Several animal models are able to reproduce at least some of the pathogenic effects of ZIKV infection of humans. Fetal pathology occurs in ZIKV-infected pregnant mice and monkeys.[20] This may allow for their use for testing vaccine candidates and therapeutic agents, with the caveat that pregnancy compromises some aspects of the immune response in normal, healthy animals and humans. Important information for ZIKV vaccine production may be drawn from an extensive history of successful vaccine development against similar flaviviruses, such as YFV, DENV, and Japanese encephalitis virus (JEV). Human vaccines have been licensed, and quantitative correlates or surrogates of protection have been developed for these other mosquito-borne flaviviruses. Neutralizing antibodies and total binding antibody responses appear to be very important protective agents in vaccine efficacy for the other flaviviruses.[20]

Building upon the above knowledge, several approaches to Zika vaccine production are under development. Virus-like particle vaccines generate neutralizing antibodies against the ZIKV E protein that, when passively transferred, significantly reduce weight loss, morbidity, and mortality in mice upon subsequent challenge with the intact virus.[49] DNA vaccines and adenovirus vectors expressing ZIKV proteins, as well as purified inactivated virus vaccines, also induce the production of virus-specific neutralizing antibodies. In preclinical trials, neutralizing antibodies protected normal mice and rhesus macaques against ZIKV challenge after one or two immunizations. Purified IgG from vaccinated animals also passively protects mice and monkeys, even at low titers.[50] It should be noted, however, that while these vaccine candidates appear promising, the above tests were performed in immunocompetent animals that do not typically develop clinical illness. Accordingly, the ability of these vaccines to prevent ZIKV-induced disease remains to be determined.[20]

One promising vaccine candidate is a recombinant chimeric virus, which expresses the ZIKV prM/E protein in a licensed, live-attenuated JEV vaccine.[51] One dose of this chimeric vaccine elicits robust and long-lasting immune responses that decrease the production of proinflammatory cytokines and chemokines, including IFN-γ, in mice and macaques following ZIKV challenge. Moreover, no viremia is detectable in the vaccinated animals. Additionally, immunization of female mice with this vaccine protects against placental and fetal neurological damage when they are challenged during pregnancy. Another chimeric vaccine candidate utilizes a recombinant chimpanzee adenovirus expressing ZIKV prM/E glycoprotein. A single immunization with this construct rapidly produces neutralizing antibodies that protect both immunocompetent and immunodeficient mice and cross-neutralizes heterologous ZIKV strains. Specific T cell responses are also induced. One vaccination also completely protects male mice against testicular damage.[52]

Using a different approach, Muthumani et al.[53] developed a DNA vaccine that also targets ZIKV prM/E and generates specific cellular and humoral immunity, including neutralizing antibodies, in mice and nonhuman primates after a single dose. The vaccine is administered by the intradermal route using low-voltage electroporation. Even mice without receptors for type I IFN are completely protected against weight loss, viral pathology in brain tissue, and death.

In a different vaccination strategy, rhesus macaques and immunocompetent mice are administered a monoclonal antibody that blocks viral anti-IFN receptor activity, followed by intravaginal or subcutaneous inoculation with a Brazilian ZIKV strain. This vaccine strategy protects against subsequent intravaginal challenge with a homologous virus strain. Protection is accompanied by high titers of ZIKV-specific neutralizing antibody in both serum and the vaginal lumen.

ZIKV-specific CD4[+] T helper cells and CD8[+] T killer cells are recruited to and retained in the females' reproductive tracts. Passive transfer of memory T cells or antibody also confers considerable protection against intravaginal infection, but fails to provide sterilizing immunity. Both B and T lymphocytes provide considerable and redundant anti-ZIKV defense against intravaginal challenge, which may reduce the risk of sexually transmitted ZIKV infection.[36] It will be important to determine whether this protection extends to challenge with heterologous virus strains.

In 2016, several Phase I clinical trials of plasmid DNA vaccine candidates began in normal men and women in the United States and Canada in order to test for safety and immunogenicity, as evidenced by the production of neutralizing antibodies. Additionally, three Phase I clinical trials have been initiated to test the safety and immunogenicity of a purified, inactivated Puerto Rican strain of ZIKV. RNA-based and purified protein subunit vaccines are also under development.[20] The efficacy of these vaccines will be difficult to test in natural settings due to the greatly diminished numbers of ZIKV infections following the initial outbreak in Brazil and other countries in the western hemisphere.

Decreased Exposure to ZIKV Vectors

Until the licensing of an effective vaccine against ZIKV, the best way for most people to avoid becoming infected should another large outbreak occur is to prevent being bitten by infected mosquitoes, as recommended on the CDC's Zika site.[5] One should also check the CDC's travel recommendations in order to avoid entering at-risk regions, especially pregnant or potentially pregnant women and their partners.

Efforts to reduce or eliminate human exposure to the ZIKV vector species of *Aedes* mosquitoes have been put into action. *Ae. aegypti* and *Ae. albopictus* lay their eggs in standing water in a wide variety of containers, including animal dishes and bird baths, old tires, flower pots, tree holes, cemetery vases, and pool or hot bath covers.[5] The extreme variety and ubiquitous nature of these mosquito-breeding sites make their elimination very challenging, especially for those living in settlements in watery environments, particularly Amazonia. Efforts to reduce the numbers of ZIKV breeding sites, nevertheless, may have played an important role in rapidly ending the ZIKV outbreak in Texas, United States. It should be noted, however, that the large Zika epidemic in Brazil also ended within a relatively short period of time, so the actual value of decreasing *Aedes* breeding sites is unknown. Removal of large numbers of sites of standing water in urban settings may also have an ad-

verse effect upon urban wild animals, such as rodents and birds, which rely on these sites for drinking water. Additionally, both *Ae. aegypti* and *Ae. albopictus* are desiccation resistant. Indeed, *Ae. aegypti* eggs require a period of drying in order to embryonate. The eggs then hatch when submerged in water.[27]

Decreasing Human-to-Human Transmission

Since ZIKV persists in semen for many months after the virus is no longer detectable in the blood, women who are, or intend to become, pregnant should avoid sexual contact with a man who has been either infected or traveled to a region with active infection within the past 6 months. Alternatively, people who chose to have sexual relations with a potentially infected partner can use a condom.[5]

TREATMENT

While no FDA-approved cure is currently available for ZIKV infection, a number of compounds targeting different viral components are either in development or in clinical trials. Some of these compounds decrease fetal and adult mice brain disorders or inhibit ZIKV from infected dams from reaching the fetuses. A number of such treatment modalities are mentioned here.

Inhibitors of Viral Nonstructural Protein Activity

Novobiocin (typically used as an antibiotic) and lopinavir–ritonavir act as ZIKV NS2B–NS3 protease inhibitors. Novobiocin significantly increases survival rate, reduces viral blood and tissue (kidney and testes) loads, and decreases severe histopathological changes in immunocompromised mice with disseminated ZIKV infection.[15]

Bromocriptine inhibits ZIKV replication in vitro by interacting with the catalytic site of the NS2B-NS3 protease.[54] Since bromocriptine acts synergistically with IFN-α, this drug combination might also be effective in vivo. Bromocriptine is safe for use by pregnant women and may be easily administered vaginally using suppositories or vaginoadhesive disks.

Sofosbuvir is a uridine nucleoside analog that inhibits the polymerase activity of ZIKV NS5, blocks viral replication in human fetal-derived neuronal stem cell cultures, and protects these cells from virus-induced apoptotic death. It also induces an increase in A-to-G mutations in the ZIKV genome. In vivo, sofosbuvir protects immunodeficient mice against lethal ZIKV challenge.[55–58] Sofosbuvir is well tolerated by pregnant mice and prevents vertical transmission of ZIKV. It should be noted, however, that this drug is prohibitively expensive for use in low-income regions, such as vast urban slums and Amazonia.

Other nucleoside or nucleotide analogs also serve as ZIKV polymerase inhibitors. Analogs of ATP also act in this manner.[59] The imino-C-nucleoside BCX4430 has broad-spectrum antiviral activity against a wide range of RNA viruses, including both the African and Asian lineages of ZIKV.[60] BCX4430 alters electrostatic interactions of the nucleoside sugar ring with the viral polymerase, leading to nonobligate chain termination during ZIKV RNA synthesis. Moreover, trials of this drug have been performed in an IFN-receptor-deficient mouse model of severe ZIKV infection, which produces conjunctivitis, encephalitis, myelitis, infection of brain and testes, and death in mice. High-dose treatment with BCX4430 resulted in the survival of 7 of 8 of these animals when administered 4 h prior to the time of infection.[61] The drug's efficacy remains to be determined when administered during active, symptomatic infection as well as whether it can prevent an asymptomatic fetus or newborn from later developing disease.

TPB (3-chloro-N-[({4-[4-(2-thienylcarbonyl)-1-iperazinyl]phenyl}amino)carbonothioyl]-1-benzothiophene-2-carboxamide) is a nonnucleoside analog that binds to and allosterically blocks the catalytic active site of the NS5 polymerase. TPB inhibits replication of both African and Asian ZIKV strains in vitro and decreases viremia in immunocompetent mice in vivo.[62] Since pregnant women, fetuses, and newborns lack normally functioning immune responses, this drug needs to be tested for protective activity in these populations as well.

7-Deaza-2′-C-methyladenosine also inhibits ZIKV polymerase activity in vitro. It decreases viremia and delays the onset of symptomatic disease and death in vivo in mice lacking IFN-α/β and IFN-γ receptors.[63] This compound also inhibits replication of DENVs, YFV, WNV, and tick-borne encephalitis virus (TBEV), as well as hepatitis C virus, another member of the Flaviviridae family.

Compounds That Target Host Cell Factors

Some drug development strategies target host cell molecules that are necessary for ZIKV activities since the mutation rate is much lower in eukaryotic cells than it is in viruses, especially RNA viruses. Host cell ER-associated functions, such as protein processing, maturation, and modification, are required during the ZIKV life cycle. The host ER-associated signal peptidase is necessary for processing viral prM and E structural proteins. Cavinafungin, a lipopeptide from the fungus

Colispora cavincola, targets this signal peptidase.[64] The ER-localized oligosaccharyl transferase protein complex is also required for successful ZIKV infection. An aminobenzamide-sulfonamide compound, NGI-1, chemically modulates these complexes and inhibits ZIKV infection of placental cells and human neural progenitor cells.[65]

ZIKV is also highly dependent upon host cell lipid metabolism. Nordihydroguaiaretic acid, a phenolic component of the desert shrub *Larrea tridentata*, and its derivatives disrupt host lipogenesis and lipid homeostasis, probably by interfering with the sterol regulatory element-binding proteins pathway. Nordihydroguaiaretic acid and other structurally unrelated inhibitors of the pathway, such as the red wine antioxidant resveratrol, PF-429242, and fatostatin, decrease ZIKV replication.[66]

Previously Described Antiviral Compounds and Interferons

A number of previously described antiviral compounds are active against ZIKV infection and disease onset. It should be noted that some antiviral drugs can cause serious side effects, even in normal people, which may be intensified in pregnant women, fetuses, and newborns. Combination drug therapy that includes one or more of these compounds is often more effective than a single-drug regimen and may allow the individual drugs to be used at lower concentrations and, perhaps, avoid the toxic effects of any one drug.

Ribavirin is a guanosine analog that inhibits RNA replication by causing RNA chain termination. Favipiravir selectively inhibits the ZIKV RNA polymerase. Favipiravir also decreases cell death in neuronal progenitor cells infected by Asian lineage ZIKV. It acts by increasing phosphorylation and activation of the prosurvival AKT pathway and expression of the antiapoptotic *BCL2* (B cell lymphoma 2) gene.[67] The AKT pathway is also required for neurogenesis. It should be noted, however, that favipiravir is contraindicated for pregnant women due to teratogenic and embryotoxic effects in monkeys and other animals.

Both ribavirin and favipiravir inhibit ZIKV replication or transcription of the viral E protein in several human cell types, including neuronal progenitor cells.[67] A separate study reports, however, that while ribavirin and favipiravir have antiviral effects in a monkey kidney cell line in vitro, they do not do so in ZIKV-infected neuronal cells.

Combining favipiravir with IFN-α improves disease outcome. Since IFN does not cross the blood–brain barrier, when administered alone, it might not protect adults from the establishment of GBS. Favipiravir can enter semen, so the combination of these two antiviral compounds may prevent sexual transmission by infected men.[68] IFN-α and IFN-β, the nucleotide analog phosphoramidate, and the polymerase inhibitor sofosbuvir act synergistically to lower ZIKV RNA by greater than 2 logs.[55] Another polymerase inhibitor, 7-deaza-20-C-methyladenosine, prevents replication of both African and Asian ZIKV in astrocytes and in cortical and motor neurons derived from human-induced pluripotent stem cells. This compound also prevents cytopathic effect in these cells.[69]

Ribavirin and IFN-β alone or in combination inhibit the replication of the African strain of ZIKV in both human and mosquito cell lines. Ribavirin also decreases viremia and prolongs survival time in vivo in immunocompromised mice that are normally highly susceptible to fatal infection. Interestingly, viral loads in the brains of treated mice remain unaffected.[70]

IFN therapy is expensive and may cause serious side effects. Chemical means of inducing IFN synthesis, however, stimulate immune activity against ZIKV both in vitro and in vivo and may circumvent some of the shortcomings of administering the IFNs themselves. The IFN-activating molecule 1-(2-fluorophenyl)-2-(5-isopropyl-1,3,4-thiadiazol-2-yl)-1,2-dihydrochromeno[2,3-c]pyrrole-3,9-dione inhibits replication of ZIKV in vitro by stimulating IRF3-dependent expression and secretion of IFN. It also activates human peripheral blood immune cells to secrete the proinflammatory cytokines TNF-α, IL-6, and IL-1β, but not the antiinflammatory IL-10.[71]

ZIKV stimulates the production of the ISG cholesterol-25-hydroxylase.[72] The normal role of this enzyme is to oxidize cholesterol to 25-hydroxycholesterol (25HC), a natural oxysterol, which regulates sterol biosynthesis. Importantly, it passes through the blood–brain barrier. A synthetic version of 25HC inhibits ZIKV entry into human cells in vitro.[13] In vivo, 25HC reduces viremia in young, immunocompetent mice as well as decreasing the number of deaths, even in IFN pathway-deficient mice. This compound additionally decreases infection of human cortical organoids derived from embryonic stem cells and reduces ZIKV-associated microcephaly in fetal mice.[13]

The anti-ZIKV activity of the IFN-stimulated, iron–sulfur protein viperin involves targeting ZIKV NS3 and, at least in part, stimulating NS3 degradation in the target cell's proteasomes. In addition to its roles as a polyprotein protease, viral helicase, and nucleoside 5'-triphosphatase, ZIKV NS3 also aids in immune evasion.[73] NS3 degradation thus is able to combat Zika infection by multiple means.

Repurposed Antiparasitic Drugs

Several antimalarial drugs, including chloroquine, amodiaquine, and mefloquine,[74–76] possess anti-ZIKV activity as well. Chloroquine reduces transmission of ZIKV from chronically infected mouse dams and sires to their offspring and decreases viral load in fetal brains by more than 20-fold.[75] Chloroquine appears to block the endosomal acidification required for endocytosis-mediated ZIKV entry into host cells. It additionally blocks viral membrane fusion prior to the escape of the nucleocapsid from endosomes into the cells' cytoplasm for reproduction. Chloroquine also inhibits ZIKV membrane fusion to human brain microvascular endothelial cells, human neural stem cells, and mouse neurospheres and partially reverses the extension of misshapen neurites from ZIKV-infected neurospheres.[77] Chloroquine has been used to treat millions of people with malaria over several decades and has an excellent safety record as long as it is administered at proper dosages. Amodiaquine is used to treat chloroquine-resistant malaria. An important characteristic of the lipophilic antimalarial compound mefloquine is that it is able to pass through the placenta into the fetus during pregnancy.[76]

Suramin is an FDA-approved glycosaminoglycan drug that blocks ZIKV infection, even when administrated up to 24 h after infection. It inhibits ZIKV adsorption, entry, and replication in kidney cells in vitro.[78] Other glycosaminoglycans or their analogs, such as highly sulfated heparin and dextran sulfate, also block ZIKV infection. Heparin sulfate is a negatively charged polysaccharide that is used as an attachment factor for several flaviviruses, including DENVs, JEV, YFV, and TBEV. The viruses bind to heparin sulfate primarily via electrostatic interactions of basic viral amino acids with the drug's negatively charged sulfate groups. Desulfated heparin analogs are not active, suggesting a major role of the sulfonate groups in inhibiting ZIKV infection. No direct interaction is seen between ZIKV and heparin, unlike the case for several other flaviviruses.[78]

The anthelmintic drug niclosamide decreases ZIKV replication in human-induced neural stem cells in vitro. It partially restores stem cell differentiation, reduces the numbers of proinflammatory immune cells, and blocks apoptotic death of these cells. In a humanized embryonic chick model system in which human neural cells are inoculated into ZIKV-infected chick embryos, niclosamide increased fetal cranial width and height and neuronal differentiation in vivo.[79]

Anti-ZIKV Effects of Nutraceuticals and Other Antioxidants

Several commonly consumed nutraceuticals have antioxidant and antiviral activities. One such nutraceutical, the green tea polyphenol epigallocatechin gallate, blocks viral binding to potential host cells.[80] It easily crosses the placenta and is found in fetal brain, eyes, and heart.[81] Curcumin is an antioxidant component present in turmeric, a popular food additive. It also blocks ZIKV from attaching to host cells.[82] The popular flavonoid antioxidant quercetin and its derivatives, present in many Chinese herbs, vegetables, and fruits, block ZIKV growth in host cells in vitro and reduce the fatality rate in ZIKV-infected immunocompromised mice in vivo.[83]

ZIKV infection of immunocompromised mice damages their testes as a result of increased oxidative stress from elevated levels of reactive oxygen species, nitric oxide, glutathione peroxidase 4, and the proinflammatory cytokines IL-1β, IL-6, and G-CSF. The antioxidant, selenium-containing compound, ebselen, decreases oxidative stress, leukocyte infiltration, and proinflammatory responses in the testes. It also blocks sexual transmission of ZIKV to female mice in a sperm transfer model system.[84] It remains to be seen if ebselen is also effective during natural sexual activity.

Other Compounds Reducing ZIKV Neurological Pathology

Hippeastrine hydrobromide and amodiaquine dihydrochloride dihydrate eliminate ZIKV in infected human neural progenitor cells. The former drug candidate also rescues ZIKV-induced growth and differentiation defects in human forebrain organoids in vitro, increases organoid size to that found in uninfected controls, and reduces virus load to undetectable levels. It completely blocks the in vivo infection of the adult mouse forebrain cortex, hippocampus, and striatum as well, without producing neurotoxic effects.[85]

Naloxone, an inhibitor of cAMP-responsive element-binding protein 1 (CREB1), decreases interactions between ZIKV and host cells. The cyclin-dependent kinase (CDK) inhibitors SNS-032, dinaciclib, PHA-793,887, AT7519, BS194, purvalanol A, RGB-286,167, and alvocidib decrease ZIKV replication in neural cells.[86] At autopsy, infected stillborn children have been found to have increased levels of caspase 3, an important component of an apoptotic pathway, in vacuolated and apoptotic neurons.[11] The same study found that emricasan, a pan-caspase inhibitor, blocks ZIKV-induced apoptosis of human cortical neural progenitors in monolayer and three-dimensional organoid

cultures. Combination treatment with emricasan and PHA-690509 has an additive anti-ZIKV effect in inhibiting caspase-3 activity and protecting astrocytes.

Synthetic Peptides of Viral Proteins

Another category of antiflaviviral compounds is comprised of synthetic peptides derived from viral proteins. Development of the peptides is more cost effective and may prove to be safer than some of the other antiviral treatment options. One such peptide, Z2, from the stem region of ZIKV E protein, inhibits in vitro infection of cells by disrupting viral membrane integrity. Importantly, Z2 passes through the placenta and enters fetal tissues. It is safe for use in pregnant mice, blocks vertical transmission of ZIKV to mice fetuses, and protects immunocompromised mice against lethal ZIKV challenge.[87]

Other Compounds With Anti-ZIKV Activity

Obatoclax, SaliPhe, and gemcitabine inhibit ZIKV-induced pathology in human retinal pigment epithelial cells.[88] All three compounds prevent the production of viral RNA and proteins, but their mechanism of action differs. Obatoclax inhibits ZIKV from entering cells via endocytosis. It also alters the expression of cellular genes that regulate cell proliferation, the mitogen-activated protein kinase cascade, and reactive oxygen species metabolism. SaliPhe targets vacuolar ATPase and prevents blocks endosomal acidification. Gemcitabine interferes with de novo pyrimidine production. It also affects the expression of cell cycle and cell division genes. Obatoclax and SaliPhe have synergistic anti-ZIKV activity.[88]

A large-scale screen of small molecules demonstrated that rolipram, preladenant, and derivatives of ASN 07115854 have anti-ZIKV activity. The most potent of these, ASN 07115873, has an inhibitory concentration$_{50}$ (IC$_{50}$) of 189.2 pM. Their antiviral activities appear to rely primarily upon their common structural features: an assembly of two or three aromatic/aliphatic rings in *para-* or *meta-*configuration and N-phenyl-substituted piperazine or a phenyl-substituted piperazine-like moiety. Similar results are seen with several previously described anti-ZIKV compounds: PHA-690509, obatoclax, fatostatin, and sertraline, some of which were mentioned previously.[89]

A different large-scale screen detected anti-ZIKV activity in ivermectin, deferasirox, sertraline, pyrimethamine, cyclosporine A, and azathioprine.[90] The anthelmintic drug ivermectin acts by increasing the permeability of cell membranes. Deferasirox alters iron metabolism, which plays an important role in the viral life cycle. Sertraline may act by perturbing neurotransmitter signaling. Pyrimethamine is a folic acid inhibitor used to treat parasite infections, including toxoplasmosis. Cyclosporine A inhibits CD4$^+$ T helper cell activity, reducing inflammation and immunopathology. Azathioprine suppresses the growth of T and B cells.

SUMMARY OVERVIEW

Diseases: Joint pain and rash, microcephaly, miscarriage, Guillain–Barré syndrome

Causative agent: Zika virus

Vectors: *Aedes*, *Culex*, *Anopheles*, and *Mansonia* species mosquitoes, especially *Ae. aegypti* and *Ae. albopictus*

Common reservoirs: Primates

Mode of transmission: Mosquito bite, transplacentally, sexually

Geographical distribution: Africa, South Pacific, South America

Year of emergence: 1947 (Africa), 2007 (South Pacific), 2014 (South America)

REFERENCES

1. Kokernot RH, Smithburn KC, Gandara AF. Neutralization tests with sera from individuals residing in Mozambique against specific viruses isolated in Africa, transmitted by arthropods. *An Inst Med Trop (Lisb)*. 1960;17:201–230.
2. Duffy MR, Chen TH, Hancock WT. ZIKV outbreak on Yap Island, Federated States of Micronesia. *N Engl J Med*. 2019;360(24):2536–2543.
3. Gatherer D, Kohl A. ZIKV: a previously slow pandemic spreads rapidly through the Americas. *J Gen Virol*. 2016;97:269–273.
4. Rasmussen SA, Jamieson DJ, Honein MA, Petersen LR. ZIKV and birth defects—reviewing the evidence for causality. *N Engl J Med*. 2016;374:1981–1986.
5. Centers for Disease Control and Prevention. *Zika Virus. Zika Virus Homepage*. Assessed February 15, 2018. https://www.cdc.gov/zika/index.html.
6. Hall NB, Broussard K, Evert N, Canfield M. ZIKV-associated neonatal birth defects surveillance—Texas, January 2016–July 2017. *MMWR*. 2017;66(31):835–836.
7. Khawar W, Bromberg R, Moor M, et al. Seven cases of ZIKV infection in South Florida. *Cureus*. 2017;9(3), e1099.
8. WHO. *Zika Virus Infection*. Accessed June 27, 2020. https://www.who.int/csr/don/archive/disease/zika-virus-infection/en/.
9. van der Linden V, Filho EL, Lins OG, et al. Congenital Zika syndrome with arthrogryposis: retrospective case series study. *Br Med J*. 2016;354, i3899.
10. Vorou R. ZIKV, vectors, reservoirs, amplifying hosts, and their potential to spread worldwide: what we know and what we should investigate urgently. *Int J Infect Dis*. 2016;48:85–90.
11. Azevedo RSS, de Sousa JR, Araujo MTF, et al. *In situ* immune response and mechanisms of cell damage in central nervous system of fatal cases microcephaly by Zika virus. *Sci Rep*. 2018;8:1.
12. Leal MC, Muniz LF, Ferreira TSA, et al. Hearing loss in infants with microcephaly and evidence of congenital Zika virus infection—Brazil, November 2015–May 2016. *MMWR*. 2016;65(34):917–919.
13. Li C, Xu D, Ye Q, et al. Zika virus disrupts neural progenitor development and leads to microcephaly in mice. *Cell Stem Cell*. 2016;19:120–126.
14. Cui L, Zou P, Chen E, et al. Visual and motor deficits in grown-up mice with congenital Zika virus infection. *EBioMedicine*. 2017;20:193–201.
15. Yuan S, Chan JF-W, den-Haan H, et al. Structure-based discovery of clinically approved drugs as ZIKV NS2B-NS3 protease inhibitors that potently inhibit ZIKV infection *in vitro* and *in vivo*. *Antiviral Res*. 2017;145:33–43.
16. Bowen JR, Quicke KM, Maddur MS, et al. Zika virus antagonizes type I interferon responses during infection of human dendritic cells. *PLoS Pathog*. 2017;13(2), e1006164.
17. Plourde AR, Bloch EM. A literature review of Zika virus. *Emerg Infect Dis*. 2016;22(7):1185–1192.
18. Dar HA, Zaheer T, Paracha RZ, Ali A. Structural analysis and insight into Zika virus NS5 mediated interferon inhibition. *Infect Genet Evol*. 2017;51:143–152.
19. Hamel R, Dejarnac O, Wichit S, et al. Biology of Zika virus infection in human skin cells. *J Virol*. 2015;89:8880–8896.
20. Barouch DH, Thomas SJ, Michael NL. Prospects for a ZIKV vaccine. *Immunology*. 2015;46:176–182.
21. Quicke KM, Bowen JR, Johnson EL, et al. Zika virus infects human placental macrophages. *Cell Host Microbe*. 2016;20:83–90.
22. Onorat M, Li Z, Liu F, et al. Zika virus disrupts phospho-TBK1 localization and mitosis in human neuroepithelial stem cells and radial glia. *Cell Rep*. 2016;16(10):2576–2592.
23. Oh Y, Zhang F, Wang Y, et al. Zika virus directly infects peripheral neurons and induces cell death. *Nat Neurosci*. 2017;20(9):1209–1212.
24. Gaburro J, Bhatti A, Harper J, et al. Neurotropism and behavioral changes associated with Zika infection in the vector *Aedes aegypti*. *Emerg Microbes Infect*. 2018;7:68.
25. Aid M, Abbink P, Larocca RA, et al. ZIKV persistence in the central nervous system and lymph nodes of rhesus monkeys. *Cell*. 2017;169:610–620.
26. Schmitt K, Charlinsa P, Veselinovic M, et al. Zika viral infection and neutralizing human antibody response in a BLT humanized mouse model. *Virology*. 2018;515:235–242.
27. Kauffman EB, Kramer LD. Zika virus mosquito vectors: competence, biology, and vector control. *J Infect Dis*. 2017;216(S10):S976–S990.
28. Althouse BM, Vasilakis N, Sall AA, Diallo M, Weaver SC, Hanley KA. Potential for ZIKV to establish a sylvatic transmission cycle in the Americas. *PLoS Negl Trop Dis*. 2016;10(12), e0005055.

29. Dupont-Rouzeyrol M, O'Connor O, Calvez E, et al. Co-infection with Zika and dengue viruses in 2 patients, New Caledonia, 2014. *Emerg Infect Dis.* 2015;21(2):381–382.

30. Monaghan AJ, Morin CW, Steinhoff DF, et al. On the seasonal occurrence and abundance of the ZIKV vector mosquito *Aedes aegypti* in the contiguous United States. *PLoS Curr.* 2016;16:8.

31. de Souza WV, de Fátima Pessoa Militão de Albuquerque M, Vazquez E. Microcephaly epidemic related to the ZIKV and living conditions in Recife, Northeast Brazil. *BMC Public Health.* 2018;18:130.

32. de Oliveira-Filho EF, Oliveira RAS, Ferreira DRA, et al. Seroprevalence of selected flaviviruses in free-living and captive capuchin monkeys in the state of Pernambuco, Brazil. *Transbound Emerg Dis.* 2018;65(4):1094–1097.

33. Buechler CR, Bailey AL, Weiler AM, et al. Seroprevalence of ZIKV in wild African green monkeys and baboons. *mSphere.* 2017;2, e00392-16.

34. Bueno MG, Martinez N, Abdalla L, dos Santos CND, Chame M. Animals in the ZIKV life cycle: what to expect from megadiverse Latin American countries. *PLoS Negl Trop Dis.* 2016;10(12), e0005073.

35. Chiu CY, Martín CS-S, Bouquet J, et al. Experimental ZIKV inoculation in a New World monkey model reproduces key features of the human infection. *Sci Rep.* 2017;7:17126.

36. Scott JM, Lebratti TJ, Richner JM, et al. Cellular and humoral immunity protect against vaginal Zika virus infection in mice. *J Virol.* 2018;92(7), e00038-18.

37. Xia H, Luo H, Shan C, et al. An evolutionary NS1 mutation enhances Zika virus evasion of host interferon induction. *Nat Commun.* 2018;9:414.

38. Sapparapu G, Fernandez E, Kose N, et al. Neutralizing human antibodies prevent Zika virus replication and fetal disease in mice. *Nature.* 2016;540(7633):443–447.

39. Reynolds CJ, Suleyman OM, Ortega-Prieto AM, et al. T cell immunity to Zika virus targets immunodominant epitopes that show cross-reactivity with other flaviviruses. *Sci Rep.* 2018;8:672.

40. Herrera BB, Tsai W-Y, Chang CA, et al. Sustained specific and cross-reactive T cell responses to Zika and dengue viruses NS3 in West Africa. *J Virol.* 2018;92(7). e01992-17.

41. Ricciardi MJ, Magnani DM, Grifoni A, et al. Ontogeny of the B- and T-cell response in a primary Zika virus infection of a dengue-naïve individual during the 2016 outbreak in Miami, FL. *PLoS Negl Trop Dis.* 2017;11(12), e0006000.

42. Paquin-Proulx D, Avelino-Silva VI, et al. MAIT cells are activated in acute dengue virus infection and after *in vitro* Zika virus infection. *PLoS Negl Trop Dis.* 2018;12(1), e0006154.

43. Badolato-Corrêa J, Sánchez-Arcila JS, de Souza TMA, et al. Human T cell responses to dengue and Zika virus infection compared to dengue/Zika coinfection. *Immun Inflamm Dis.* 2018;6(2):194–206.

44. Sun X, Hua S, Chen H-R. Transcriptional changes during naturally-acquired Zika virus infection render dendritic cells highly conducive to viral replication. *Cell Rep.* 2017;21(12):3471–3482.

45. Kumar A, Hou S, Airo AM, et al. Zika virus inhibits type-I interferon production and downstream signaling. *EMBO Rep.* 2016;17:1766–1775.

46. Glasner A, Oiknine-Djian E, Weisblum Y, et al. Zika virus escapes NK cell detection by upregulating major histocompatibility complex class I molecules. *J Virol.* 2017;91, e00785-17.

47. Wang J, Liu J, Zhou R, et al. Zika virus infected primary microglia impairs NPCs proliferation and differentiation. *Biochem Biophys Res Commun.* 2018;497(2):619–625.

48. Luo H, Winkelmann ER, Fernandez-Salas I, et al. Zika, dengue and yellow fever viruses induce differential anti-viral immune responses in human monocytic and first trimester trophoblast cells. *Antiviral Res.* 2018;151:55–62.

49. Espinosa D, Mendy J, Manayani D, et al. Passive transfer of immune sera induced Zika virus-like particle vaccine protects AG129 mice against lethal Zika virus challenge. *EBioMedicine.* 2018;27:61–70.

50. Abbink P, Larocca RA, de la Barrera RA, et al. Protective efficacy of multiple vaccine platforms against ZIKV challenge in rhesus monkeys. *Science.* 2016;353(6304):1129–1132.

51. Li X-F, Dong H-L, Wang H-J, et al. Development of a chimeric Zika vaccine using a licensed live-attenuated flavivirus vaccine as backbone. *Nat Commun.* 2018;9:673.

52. Xu K, Song Y, Dai L, et al. Recombinant chimpanzee adenovirus vaccine AdC7-M/E protects against Zika virus infection and testis damage. *J Virol.* 2018;92(6), e01722-17.

53. Muthumani K, Griffin BD, Agarwal S, et al. *In vivo* protection against ZIKV infection and pathogenesis through passive antibody transfer and active immunization with a prMEnv DNA vaccine. *NPJ Vaccines.* 2016;1:16021.

54. Chan JF-W, Chik KK-H, Yuan S, et al. Novel antiviral activity and mechanism of bromocriptine as a Zika virus NS2B-NS3 protease inhibitor. *Antiviral Res.* 2017;141:29–37.

55. Snyder B, Goebel S, Koide F, Ptak R, Kalkeri R. Synergistic antiviral activity of sofosbuvir and type-I interferons (α and β) against ZIKV. *J Med Virol.* 2018;90:8–12.

56. Bullard-Feibelman KM, Govero J, Zhu Z, et al. The FDA-approved drug sofosbuvir inhibits Zika virus infection. *Antiviral Res.* 2017;137:134–140.

57. Mesci P, Macia A, Moore SM, et al. Blocking Zika virus vertical transmission. *Sci Rep.* 2018;8:1218.

58. Sacramento CQ, de Melo GR, de Freitas CS, et al. The clinically approved antiviral drug sofosbuvir inhibits Zika virus replication. *Sci Rep.* 2017;7:40920.

59. Hercík K, Kozak J, Šála M, et al. Adenosine triphosphate analogs can efficiently inhibit the Zika virus RNA-dependent RNA polymerase. *Antiviral Res.* 2017;137:131–133.

60. Eyer L, Zouharová D, Širmarová J, et al. Antiviral activity of the adenosine analogue BCX4430 against West Nile virus and tick-borne flaviviruses. *Antiviral Res.* 2017;142:63–67.

61. Julander JG, Siddharthan V, Evans J, et al. Efficacy of the broad-spectrum antiviral compound BCX4430 against Zika virus in cell culture and in a mouse model. *Antiviral Res.* 2017;137:14–22.

62. Pattnaik A, Palermo N, Sahoo BR, et al. Discovery of a non-nucleoside RNA polymerase inhibitor for blocking Zika virus replication through *in silico* screening. *Antiviral Res.* 2018;151:78–86.

63. Zmurko J, Marques RE, Schols D, Verbeken E, Kaptein SJF, Neyts J. The viral polymerase inhibitor 7-deaza-2′-C-methyladenosine is a potent inhibitor of in vitro Zika virus replication and delays disease progression in a robust mouse infection model. *PLoS Negl Trop Dis.* 2016;10(5), e0004695.

64. Estoppey D, Lee CM, Janoschke M, et al. The natural product cavinafungin selectively interferes with Zika and dengue virus replication by inhibition of the host signal peptidase. *Cell Rep.* 2017;19:451–460.

65. Puschnik AS, Marceau CD, Ooi YS, et al. A small molecule oligosaccharyltransferase inhibitor with panflaviviral activity. *Cell Rep.* 2017;21(11):3032–3039.

66. Merino-Ramos T, de Oya NJ, Saiz J-C, Martín-Acebes MA. Antiviral activity of nordihydroguaiaretic acid and its derivative tetra-*O*-methyl nordihydroguaiaretic acid against West Nile virus and ZIKV. *Antimicrob Agents Chemother.* 2017;61, e00376-17.

67. Kim J-A, Seong R-K, Kumar M, Shin OS. Favipiravir and ribavirin inhibit replication of Asian and African strains of ZIKV in different cell models. *Viruses.* 2018;10:72.

68. Pires de Mello CP, Tao X, Kim TH, et al. ZIKV replication is substantially inhibited by novel favipiravir and interferon alpha combination regimens. *Antimicrob Agents Chemother.* 2018;62, e01983-17.

69. Lanko K, Eggermont K, Patel A, et al. Replication of the Zika virus in different iPSC-derived neuronal cells and implications to assess efficacy of antivirals. *Antiviral Res.* 2017;145:82–86.

70. Kamiyama N, Soma R, Hidano S, et al. Ribavirin inhibits Zika virus (ZIKV) replication *in vitro* and suppresses viremia in ZIKV-infected STAT1-deficient mice. *Antiviral Res.* 2017;146:1–11.

71. Pryke KM, Abraham J, Sali TM, et al. A novel agonist of the TRIF pathway induces a cellular state refractory to replication of Zika, Chikungunya, and dengue viruses. *mBio.* 2017;8, e00452-17.

72. Chen Y, Wang S, Yi Z, et al. Interferon-inducible cholesterol-25-hydroxylase inhibits hepatitis C virus replication via distinct mechanisms. *Sci Rep.* 2014;4:7242.

73 Panayiotou C, Lindqvist R, Kurhade C, et al. Viperin restricts ZIKV and tick-borne encephalitis virus replication by targeting NS3 for proteasomal degradation. *J Virol.* 2018;92(7), e02054-17.

74. Han Y, Mesplède T, Xu H, Quan Y, Wainberg MA. The antimalarial drug amodiaquine possesses anti-Zika virus activities. *J Med Virol.* 2018;90(5):796–802.

75. Shiryaev SA, Mesci P, Pinto A. Repurposing of the antimalaria drug chloroquine for ZIKV treatment and prophylaxis. *Sci Rep.* 2017;7:15771.

76. Barbosa-Lima G, Moraes AM, da S Araújo A, et al. 2,8-Bis(trifluoromethyl)quinoline analogs show improved anti-Zika virus activity, compared to mefloquine. *Eur J Med Chem.* 2017;127:334–340.

77. Delvecchio R, Higa LM, Pezzuto P. Chloroquine, an endocytosis blocking agent, inhibits Zika virus infection in different cell models. *Viruses.* 2016;8:322.

78. Tan CW, Sam I-C, Chong WL, Lee VS, Chan YF. Polysulfonate suramin inhibits Zika virus infection. *Antiviral Res.* 2017;143:186–194.

79. Cairns DM, Boorgu DSSK, Levin M, Kaplan DL. Niclosamide rescues microcephaly in a humanized *in vivo* model of Zika infection using human induced neural stem cells. *Biol Open.* 2018;7, bio031807.

80. Carneiro BM, Batista MN, Braga ACS, Nogueira ML, Rahal P. The green tea molecule EGCG inhibits ZIKV entry. *Virology.* 2016;496:215–218.

81. Chu KO, Wang CC, Chu CY, Choy KW, Pang CP, Rogers MS. Uptake and distribution of catechins in fetal organs following *in utero* exposure in rats. *Hum Reprod.* 2007;22:280–287.

82. Mounce BC, Cesaro T, Carrau L, Vallet T, Vignuzzi M. Curcumin inhibits Zika and Chikungunya virus infection by inhibiting cell binding. *Antiviral Res.* 2017;142:148–157.

83. Wong G, He S, Siragam V, et al. Antiviral activity of quercetin-3-B-O-D-glucoside against ZIKV infection. *Virol Sin.* 2017;32(6):545–547.

84. Simanjuntak Y, Liang JJ, Chen SY, Li JK, Lee YL, Wu HC. Ebselen alleviates testicular pathology in mice with Zika infection and prevents its sexual transmission. *PLoS Pathog.* 2018;14(2), e1006854.

85. Zhou T, Tan L, Cederquist GY, et al. High-content screening in hPSC-neural progenitors identifies drug candidates that inhibit Zika infection in fetal-like organoids and adult brain. *Cell Stem Cell.* 2018;21:274–283.

86. Xu M, Lee EM, Wen Z, et al. Identification of small molecule inhibitors of Zika virus infection and induced neural cell death via a drug repurposing screen. *Nat Med.* 2016;22(10):1101–1107.

87. Yu Y, Deng Y-Q, Zou P, et al. A peptide-based viral inactivator inhibits ZIKV infection in pregnant mice and fetuses. *Nat Commun.* 2017;8:15672.

88. Kuivanen S, Bespalov MM, Nandania J, et al. Obatoclax, saliphenylhalamide and gemcitabine inhibit Zika virus infection *in vitro* and differentially affect cellular signaling, transcription and metabolism. *Antiviral Res.* 2017;139:117–128.

89. Micewicz ED, Khachatoorian R, French SW, Ruchala P. Identification of novel small-molecule inhibitors of ZIKV infection. *Bioorg Med Chem Lett.* 2018;28:452–458.

90. Barrows NJ, Campos RK, Powell S, et al. A screen of FDA-approved drugs for inhibitors of Zika virus infection. *Cell Host Microbe.* 2016;20(2):259–270.

CHAPTER 4

West Nile Virus

INTRODUCTION

West Nile virus (WNV) was first isolated in 1937 in the West Nile district of Uganda[1] and was subsequently reported in other areas of Africa, the Middle East, Europe, South Asia, and Australia. For decades, infections with WNV were generally mild and infrequent. This changed in the 1990s as severe disease became increasingly common and widespread, due at least in part, to commerce and the dispersal of *Culex pipiens* mosquitoes, the introduction of WNV into house sparrows, and climate warming.[2]

Bird and, later, human infections were first seen in the Western Hemisphere in the United States in 1999 and the virus began to overwinter in *Culex* mosquitoes in New York City in early 2000. WNV is now endemic throughout North, South, and Central America.[3] Between 1999 and 2016, California, Colorado, and Texas reported greater than 5000 cases of WNV disease, with over 3000 cases of neuroinvasive disease in California and Texas alone. It should be noted that WNV had, essentially, not reached these Western states until 2002. In the United States in 2017, WNV infected people, birds, or mosquitoes in 47 states and the District of Columbia. Reported human disease incidence in that year was 2002. Of these, 1339 (67%) were neuroinvasive disease and 663 (33%) were nonneuroinvasive.[4,5] These figures likely underestimate the true number of infections since most WNV infections in humans are asymptomatic.

In approximately 20% of those infected, a mild, self-limiting form of febrile illness ensues. A small number of those infected (less than 1%) develop the severe, potentially fatal neuroinvasive disease. Some survivors have long-term or permanent neurological damage.[5] The recent rapid geographical spread of the virus and the increase in disease incidence and severity have brought WNV to the attention of both the healthcare community and the general public.

HISTORY

Infection with WNV typically resulted in occasional cases of mild, febrile illness from its discovery in 1937 until 1957, when an outbreak produced severe neurological symptoms in residents of Israeli nursing homes. This Israeli strain had a high mortality rate in geese.[6] Such serious disease manifestations remained uncommon until the mid-1990s through the early 2000s. During that time period, large outbreaks of severe disease occurred in Algeria (1994), Romania (1996), Tunisia (1997), Russia (1999), the United States (1999–2005), Israel (2000), Sudan (2002), and Canada (2003–2004).[7–9] Up to 60% of hospitalized patients developed the neuroinvasive disease, with a mortality rate of 4%–7%.[10]

The Israeli strain of WNV is believed to have entered the United States during the late summer of 1999 from mosquitoes carried aboard cargo ships docking in New York Harbor or from infected exotic imported or migratory birds.[6,11] Evidence suggests that the resulting outbreak in New York was amplified in house sparrows.[12] A mutation in the WNV helicase gene led to high levels of viremia and mortality in American crows[13] and a large number of crows were found dead in the affected region of New York. Several exotic zoo birds are also susceptible to severe infection. In the United States during that August, 62 cases of human West Nile disease, 59 of which were severe and resulted in hospitalization, and 7 deaths, occurred coincidentally with an epizootic outbreak in birds. The reported infections were all found in the vicinity of New York City, initially in a small area of the northern portion of the borough of Queens. Genetic sequencing suggests that the strain (NY99) originated in the Middle East, with close similarity to that circulating in Israel at the time.[6] Both NY66 and the Israeli isolates are unusual in their ability to cause a high mortality rate in birds. Prior to this flavivirus outbreak, most cases of viral meningitis were caused by an enterovirus and primarily involved young children. Enteroviruses are transmitted by contact with contaminated fecal material. The people infected during the 1999 American outbreak did not know each other and had no common exposure history, but all spent time outdoors, particularly in the evenings. Serological testing of serum and cerebrospinal fluid (CSF) samples indicated that the causative agent was antigenically similar to Saint Louis encephalitis virus. WNV was later identified as the responsible virus for human disease.[4]

In 2000, there were 21 reported cases in humans with 2 deaths, again occurring around New York City, particularly Staten Island. The epizootic in birds, however, had by this time spread to 12 states, ranging from Vermont to South Carolina, and the District of Columbia. That year also witnessed 63 cases of infection in horses from 7 states, with a 39% fatality rate. In 2001, 66 human cases and 9 deaths were reported. In 2002, the number of human cases increased to 4156 with 284 deaths, and in 2003, 9862 human cases with 264 deaths were reported in the United States. By this time, the disease had spread through much of the country. By 2004, West Nile disease had spread westward and was reported in almost all of the states in the continental United States as well as Canada. The state with the highest number of cases at that time was California. Significantly, the numbers of cases of human West Nile disease in the United States as a whole fell in 2004 and 2005 to less than 33% of the level found in 2003, perhaps due to the establishment of immunity in asymptomatic people.[4,5] As WNV spread across the United States, it infected other highly competent avian hosts, including blue jays and American robins, which served as important amplification hosts.[14] The original WNV NY99 strain was also replaced by the WN02 strain, which is transmitted more efficiently by the mosquito vectors, especially at high temperatures.[2,15,16]

Over the last few years, West Nile disease incidence in the United States has fallen. From January 1 to December 16, 2008, the CDC was notified of 1370 cases of confirmed West Nile disease in the United States. Of these, 679 (49.6%) were West Nile fever, 640 (46.7%) were encephalitis or meningitis, 51 (3.7%) led to other/unspecified clinical manifestations, and 37 (2.7%) were fatal. The state with the highest number of cases (411 with 13 deaths) was California and accounted for 30% of the total number of cases in the country. Two other Western states, Arizona and Colorado, also had a high number of cases of West Nile disease (109 and 95, respectively), while nearby Utah, Nevada, and New Mexico had lower numbers (26, 16, and 9 cases, respectively). Mississippi, with a greatly different climate, reported 99 cases. The states with the highest incidence rates of human West Nile encephalitis/meningitis in 2008 were South Dakota, Kansas, and Nebraska. California, Arizona, and Nebraska also had the highest number of infected blood donors in 2008 (68, 26, and 13 positive donors, respectively).[5] From 2009 to 2011, case numbers for the country as a whole were lower than those reported in 2008, but they resurged again in 2012. In that year, over 5500 WNV infections were reported, with the largest increase in Texas (1868 as opposed in 27 in 2011). The number of neuroinvasive disease cases also increased greatly,

from 486 in 2011 and over 2800 in 2012. Fatal disease also increased in 2012, from 43 in 2011 to 286 in 2012. From 2013 to 2018, the total number of infections in the United States has remained steady, ranging from 2011 to 2700, and the number of deaths ranging from approximately 100 to 170.[17]

A study of the influence of climate on human West Nile disease incidence in California, conducted on a monthly basis per county from 2006 to 2011, found only a weak correlation between human case numbers and temperatures (average, minimum, and maximum temperatures), while no such correlation existed between case numbers and either precipitation or drought (unpublished data). However, strong correlation coefficiencies (exceeding 0.8) were found between the reported numbers of infections in humans and birds and humans and mosquitoes on a per county basis by year in California from 2003 to 2014 in some, but not all counties (unreported data). Importantly, the reports of infection in both mosquitoes and birds preceded reported human cases by weeks. Monitoring numbers of infected mosquitoes may thus permit preventative measures to be implemented in only those counties where such strong correlations are found, while the public health funds could be put to other uses in counties with weak correlation or very low numbers of human cases over time. A low number of counties in several other states also have strong correlation coefficients between numbers of infected humans and mosquitoes, but this is not the case for most counties in most states (unpublished data).

West Nile disease appeared south of mainland United States in 2001, when a case of encephalitis was reported in the Cayman Islands. Surveillance of bird and horse blood found that antibodies to the virus were also present in Columbia, Cuba, the Dominican Republic, Jamaica, Guadeloupe, El Salvador, Mexico, and Puerto Rico, although disease incidence or death of animals or humans was rare.[18,19] The lack of significant disease in these areas may indicate the presence of a less virulent viral strain or false-positive test results due to cross-reactivity with other flaviviruses.

West Nile disease among humans in Canada was first noted in 2002 as 426 people in Quebec and Ontario became ill and 20 died. As the number of cases in the United States peaked in 2003, 1494 cases with 10 deaths occurred in Canada. As in the United States, disease incidence in Canada fell in subsequent years. West Nile disease during 2008 was found in the southern portions of the Canadian provinces of Manitoba, Saskatchewan, and Ontario, while British Columbia and Alberta reported travel-related cases.[5]

THE DISEASES

WNV disease is currently endemic in many areas of the world, including Africa, the Middle East, Southwestern Asia, Europe, and the Americas. In temperate regions (latitudes 23.5°–66.5°), the reported numbers of cases are most common during the late summer and fall, in accordance with the biting habits of its mosquito vectors. In warmer climates, such as the American South, the disease occurs year-round. See Davis et al.[10] for an excellent review of WNV-induced disease.

Mild West Nile Infection

Most infected individuals remain asymptomatic, with no illness occurring in approximately 80% of those infected. West Nile fever is a mild illness, arising in about 20% of those infected by WNV and occurs in all age groups. It is characterized by fever and chills, severe frontal headache, ache in the eyes upon movement, pain in the chest and lumbar regions, tiredness, nausea and vomiting, swollen lymph nodes, and a non-itching skin rash. This condition may last from several days to several weeks. No permanent ill effects are associated with West Nile fever.[5,20]

Neuroinvasive Disease

Serious disease symptoms occur in 0.75% of those infected with WNV. The fatality rate among those affected is 3%–15% and over half of those with neuroinvasive illness develop long-term nervous system disorders. Most of the damage occurs in the brain stem, hippocampus, cerebellum, and anterior horn of the spinal cord.[21] Following a 3–4-day incubation, a small percentage of infected individuals develop at least one of the following symptoms: severe headache, high fever, stiff neck, stupor, disorientation, confusion, coma, tremors, convulsions, muscle weakness, parkinsonism, loss of vision, numbness, or paralysis.[22,23] These symptoms may persist for several weeks. The CSF contains WNV-specific IgM antibodies and pleocytosis, composed primary of neutrophils, in approximately half of the patients.[10] Frequently, long-term sequelae, such as weakness, myalgia, persistent movement disorders, and cognitive deficits, follow recovery from acute West Nile neuroinvasive disease.[7,24,25] Neuroinvasive disease may be manifested in several forms, as described later.

West Nile Encephalitis or West Nile Meningitis

West Nile encephalitis and meningitis are inflammations of the brain or meninges, respectively, after infection. West Nile meningoencephalitis may also occur. These conditions are found most commonly in those who are over the age of 50 years or are immunosuppressed. The latter group includes the recipients of organ transplants, 40% of who develop neuroinvasive disease.[26] Among those with severe encephalitis, WNV may be present in the basal ganglia, thalamus, substantia nigra, and pons.[27] Half of the WNV-associated deaths in 2002 were reported in people older than 77 years. Meningitis is more common among younger people, while encephalitis is more prevalent in older individuals. Severe disease manifestations are rare in children under the age of 1 year. Diabetes is a risk factor for death from WNV infection.

The symptoms of West Nile meningitis are similar to those seen in other viral meningitis cases and include abrupt onset of fever, severe headache, Kernig's and Brudzinski's signs, and sensitivity to light and noise. Gastrointestinal upset may lead to dehydration. The outcome is usually favorable, although headache, fatigue, and muscle ache may persist in some people. The fatality rate from WNV meningitis in the United States is approximately 2%.

West Nile encephalitis varies widely in severity and may manifest as a mild state of confusion to a severe form resulting in coma or death. The overall mortality rate for this form of encephalitis is 12%–15%, reaching 35% in elderly patients.[28] A coarse tremor of the upper extremities is common and may be associated with movement. Parkinson's-like symptoms may also be seen, as well as abnormal movement or cerebellar ataxia with gait impairment. These generally resolve over time, but may persist in those with severe disease. Impaired movement appears to result from an attraction of the virus to the neurons in the areas of the brain involved in motor control, including the brain stem, the substantia nigra, and the cerebellum. Fatigue, headache, and cognitive dysfunction may continue for over a year. The latter includes difficulties in concentration, decreased attention span, apathy, and depression.[27]

West Nile Poliomyelitis

West Nile poliomyelitis or acute flaccid paralysis results from inflammation of and damage to the spinal cord, especially the anterior horn motor neurons.[28] Beginning with limb weakness, the disease often progresses rapidly during the next 48 h. Many patients are left with permanent limb weakness.[27]

West Nile poliomyelitis is manifested by a sudden onset of weakness of the muscles of the limbs or the breathing muscles, similar to the symptoms seen during infection with the poliovirus. This weakness may be rapidly progressive and tends to affect one side of the body more than the other. Severe disease may lead to a more symmetric dense quadriplegia. Weakness may also affect the facial muscles. Numbness or loss of sensation usually does not occur, but affected individuals may experience great pain. Respiratory failure may result from the inflammation of the high cervical region of the spinal cord or the lower brain stem, paralyzing the diaphragm and intercostal muscles. This disease manifestation is associated with high morbidity and mortality. Survivors may require extended ventilation support.[5]

West Nile poliomyelitis was first widely observed in the United States in 2002. This condition occurs less commonly than encephalitis or meningitis and is seen in younger persons, with the peak incidence occurring between the ages of 35 and 65 years. People with this disease may recover limb strength completely or may not recover it to any significant extent. Recovery of those people experiencing quadriplegia or respiratory failure is slow and is rarely complete.[5]

Other Neuroinvasive Disease Due to WNV

Another serious neuroinvasive manifestation of WNV infection is the inflammation and demyelination of peripheral nerves, leading to a condition similar to Guillain–Barré syndrome. Affected persons have a sense of fatigue and generalized weakness and sensory and autonomic dysfunction.[5] The CSF may contain elevated protein levels.

THE VIRUS

WNV Structure

Similar to other flaviviruses, WNV is transcribed as a single polyprotein that is subsequently cleaved to produce three structural and seven nonstructural proteins (NS1–NS7). The structural proteins are the capsid protein, prM (premembrane), and E protein found in the viral envelope. The binding of the E protein to the natural killer cell (NK cell) activation receptor NKp44 on NK cells plays an important role in WNV-mediated NK activation, degranulation, interferon (IFN)-γ secretion, and NK cell cytolytic activity. Recombinant NKp44 binds directly to purified WNV E protein as well.[29] N-linked glycosylation of either E protein or NS1 increases viral virulence, as discussed later.

The NS5 polymerase is part of the WNV replication complex. NS5 has been reported to be expressed only after the virus is released into the cytoplasm and is located within flavivirus-induced membranes. However, while WNV replication occurs within the cytoplasm, NS5 normally transits into the nucleus of both WNV-infected and NS5-transfected host cells. A

point mutation in the nuclear localization sequence of the viral NS5 gene in the attenuated Kunjin strains from Australia abrogates NS5 nuclear entry. (Kunjin virus is the subject of a separate chapter.) Inability of NS5 to enter the nucleus results in virtually complete cytoplasmic accumulation of NS5, which decreases the replication and survival of the mutated virus. Nuclear trafficking is thus vital for at least the Kunjin virus WNV variant replication.[30] Since NS5 also functions as a methyltransferase and interferes with host immune responses, NS5 nuclear localization may also be vital to one or more of those activities.

WNV is cytolytic: both the NS3 and capsid proteins stimulate caspase 3 activation and rapid apoptosis in mouse brains and neurons in vivo.[21] Apoptosis is a common form of cell self-destruction that serves as a cellular defense mechanism that limits viral spread by killing infected host cells. Apoptosis may be pathogenic when it occurs in nondividing or noninfected cells, such as normal neurons, which are then eliminated. Infected mice with defective caspase 3 have reduced neuronal death in the cerebral cortex, brain stem, and cerebellum.[21] WNV can also cause cell death by necrosis. Interestingly, in mice, apoptosis is much more common in the spinal cord than in the brain.[31]

WNV and MicroRNA/Small Interfering RNA

NS4B acts together with subgenomic flavivirus RNA (sfRNA) to control WNV protein production by blocking the actions of the host's protective RNAi pathways, leading to increased viral virulence.[32] The small interfering RNA (siRNA) siFvEJW acts upon a conserved sequence in the WNV E protein. Using a targeting system to deliver this siRNA intranasally to the CNS during the late stage of neuroinvasive disease in WNV-infected mice decreases viral load in the brain as well as neuropathology, increasing survival time.[33] By blocking the E protein production, siFvEJW gives the mice time to develop humoral and cell-mediated immunity, both of which help in virus clearance from the CNS and peripheral tissues. It should be noted, however, that intranasal delivery of WNV into the human CNS faces difficulties due to differences in mouse and human noses that must be overcome before this treatment can be used in humans.

A variety of host cell microRNAs (miRNAs) inhibits the replication of flaviviruses, including members of the miRNAs miR-34, miR-15, and miR-517 families. Members of the miR-34 family have strong antiflaviviral effects against WNV, Japanese encephalitis virus (JEV), dengue virus (DENV)-2, and Zika virus (ZIKV).[34] The miR-34 family normally represses the Wnt/β-catenin signaling pathway and enhances interferon response factor (IRF)-3 phosphorylation and nuclear translocation, followed by the extracellular release of type I IFN (IFN-α and IFN-β). Exposure of host cells to viral double-stranded RNA (dsRNA), including that found in WNV, reduces the miR-34-mediated inhibition of the Wnt signaling pathway, leading to antiviral type I IFN release by cells.[34]

Another miRNA, miR-532-5p, is upregulated by the WNV Kunjin variant after a viral infection of the brains of infected mice in vivo. This siRNA downregulates expression of the cellular genes SEC14 and spectrin domain (SESTD1) and TAK1-binding protein 3 (TAB3) in a human kidney cell line as well as in infected mouse brains.[35] Both SESTD1 and TAB3 are required for efficient Kunjin replication. SESTD1 normally inhibits Ca^{2+}-mediated signals, while TAB3 helps to regulate the activation of transforming growth factor-β-activated kinase 1 (TAK1) phosphatase, whose actions are required for target cell survival.[36] It should be noted that WNV lineage 1 Kunjin strains cause little pathology in humans, but may cause severe pathology in horses. Further studies using more pathogenic WNV strains are needed in order to test the efficacy of this miRNA in humans. Human miR-6124 is also upregulated during in vitro WNV infection in a neuronal epithelioma cell line. This miRNA increases apoptosis by decreasing the expression of the antiapoptotic proteins CCCTC-binding factor (CTCF) and EGFR-coamplified and EGFR-overexpressed protein (ECOP).[37]

RNA interference (RNAi) also plays a protective role in mosquito immune responses to WNV. Both *C. quinquefasciatus* mosquito cells infected in vitro and orally infected *C. quinquefasciatus* mosquitoes (Kunjin strain) produce viral noncoding sfRNA that interact with the RNAi-processing enzymes Dicer and Argonaute 2, whose actions are required for cleavage and production of host miRNAs.[38] Additionally, in WNV Kunjin-infected mosquito cells, the miRNA aae-miR-2940-5p is downregulated. This miRNA normally suppresses the production of a host metalloprotease that is required for virus replication.[39]

The WNV Life Cycle

WNV typically enters its vertebrate host during an infected mosquito's blood meal as the mosquito inoculates the virus into the host's skin. WNV first infects the keratinocytes in the skin's epidermal layer. WNV is found in the skin for up to 4 months in experimentally infected mice in vivo and for approximately a month in human keratinocytes in vitro.[40] WNV then enters the skin's Langerhans cells, a form of dendritic cell (DC)

in the skin, before infecting and multiplying to high levels in neutrophils that are recruited to the area. The infected Langerhans cells and neutrophils migrate to regional lymph nodes and, from there, into the bloodstream, leading to a primary viremia.[7,41] This virus then goes to the spleen where it is amplified, causing a secondary viremia, which persists for up to a week and then drops as the host begins to produce and release IgM neutralizing antibodies into the blood serum. Viremia only reaches a low level in human blood.[10] After the secondary viremia, WNV invades the CNS. The replication typically only occurs in an interleukin-1β (IL-1β)-dependent manner in the skin, draining lymph nodes, spleen, and CNS in humans.[20,42] In nonneural cells, the WNV cellular receptor is believed to be the integrin $\alpha_v\beta_3$.[43] After binding to its receptor, WNV stimulates a rapid and sustained Ca^{2+} influx through Ca^{2+} channels in the cell's plasma membrane. The presence of cytoplasmic Ca^{2+} is believed to play an important role during the early stages of virus replication by its action on the endoplasmic reticulum (ER) membrane. Increased cytoplasmic Ca^{2+} levels also influence the later stages of cellular infection by activating the cleavage of caspase 3.[44] WNV replication is independent of WNV-induced autophagy in cultured neurons, unlike the replication of other flaviviruses, including DENV, tick-borne encephalitis virus (TBEV), and JEV.[45]

The infection of the spleen is followed by the migration of WNV to the CNS. In mice, mortality is greater in the absence of splenic macrophages, but no change in mortality occurs in the absence of the lymph node draining-macrophages after footpad inoculation. After entering into the spleen, WNV infects not only tissue macrophages, but also the immature blood monocytes, some populations of DC, and neutrophils. The increase in viral load quickens WNV spread to the brain.[46] Afterward, the infected mice retain normal amounts of WNV-specific antibodies and CD8+ T killer cells, but the number of NK cells and CD4+ T helper cells is increased in comparison with those found in normal mice. Infected splenic monocytes express the high levels of the *IL18* gene, whose protein product is vital for the production of the protective, antiviral NK cells.[46]

Unlike other splenic myeloid cell types, such as neutrophils, splenic macrophages have high levels of mRNAs for the complement protein C1q, the apoptotic cell clearance protein Mertk, IL-18, and the cellular IgG receptor FcγR1. Splenic macrophages may also be a major source of the C4 and C1 complement molecules. The cellular expression of proapoptotic caspase 12 is restricted to splenic macrophages and appears to stimulate anti-WNV responses. This is in accord with the increased WNV susceptibility of splenic macrophage-deficient mice.[46] Taken together, splenic macrophages may exert their anti-WNV activity by enhancing both the apoptotic and complement cascades, both of which destroy virally infected cells. In addition to the spleen, low but similar levels of viral infection are also present in the lung, kidney, heart, pancreas, skeletal muscles, and thymus, but, unlike the case in birds, not in the liver.[47]

WNV typically has a defined tissue tropism, infecting cells of the CNS, splenic macrophages, B cells, and T cells. The RIG-I-like receptor (RLR) and type I IFN pathways (discussed later) are at least partially responsible for this tropism since mice with defective RLR or IFN signaling pathways have expanded tissue tropism and infect cells that are not normally hosts of WNV due to inflammatory responses that block early WNV replication in the liver.[48,49] WNV also induces the genes associated with NK cell activation and receptor signaling, as well as their production of proinflammatory cytokines. The activation of these genes, in addition to stimulation by the RLR and IFN pathways, is important to limiting WNV infection of nonpermissive tissue.[49]

WNV and the CNS

Viral entry into and spread within the CNS relies, in part, upon axonal transport in both retrograde and anterograde directions by extracellular secretion of WNV from axons, seen in vitro in compartmentalized neuron cultures and during in vivo infection of the intrasciatic nerve in mice.[50] The proinflammatory chemokine migration inhibitory factor (MIF) plays an important role in speeding viral entry into the CNS by reducing the integrity of the blood–brain barrier (BBB). During acute infection, increased MIF levels are present in both the plasma and the CSF. WNV infection of mice induces MIF in vivo and blocking its activity decreases the mortality rate. Additionally, mice lacking a functional *MIF* gene have both a lower viral load and less inflammation in the brain than wild-type infected animals.[51] MIF increases the levels of tumor necrosis factor-α (TNF-α) and matrix metalloproteinases (MMPs). MMPs are responsible for the disruption of the BBB. MIF also elevates the levels of the proinflammatory compounds nitric oxide and the cyclooxygenase-2 (COX-2) enzyme as well as its product, the proinflammatory lipid prostaglandin E2 (PGE$_2$).[52]

Although neurons are the primary target of WNV in the brain, monocytoid cells and human cortical astrocytes are also infected by WNV in vitro and ex vivo.[53] The latter produce COX-1, COX-2, and PGE$_2$ and stimulate the production of toxic reactive oxygen species and ni-

tric oxide. JEV also stimulates the production of COX-2 and PGE$_2$, but not COX-1, in astrocytes.[54] In response to COX-2, WNV-infected human brain microvascular endothelial cells (HBMECs) and cortical astrocytes increase their production of some MMPs—MMP-3 and MMP-9, while decreasing the activity of MMP-2.[55] These changes increase BBB permeability, since this barrier is composed of endothelial cells, perivascular astrocytes, and the basement membrane. The basement membrane is attacked by MMPs, allowing gaps to appear between the cells in the BBB. Experimentally inhibiting COX-2, but not COX-1, activity abrogates the production of PGE$_2$; MMP-1, MMP-3, and MMP-9; and the proinflammatory cytokines IL-1β, IL-6, and IL-8. WNV-infected astrocytes secrete much higher levels of the chemokines CXCL10, CCL2, and CCL5 and cytokines than do infected neurons, and do so later during the course of infection.[56] Additionally, the activation of the COX-2/PGE$_2$ pathway by WNV induces the plasmin/urokinase plasminogen activator (uPA) which, like the MMPs, disrupts the BBB. Increased levels of uPA occur in other neurological diseases as well.[57]

Interactions between the tight junction proteins on the apical side and the adherens junction proteins on the basolateral side of HBMECs maintain a functional BBB. WNV, as well as TBEV and JEV, infects and multiplies in HBMECs. WNV then increases the expression of the cellular adhesion molecules vascular cell adhesion molecule-1 (VCAM-1) and E-selectin, which will be further discussed later in this chapter. WNV initially enters the CNS using a transcellular pathway,[58] without altering BBB integrity. Afterward, the levels of the BBB tight junction proteins, zona occludens, claudin-1, occludin, and junctional adhesion molecule-A (JAM-A), and the adherens junction proteins, β-catenin and vascular endothelial cadherin, decrease in infected mice as the levels of MMP-1, MMP-3 and MMP-9 increase. In the presence of supernatants of infected astrocyte cultures in vitro, some of the tight junction HBMEC proteins are lost in a process that is reversible by MMP inhibitors.[55] Elevated levels of the MMPs listed already increase BBB permeability and allow monocytes and lymphocytes to infiltrate the brain.[59,60] The infected leukocytes enhance WNV neuroinvasion by acting as "Trojan horses" that carry the virus past the BBB and into the CNS.[59]

Infected astrocytes play an important role in WNV-induced neuroinflammation and neuron death. The WNV capsid proteins increase the expression of the astrocyte genes encoding the proinflammatory proteins CXCL10, IL-1β, and indolamine-2',3'-deoxygenase. WNV additionally alter the expression of ER stress genes, including growth arrest/DNA damage-inducible gene 153, eukaryotic translation initiation factor 2 alpha kinase 3, and glucose-regulated protein 78 kDa. These proteins are produced in response to the accumulation of large amounts of unfolded or misfolded proteins.[53] DENV, TBEV, and JEV also modulate the unfolded protein response, thus allowing greater production of viral RNA and proteins.[61] Both WNV and JEV increase the expression of CCAAT-enhancer-binding protein homologous protein, a transcription factor induced by the unfolded protein response.[62] Additionally, the protective astrocyte-specific ER stress sensor gene OASIS (old astrocyte specifically induced substance) is reduced. This leads to the induction of the afore-mentioned ER stress genes and apoptosis in neurons, but not astrocytes. Cytotoxic factors for neurons are also induced in WNV-infected astrocytes.[53]

The infection of astrocytes and neurons stimulates the production of the WNV capsid protein, which, in turn, alters the expression of the chemokine CXCL10 by regulating the inducible nitric oxide synthetase enzyme activity and, subsequently, increasing nitric oxide production.[53] CXCL10 recruits $CD8^+$ T killer cells into the CNS via the chemokine receptor CXCR3.[10] Deficiency in either CXCL10 or CXCR3 raises the viral load in the brain and increases morbidity and mortality.[63] The chemokine receptor CCR5 also is involved in WNV infection of the CNS since people with defective CCR5 genes are at greater risk for developing fatal WNV disease.[64] Approximately 1% of Caucasians are homozygous for this faulty gene.[10]

WNV Strains—Locations and Virulence

WNV is common in Africa, Southern Asia, and the Middle East and is found throughout Europe, Australia, and North, Central, and South America as well. Viral strains have been assigned to 6–9 lineages, based upon the sequence analysis of either the E protein gene or the complete WNV genome. Lineage 1 viruses are found in North Africa, the Middle East, Europe, India, Asia, the Americas, and Australia, with the Australian strain being designated as the Kunjin virus. Lineage 2 viruses are found only in southern Africa and Madagascar. Lineage 1 viruses have been viewed as being more pathogenic than lineage 2 viruses,[65] but highly virulent neuroinvasive and less virulent strains exist in both of these WNV lineages. Lineage 3, the "Rabensburg" strain, was isolated from *Cx. pipiens* in the Czech Republic in 1997. Lineage 4, the "Krasnodar" strain, was isolated from ticks in southern Russia. Lineage 5 contains WNV in humans and mosquitoes from India, and the other putative lineages are composed of the KUNV MP502–

66, the "Sarawak" strain, from Malaysia; the "Koutango isolate" from Senegal; a lineage detected but not isolated from mosquitoes in Spain; and a potential lineage detected in *Uranotaenia* species mosquitoes from Austria.[66] Other than lineages 1 and 2 strains, only one lineage 5 strain and the Koutango isolate are known to cause human disease.

In the New World, the original lineage 1 WNV genotype, NY99, was isolated in New York and was the predominant, if not only, genotype found in the United States from 1999 to 2005. It has now been displaced by a newer genotype, NA/WN02, first found in Texas in 2002. It has 13 nucleotide changes from NY99 and is able to disseminate more readily in the local mosquito populations.[67] Since 2003, NA/WN02 has spread throughout the Upper Texas Gulf Coast and into other parts of the United States, including California, Illinois, New York, and North Dakota. Another genotype, SW/WN03, was first reported in Arizona, Colorado, and northern Mexico in 2003. It is now found in the Upper Texas Gulf Coast region as well. Since then, some other Texas isolates, groups 4–6, have major differences, suggesting that WNV is continuing to mutate.[67]

Outbreaks in humans are confined to WNV lineage 1 strains, while lineage 2 strains are maintained in enzootic cycles, predominately in Africa. The Kunjin virus in Australia has now been classified as a lineage 1 WNV and is the subject of a separate chapter. Lineage 2 strains are often considered to be of low virulence; however, lethal linage 2 epidemics in Central Europe and elsewhere have led to hundreds of severe cases of human disease or death.[68]

A recent report examined pathogenicity in 10 old or new lineages 1 and 2 strains, a putative lineage 6 strain from Malaysia, and the proposed Koutango lineage 7 strain. Virulence in mice was based on the lethal dose$_{50}$ (LD$_{50}$), median survival times, infectious dose$_{50}$ (ID$_{50}$), replication in neural and extraneural tissues, and antibody production. All lineage 1a strains, recent lineage 2 strains, and the Koutango strain are classified as highly virulent. The B956 strain (lineage 1) is classified as moderately virulent and the Kunjin strain (lineage 1) and Malaysian isolates (lineage 6) as having low virulence.[66] Almost all mice infected with the highly virulent strains contain the virus in the liver and spleen plus high viral loads in the heart and kidney. By contrast, no infection of peripheral organs is seen in almost any of the moderate or low-virulent strains. It should be noted that these results were obtained in mice and may not completely reflect virulence in humans. While virulence may not correlate with lineage or geographic origin, human WNV cases from India,

Africa, and the Middle East tend to be more frequent in children and younger adults. In these regions, infection typically presents as a mild, childhood disease. Most of the adults in the region are seropositive for WNV and immune to infection.[65,66]

The neuroinvasive potential of WNV is strain-dependent. Most of the strains of WNV are neurovirulent when experimentally inoculated intracranially into mice, but only some strains are neuroinvasive when inoculated peripherally, in a manner that is similar to natural transmission.[69] The occurrence of the large outbreaks of severe neuroinvasive disease in the 1990s is believed to be due to the emergence of new, more virulent, lineage 1 viral variants. One of the differences between an avirulent lineage 2 (WNV-MAD78) and a highly virulent lineage 1 viral strain (WNV-NY99) is that the replication of the WNV-MAD78 strain in astrocytes is delayed. The lower number of WNV-MAD78 in these glial cells when compared to those of WNV-NY is due to an IFN-independent reduction in cell-to-cell spread. Interestingly, both strains replicate in HBMECs and neurons in a similar fashion and both enter the CNS by traversing endothelial cells.[70]

Several other differences are found between highly virulent and less virulent strains of WNV.[7] The highly virulent lineage 1 NY99 strain has an N-linked glycosylation site on the viral E protein that correlates with its ability to enter the CNS. This site is not present in less virulent lineages 1 and 2 strains. The attenuated lineage 2 WNV-MAD78 strain from Madagascar, which is less neuroinvasive, lacks this glycosylation site, leading to altered stability at mildly acidic pH.[71] The attenuated phenotypes of the Kunjin and MAD78 strains from Australia and Madagascar, respectively, might be also be explained by these strains' higher degree of sensitivity to type I IFNs. These strains are defective in their ability to suppress the Janus kinase/signal transducer and the activator of transcription (JAK/STAT) pathway of IFN signaling. They are unable to block the nuclear translocation of STAT, leading to the accumulation of STAT proteins in the cytoplasm. MAD78 only produces low numbers of virus in cell culture and fails to cause disease in mice in vivo. MAD78 is, however, able to grow in human cell lines that lack the IFN receptor.[72] Examination of mild and severe neuroinvasive disease caused by lineage 2 WNV revealed a similar potential glycosylation motif at this E protein site. Other flaviviruses, JEV, DENV, and TBEV, also possess this potential glycosylation site.[73] N-linked glycosylation, nevertheless, is not the sole determinate of virulence, since at least some virulent WNV strains are not glycosylated at this site. In fact, some low-virulence WNV strains have

additional deletions in their 3′-noncoding regions.[74] Some low-virulence WNV lineages 1 and 2 strains also differ in the expression or accessibility of E protein epitopes.[69]

The N-linked glycosylation site in the E protein effects WNV lineage 1 transmission by mosquito vectors. Lack of glycosylation decreases viral load in mosquito midguts and salivary glands. Most WNVs found in salivary secretions do contain this glycosylation site, indicating a reversion to the wild-type glycosylation pattern. The transmission of WNVs lacking this glycosylation site is decreased in *Cx. pipiens* and, to a lesser extent, in *Culex tarsalis*, mosquitoes.[75] It should be noted that *Cx. tarsalis* has a higher midgut pH than *Cx. pipiens*. Interestingly, lack of this glycosylation site in some lineage 1 WVN has also been reported to not affect peak virus titer in mosquito cells, even though some minor differences were found in infected vertebrate cells.[38] This is in contrast to the reports mentioned previously, perhaps due to the usage of different virus strains or mosquito cell types. In support of this contention, glycosylated WNV infects a greater amount of *Cx. pipiens* mosquitoes than does a mutated WNV strain that lacks glycosylation, but the opposite is true for the infection of *Cx. tarsalis*.[75] Of note, one study found that dual infection with the endosymbiont bacterium *Wolbachia* increases mosquito's resistance to WNV, while another study reported that *Wolbachia* increases WNV titer in *Cx. tarsalis*.[76,77]

Many variations in NS genes are present among WNV lineage 1 strains that vary in virulence. These include a variation in NS1,[78] NS2A,[79] NS3,[13] NS4B, and NS5.[73-75,80] While many of these genetic alterations were discovered by mutation analysis, some of them have been detected in human or bird populations. Alteration of the NS4B gene may change virulence in mice by controlling temperature sensitivity and the attenuation of neuroinvasive and neurovirulent phenotypes.[81] Such differences exist between NY99 and KEN-3829 strains that are much more or less virulent in American crows, respectively. This suggests that the ability to replicate efficiently at the higher body temperatures found in the crows is an important virulence factor.[82] At least one alteration of the NS1 gene of WNV lineage 2 also alters virulence.[68]

WNV Infection of Animals

Among vertebrates, WNV primarily infects over 200 species of birds in addition to humans and horses, but may also infect other mammals, such as cats, dogs, squirrels, chipmunks, bats, skunks, bears, and domestic rabbits. Birds are the most important WNV reservoir host species. The virus infects their brains, livers, lungs, spleens, adrenal glands, hearts, and kidneys.[20] Horses usually recover after the infection with WNV; however, 10% of the infected horses develop encephalitis or myelitis with a mortality rate of 28%–45%.[83] A vaccine is currently available for use in horses, but not in humans. Experimentally infected cats develop a mild fever and are slightly lethargic for approximately 1 week, while dogs remained asymptomatic. The low levels of virus in the blood of these animals suggest that they may not be able to transmit WNV to mosquitoes and, therefore, are unlikely to serve as reservoirs for human infection.

WNV Transmission

Several species of mosquitoes serve as vectors for WNV. Most of these belong to *Culex* genus, particularly ornithophilic mosquitoes that feed primarily on birds, such as *Cx. pipiens*, *Cx. restuans*, and *Culex univittatus*.[84,85] The former species generally feed between dusk and dawn and are able to survive the winter in temperate areas, such as New York City. Fifty-eight species of WNV-infected mosquitoes have been identified in North America; the most important of these are *Cx. pipiens* and *Cx. restuans* in the northeastern United States and Canada, *Cx. quinquefasciatus* in the southern United States, *Cx. tarsalis* in the western United States and Canada, and *Cx. nigripalpus* in Florida in the extreme southeastern United States (see Fig. 4.1).

Of these, *Cx. restuans* is more prevalent in urban and metropolitan areas since their larvae are best adapted to tolerate pollution, although *Cx. pipiens* are also associated with urban and suburban outbreaks and, subsequently, with human infections.[2,38] Other species of infected mosquitoes include *Ochlerotatus triseriatus*, *Ochlerotatus japonicus*, *Ochlerotatus vexans*, *Aedes albopic-

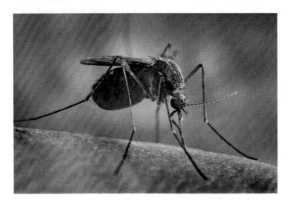

FIG. 4.1 *Culex quinquefasciatus* mosquito. (Credit: CDC—content provider/James Gathany; James Gathany—photo credit.)

tus, and *Cx. salinarius*, which are more likely to bite humans than birds.

The primary route of human infection is via the bite of a mosquito that had previously fed on an infected bird, which served as the amplifying host. Different species of mosquitoes often transmit WNV between birds as opposed to transmitting the virus from birds to humans.[10] *Cx. restuans* and *Cx. pipiens* tend to feed on birds, suggesting that these mosquitoes may be important species for enzootic infection. *Cx. salinarius* is apt to feed on both vertebrates and birds and thus may serve as an important bridge for zoonotic transmission from birds to humans.[38]

In vitro infection of cells with a newly discovered Australian flavivirus, Bamaga virus, significantly reduces the growth of Kunjin and Murray Valley encephalitis viruses, all of which are present in Australia.[86] Bamaga virus also reduces WNV transmission by dual-infected *Culex* mosquitoes. Further studies are needed to determine whether Bamaga virus may be used as a biological weapon that can significantly decrease the transmission of WNV to humans as well as whether it causes any pathology in immunocompetent or immunocompromised people.

The duration and magnitude of viremia vary greatly among the many species of birds in North America that are able to host WNV.[10] High levels of the virus may circulate in the blood of some species for greater than 100 days. Passeriformes birds, such as crows, jays, grackles, finches, and sparrows, have the highest levels of viremia, which may exceed 10^{10} plaque-forming units/mL in blood and result in transmission to more than 80% of the mosquitoes feeding upon them.[10] The widespread and aggressively invasive house sparrow is also an important viral reservoir since it is a highly competent host for WNV and also produces multiple broods yearly.[2] Besides the transmission to birds by mosquito bite, bird-to-bird infection may also occur due to viral release from the cloaca and the nasopharynx.[10] One of the first outbreaks of severe WNV-associated disease in birds and humans occurred in 1989 in Israel. During this outbreak, high mortality rates were reported among birds as was later true during the first outbreak of WNV-associated disease in New York.

Once within the mosquito, WNV travels to the salivary glands from where it is injected into the next vertebrate host during a blood meal. The virus then enters into the mosquitoes' blood and crosses the BBB and causes noncytolytic inflammation of the central or peripheral nervous system that persists in the insect for the remainder of its life. An infected *Culex* species mosquito injects approximately 10,000 viable WNVs into its vertebrate host during one feeding.[10] Humans and other mammals are dead-end hosts since they fail to develop high enough bloodstream levels of WNV to play a significant role in the transmission of the virus to mosquitoes. Several species of WNV-infected mosquitoes are able to survive in a dormant form during the winter, enabling viral persistence in the mosquito vector and reemergence each spring. WNV is also transmitted vertically between mosquitoes by the transovarian route.[10,28] In parts of Asia and Africa, WNV has also been reported in ticks; however, it is not known whether or not these insects play a role in transmission to humans.

Human-to-human transmission has been shown to occur very rarely and by several routes, including blood transfusion and organ transplantation. In 2003, two instances of WNV transmission from contaminated blood were reported among the 4.5 million transfusions in the United States. Both donor blood and organs are now screened for the presence of the virus using nucleic acid testing. Slightly over 1000 viremic, but asymptomatic, blood donors were found. A very small number of infections have also occurred due to breastfeeding or transplacental transmission to the fetus. Transmission may have occurred on at least one occasion from a contaminated dialysis machine.[28]

Infection with WNV has not been found to result from casual contact with infected humans or other mammals. Zoonotic transmission has not been reported following contact with infected horses or live or dead birds or from eating infected birds or other animals. Hunters dressing wild game birds, such as turkeys and ducks, may perhaps decrease their risk of infection by using gloves to prevent contacting the birds' blood.

THE IMMUNE RESPONSE
WNV and Interferon

The immune system produces several types of IFN in response to viral infections. WNV replication is decreased in neurons pretreated with IFN-α or IFN-β in vitro, but these cytokines are less effective if they are added to the cultures after the cells have been infected. IFN-β increases neuronal cell survival in primary sympathetic motor neurons that are infected ex vivo and does so in a manner that is independent of viral replication.[48] IFN-β regulates the BBB in vitro by helping to control endothelial permeability and tight junction formation using the guanosine triphosphatases Rac1 and RhoA.[87]

Toll-like receptor 3 (TLR3) is a pathogen recognition molecule found on macrophages. It is also constitutively expressed in neurons, astrocytes, and mi-

croglia (macrophages of the CNS). Viral engagement with TLR3 and the melanoma differentiation-associated gene 5 (MDA5) leads to the activation of transcription factors, including IRF-3 and IRF-7, and the subsequent expression of IFN-stimulated genes (ISGs).[88] In in vitro cultures of primary cortical neurons, TLR3 deficiency increases viral load.[89] Moreover, the lack of TLR3 expression also increases viral load in the brain, including in the neurons, as well as the mortality rate of mice inoculated with WNV intraperitoneally or subcutaneously. The absence of TLR3 only results in small changes in the peripheral viral load, however. Nevertheless, TLR3 may also produce detrimental effects, such as increasing endothelial cell permeability, permitting viral entry into the brain parenchyma[90] (described later). The role of TLR3 in WNV pathogenicity in mice may thus depend on complex interactions involving the host genetic predisposition and general health, viral serotype and strain, and route of infection. In humans, the latter is not a factor, since virtually all infections are via mosquito bite.

IRF-3 and IRF-7 are the master transcriptional factors that regulate IFN-α and IFN-β gene expressions and resistance to WNV-induced disease. For WNV and other positive-strand RNA viruses, TLR3, MDA5, and retinoic acid-inducible gene-I (RIG-1) recognize the intermediate viral dsRNA that is present in the endosomes and cytoplasm during replication. These host molecules then trigger the nuclear localization and activation of IRF-3. IRF-3 decreases in vitro infection of two critical cell types, macrophages and cortical neurons.[91] Interestingly, both type I IFNs fail to inhibit WNV infection in primary macrophages and cortical neurons, but not in the peripheral neurons of the superior cervical ganglia.

In infected macrophages, IRF-3 is associated with the cellular defense proteins MDA5, ISG54, and ISG56, which together lower the extent of WNV infection. IRF-3 also promotes the production of IFN-β by WNV-infected cells early during the course of infection.[92] Macrophages without the functional IRF-3 receptor-γ lack basal expression of MDA5, ISG54, and ISG56. Additionally, the production of IFN-α and IFN-β is decreased in these cells, resulting in increased WNV infection. By contrast, while neurons lacking functional IRF-3 also do not induce the expression of the cellular defense genes mentioned earlier and have reduced levels of type I IFNs, they only have a small increase in viral titers. In vivo, IRF-3-negative mice develop fatal WNV infection that is associated with higher viral loads in both peripheral and central nervous system tissues in spite of possessing fairly normal IFN responses in the periphery.[91] IRF-3 thus appears to protect different cell types by either IFN-dependent or IFN-independent mechanisms. IRF-7, IRF-5, and IRF-8 may also induce IFN gene expression in WNV-infected macrophages.

IFN-β activates the production of several ISGs, including IRF-7. IRF-7 is part of a positive feedback loop that stimulates the production of additional IFN-β as well as IFN-α production.[92] While inactivation of either the IRF-7 or the IRF-3 transcription factors separately increases susceptibility to severe West Nile disease in mice, loss of both factors results in rapid mortality.[93] This was accompanied by the complete loss of IFN-α responses in fibroblasts, macrophages, DCs, and cortical neurons. IFN-β responses are also reduced in fibroblasts and cortical neurons, but not in macrophages or DCs. These results highlight the importance of IFN-α and IFN-β in controlling WNV infection as well as differences between the relative activities of the different IFN-producing cell types. The induction of IFN-α in the cerebral cortex and primary cortical neurons is IRF-7-dependent, suggesting that IRF-7 plays an important role in the CNS, while IFN-β gene expression by cortical neurons is not regulated by IRF-7.[92]

2-5-Oligoadenylate synthase (OAS) is another ISG used by both mammalian and bird cells. This enzyme produces 2-5-linked oligoadenylates that, in turn, activate RNase L. This RNase enzyme cleaves both cellular and viral RNAs. In experimentally infected mice, lack of functional RNase L, OAS1b, or protein kinase R (PKR) increases their susceptibility to WNV infection and elevates viral burden in the draining lymph nodes, serum, and spleen, as well as in neural tissues.[94]

IFN-γ (type II IFN) is produced by several types of leukocytes early during WNV infection, including CD4+ Th1 helper cells, CD8+ T killer cells, γδ T cells, and NK cells. IFN-γ then binds to its receptor, which is preferentially expressed on epithelial cells. IFN-γ has no direct effect on WNV replication in mouse keratinocytes and DC in vitro, despite enhancing expression of some ISGs.[95] In mice lacking its receptor, IFN-γ has no effect on WNV load in the draining lymph nodes, spleen, or blood; however, mice treated with IFN-λ have improved survival rates. IFN-λ reduces the early dissemination of WNV to the brain and spinal cord by decreasing the permeability of the BBB without altering levels of proinflammatory cytokines. It does so by increasing transendothelial electrical resistance and increasing colocalization of two tight junction proteins, zonula occludens-1 and claudin-5, in vitro and in vivo tightening the BBB. This process is independent of the STAT1 pathway and protein synthesis.[95] Loss of IFN-γ signaling in WNV-infected mice increases the mortality rate from 30% in wild-type mice to 60%–90% in mice

lacking IFN-γ. The increase in fatal disease is linked to a 3- to 5-log greater amount of viral replication in the CNS as well as higher viremia and viral replication in the spleen and lymph nodes in the absence of IFN-γ.[96] This cytokine also plays an important role in reducing WNV production and dissemination by primary DCs and γδ T cells. IFN-γ also increases the expression of MHC-I on the surface of infected cells, making such cells better targets for destruction by CD8+ T killer cells. Additionally, IFN-γ activates phagocytic myeloid cells.[96]

Several WNV proteins interfere with IFN-α, IFN-β, and IFN-γ signaling.[7] Viral NS2A inhibits IFN-β transcription. NS2A, NS4B, NS3, NS4A, NS4B, and NS5 inhibit the phosphorylation and nuclear translocation of STAT1 and STAT2, JAK1, and tyrosine kinase 2.[97–100] Interestingly, only one of the earlier discussed differences in IFN signaling is found between the relatively low-virulent Australian KUNV and the highly virulent NY99 WNV strains.[97,100]

WNV and Other Aspects of the Innate Immune Response

The innate immune response in WNV-infected fibroblasts may be divided into two stages that rely upon several members of the RLR family of cytoplasmic microbial pattern recognition receptors, including RIG-1 and MDA5, as well as type I IFNs and associated molecules. The RIG-1-like receptors contain several functional domains, including a C-terminal repressor domain. RIG-1 is active early during the course of infection and primarily recognizes 5′-triphosphate RNA encoding a short dsRNA motif or single-stranded polyuridine or polycytosine. MDA5 is active at a much later time and targets longer dsRNA motifs.[101] Binding of RNA to their repressor domains leads to conformational changes in RIG-1 and MDA5. These changes trigger their translocation from the cytosol to mitochondria where they interact with a mitochondrion-localized adaptor molecule, mitochondrial antiviral signaling protein (MAVS; also known as IFN-β promoter stimulator 1), and initiate a signaling cascade that activates the IFN responses.[101]

The early immune response to WNV involves the production of both IFN-α and IFN-β and the expression and nuclear translocation of IRF-3, ISG54, and ISG56. IFN-β binds to its receptor and amplifies the antiviral response via the activation of the JAK/STAT signal transduction pathway, which, in turn, induces the expression of other ISGs. This pathway is also used during the mosquitoes' immune response to WNV.[38]

The second phase of IFN-dependent antiviral gene expression occurs very late in infection and involves at least 25 more antiviral mediators, including IRF-7, which is responsible for extensive remodeling of the cell's transcriptional activity. In fibroblasts lacking RIG-I, both the JAK/STAT and the TLR signal transduction pathways are delayed, indicating a major role for RIG-I in initiating innate immunity against WNV. MDA5 increases and maintains the RIG-I-mediated response.[102] While lack of either RIG-I or MDA5 alone reduces innate immune signaling and virus load in primary cells in vitro and increases mortality in mice in vivo, the lack of both completely eliminates innate gene expression in infected cells, causing severe pathogenesis. RIG-I and MDA5, therefore, recognize distinct WNV components in the cytoplasm.[103] MDA5 also appears to regulate optimal CD8$^+$ T killer cell activation and viral clearance from the CNS. Additionally, MDA5 decreases the replication of WNV in human hepatoma cells and fibroblasts.[101]

The microbial pathogen recognition molecules mentioned earlier depend on adaptor proteins to relay their signals. MAVS serves as an adaptor protein for RIG-I and MDA5. It activates the transcription factors IRF-3, IRF-5, IRF-7, and nuclear factor κ of B cells (NF-κB) to induce the expression of genes that limit WNV division.[103] The levels of MAVS are higher in WNV-infected cerebellar granule cell neurons than in cortical neurons.[104] Loss of MAVS leads to severe disease due to uncontrolled WNV infection of bone marrow-derived DCs, macrophages, and cortical neurons. Mice lacking MAVS or MDA5 develop excessive inflammation that involves elevation of the levels of type I IFNs, proinflammatory cytokines and chemokines, and the numbers of inflammatory DCs and pathogenic virus-specific CD8$^+$ T killer cells.[101] These pathogenic responses are associated with decreased T regulatory cell (Treg) activity.[105]

Treg levels almost double during the first 3 months of infection, but their frequency is lower in symptomatic than asymptomatic WNV-positive people for at least 1 year after infection.[106] Underscoring the importance of Treg in controlling WNV infection, while all WNV-infected blood donors in one study ($n=32$) experienced a peripheral expansion of Treg numbers, the symptomatic infection was associated with lower Treg levels. Treg-deficient mice are also more likely to develop severe disease.[106] Mice with higher Treg levels also have lower numbers of WNV-specific CD8$^+$ T killer cells, suggesting that an overactive T killer cell response may be detrimental. Nevertheless, one of the Treg cytokines, IL-10, also contributes to WNV-induced pathology. CD4$^+$ T cells produce copious amounts of IL-10 during WNV infection in vitro and in vivo. The absence of this cytokine increases the survival of infected mice.[107] Thus, the role of Treg cytokines during WNV

infection is complex and may, at times, increase rather than decrease viral disease severity.

The following ISGs control specific stages in the viral life cycle in vitro[104,105]: members of the IFN-induced proteins with tetratricopeptide repeat (IFIT) family, C6 orf150, Hpse, Nampt, Phf15, IFITM2, IFITM3, and ISG20.[94,106,108–110] PKR (an inhibitor of protein synthesis), viperin (an ER-associated protein that inhibits lipid raft formation and viral budding), and RNase L (a RNA endonuclease) reduce pathology in vivo and in vitro in a tissue- and cell-type-specific manner.[94,110] Viperin also inhibits the growth of ZIKV, but not JEV, in cultured cortical neurons, demonstrating different reactions to infection among flaviviruses.[111] Other cellular-specific restriction factors help in the control of WNV infection and pathogenesis, including pattern recognition receptors (RIG-I, MDA5, TLR3, and TLR7), RSAD2, transcription factors (IRF-7, IRF-9, STAT-1, and STAT-2), and proinflammatory cytokines (type I IFNs, IFN-γ, TNF-α, CXCL10, and IL-10).[20,49,102,107,112,113] Signaling via the RLR together with its MAVS adaptor protein also regulates inflammation and B and T cell responses during WNV infection.

Sterile alpha and HEAT/Armadillo motif (SARM; also known as Myd88-5) is a highly conserved Toll/IL-1 receptor-containing adaptor molecule that downregulates signaling by TLR3 and TLR4, as well as NF-κB or IFN-β gene expression. It is preferentially located in the CNS and protects neurons. In WNV-infected mice lacking SARM, viral replication in the brain stem and neuronal death is increased along with decreased levels of TNF-α and microglia activation, but no change is seen in lymphocyte functioning.[114] The extent of infection in various brain regions together with the magnitude of TNF-α production affects whether TNF-α is neurotoxic or neuroprotective. Additionally, since the actions of SARM differ among species, it will be necessary to test its activity in human brain stem cells.

Viperin deficiency in primary cultures of macrophages and DCs only results in a small increase in WNV replication. No differences are found between wild-type and viperin-deficient embryonic fibroblasts or cortical neurons. The case is much different for WNV-infected adult mice in which mortality rates and viral replication in the CNS and peripheral tissues is significantly higher in viperin-deficient mice than is present in normal mice. In the CNS of infected animals, viperin expression is induced by infected, as well as surrounding, cells. Rather than possessing direct antiviral activity, viperin may act indirectly by modulating host cell survival. Taken together, viperin restricts infection by WNV in a tissue- and cell-type-specific manner in adult mice.[110]

IL-1β maturation in the NLRP3 inflammasome helps to control CNS disease during WNV infection.[115] WNV-infected mice have increased levels of IL-1β in their plasma during the course of infection. Mice without a functional IL-1 receptor or components of the inflammasome signaling complex have increased susceptibility to WNV pathogenesis, associated with higher levels of WNV in the CNS, but not the periphery. Within the CNS, infection alters the kinetics and magnitude of inflammation and reduces the quality of effector CD8[+] T killer cell actions. WNV infection triggers the production of IL-1β from cortical neurons. This proinflammatory cytokine suppresses viral replication in neurons and recruits protective CD45[+] monocytes and T lymphocytes.[115] JEV also triggers IL-1β secretion by astrocytes and microglia in a manner that relies on the NLRP3 inflammasome.[116] IL-1β also is involved in increased expression of the IFIT family members IFIT1, IFIT2, and IFIT3.

The importance of IFIT2 in decreasing CNS infection is seen in mice infected by a virulent lineage 1 North American WNV strain. IFIT2 inhibits the activity of the subunits of elongation initiating factor 3 in mammalian cells, which accordingly decreases protein production, viral proliferation, and WNV disease.[104] The NS5 methyltransferase of the highly virulent emergent North American WNV-TX allows the virus to evade IFIT2 activity by modifying the WNV's 5′-untranslated region.[117] Mice without functional *IFIT2* genes have a higher than normal WNV load, with preferential replication in the CNS. In vitro cultured myeloid cells, embryonic fibroblasts, and cerebellar granule cell neurons, but not in cortical or spinal cord neurons or cells in the spleen or kidney in vivo, are more readily infected in the absence of a functional *IFIT2* gene.[104] Cellular IFIT2 production is mediated by STAT1-induced serine phosphorylation of the inhibitor of κB kinase ε (IKKε).[112] WNV infection and pathogenesis are also enhanced in vitro in cells from mice lacking either IKKε or IFIT2.

The viral NS5 methyltransferase activity also interacts with host cell protein kinase G1 (PKG1). Multiple sites in NS5 are phosphorylated during infection and at least one conserved N-terminal site is serine-phosphorylated by PKG1 in cultured cells.[118] Expressing PKG1 production in these cultures enhances viral production. Furthermore, the NS5 methyltransferase domain stably interacts with the pathogenic PKGIβ WNV, but not with the mildly pathogenic Langat virus.[118]

The complement cascade is also important in host defense against WNV. WNV activates all three complement cascades in vivo. Mice without functional C3 or complement receptors 1 and 2 have higher CNS viral loads and are more likely to develop the fatal disease at lower levels of WNV. Loss of the alternative pathway decreases antiviral CD8[+] T killer cell responses, but not B cell activity. Lack of the classical or lectin pathways leads to dysfunctional T and antigen-specific B cell activities, including delayed production of virus-specific IgM and IgG.[118,119]

Human monocyte-derived (mDCs) and plasmacytoid dendritic cells (pDCs) produce different cytokines and respond differently to WNV propagated in mammalian or mosquito cell cultures.[120] WNV grown in a primate kidney cell line are 10-fold more powerful inducers of IFN-α in pDC than in mDCs. IFN-α secretion by pDCs does not require WNV replication and appears to depend on the recognition of the virus by TLRs within acidified endosomes, while IFN-α production by mDCs relies upon viral replication, nuclear translocation of IRF-3, and viral antigen expression. This production appears to be activated by the RIG-I/MDA5 or TLR3 pathway. Importantly, WNV grown in mosquito cells do not induce pDCs to secrete IFN-α, but the mDCs respond similarly to WNV produced in either mammalian or mosquito cell lines. High levels of the IFN-dependent chemokine interferon gamma-induced protein 10 are found in pDCs exposed to WNV grown in mammalian, but not mosquito, cell cultures, while mDCs production of a neutrophil-attractant chemokine, IL-8, is greater in response to WNV propagated in mosquito, rather than mammalian, cells.[120] The presence of IL-8 may help to explain CNS neutrophilia during human WNV infection.[121]

WNV, the Adaptive Immune Response, and Cytokines

Adaptive immunity is vital for protection against WNV. Mice lacking functional T and B lymphocytes, severe combined immunodeficiency disease or *RAG1* mice, all die following infection. Experimentally infected mice lacking only antibody-producing B lymphocytes also die and have a 500-fold higher serum viral load compared to infected wild-type mice 4 days after infection.[122,123] Neutralizing antibodies, particularly IgM, target the exposed viral E protein and, to a lesser extent, the prM protein, in both mammals and birds. These antibodies are important for the clearance of WNV from the bloodstream.[38] WNV-infected mice lacking secreted, but not cell surface, IgM, together with normal production of all other antibody classes, have higher levels of viremia and viral load in the CNS plus a blunted anti-WNV IgG response compared to mice producing both secreted and cell-surface IgM. Diamond et al.[123] suggested that the levels of WNV-specific IgM at day 4 postinfection may be used to predict disease outcome. IgM-mediated complement activation may not, however, be involved in viral clearance since in vitro studies show that nonneutralizing IgM increases WNV infection of macrophages, perhaps by enhancing viral entry via complement receptor 3.[124] IgG produced in the later stages of infection reduces viral dissemination and help to clear WNV from infected cells.[123] Antibodies directed against NS1 are also protective. CD4$^+$ T helper cells increase the production of antiviral antibodies by B cells, and depletion of T helper cells increases the mortality rate. Perforin produced by CD8$^+$ T killer cells also destroys lineage 1 WNV and reduces viral load in the brain.[125]

TLR7 helps in the development of protective IL-23-mediated immune responses against WNV infection in mice.[126] IL-23 has at least two roles in WNV infection: it recruits CD11b$^+$ monocytes and macrophages into the CNS and it serves as a major regulator of the stability and maintenance of the CD4$^+$ T helper 17 (Th17) cells that produce IL-17A late during the course of infection.[126] Both IL-17A and another Th17 cytokine, IL-22, affect the course of WNV neuroinvasive disease. Both of these cytokines are typically associated with inflammation and autoimmune responses. Nevertheless, IL-17A can be either beneficial or harmful in host defense against viral, as well as bacterial and fungal, infections. In the case of WNV infection, IL-17A appears to be protective during late infection by stimulating anti-WNV CD8$^+$ T killer cell cytotoxicity in infected mice.[127] WNV infection induces IL-17A expression in mice. Treatment of WNV-infected mice with exogenous IL-17A, even at day 6 postinfection, decreases the viral load and increases their survival. Mice lacking functional IL-17A are more susceptible to WNV infection; have lower levels of CD8$^+$ T killer cell activity; and express less perforin-1, granzyme A, granzyme B, and Fas ligand, all of which are involved in the destruction of infected cells by CD8$^+$ T killer cells.[20,127] An unusual subset of T cells, the γδ cells, produces IL-17A early after infection. The role of IL-17A at that time may differ from its role later in infection. Fewer mice survive primary WNV infection in animals lacking functional γδ T cells and the survivors are more susceptible to subsequent viral challenge.[128] γδ T cells appear to act by increasing the numbers and activity of CD8$^+$ memory T killer cells.

The exact role of CD8$^+$ T killer cells in decreasing WNV neuropathology is uncertain, since neurons do not express the MHC class I molecules that are necessary for recognition by this type of T cell. As discussed previously, infected neurons secrete the chemokine CXCL10 early after infection. CXCL10 recruits effector T killer cells into the CNS, where they may function by killing infected nonneuronal cells, such as astrocytes.[63] Levels of another chemokine, RANTES, are increased in both the CNS and peripheral tissues of WNV-infected mice lacking IL-17A. RANTES protects against WNV infection by promoting leukocyte trafficking to the infected tissues. It has been shown to maintain CD8$^+$ T killer cell responses during a variety of other viral infections as well.[127]

During WNV infections, IL-22 plays a causative role in the development of chronic inflammatory conditions, including multiple sclerosis and lethal encephalitis.[129] Experimentally infected mice that are genetically deficient in this cytokine produce less proinflammatory cytokines and apoptotic cells and have lower viral loads in the CNS, but not in the peripheral tissues, than do infected mice that produce this cytokine. The levels of CXCR2, a chemokine receptor that mediates neutrophil migration, and its ligands, CXCL1 and CSCL5, are also reduced in the absence of IL-22, leading to decreased neutrophil migration into the brain.[128] It should be noted that CXCR2 ligands are expressed on endothelial cells and thus may be important for the proper functioning of the BBB. IL-22 thus appears to increase inflammation in the CNS of infected mice, at least in part, by inducing early neutrophil entry into the CNS, resulting in the development of encephalitis.

Macrophages are also involved in neutrophil localization, perhaps by affecting the expression of the *CXCL1* and *CXCL2* genes in the same manner as IL-22. The levels of these chemokines are quickly elevated to high titers in WNV-infected macrophages. Neutrophils that are rapidly recruited to the site of infection also become infected as well and serve as efficient hosts for WNV replication. Accordingly, viremia is reduced in mice whose neutrophils are depleted prior to infection. Survival of these animals is increased as is also the case for mice deficient in CXCR2.[107] Despite some of their negative roles, neutrophils still are important in host defense against WNV in mice. Their absence eventually leads to higher levels of viremia and earlier death, suggesting that neutrophils may also play a protective role in some situations. Taken together, these findings suggest that neutrophils have a biphasic response to WNV infection, hosting viral replication and dissemination during early infection, while later contributing to viral clearance.[41]

WNV influences neuronal apoptosis, a form of cellular self-destruction. CD8$^+$ T killer cells are vital in controlling WNV in the CNS. They do so by secreting perforin, which produces pores in the plasma membrane of infected cells, and granzymes, which enter the cells through the pores and, once there, induce cellular apoptosis. Additionally, another cytolytic pathway induces the binding of Fas on the surface of WNV-infected cells to Fas ligands on CD8[+] T killer cells or NK cells, resulting in the infected cell's death. While neurons do not typically express cell-surface Fas, WNV infection induces its expression on cortical neurons both in vitro and in vivo. The perforin and Fas/Fas ligand pathways are important in the defense of neurons since mice with genetic deficiencies in perforin or Fas ligand have a higher viral burden in the CNS, with a longer persistence time period, than do normal mice infected with the highly virulent lineage 1 NY99 isolate.[130,131] Viral load is also increased in the spleens of these mice, leading to their inability to clear infectious virus. Mice genetically deficient in the Fas/Fas ligand cytolytic pathway or in the exocytosis of perforin and granzymes A and B from CD8[+] T killer cells or NK cells also have as a greater rate of encephalitis when infected by the lineage 2 Sarafend WNV strain.[90] Interestingly, the opposite is true for mice infected with Murray Valley encephalitis virus, another pathogenic flavivirus.

The production of tumor necrosis factor-related apoptosis-inducing ligand (TRAIL) is induced by DENV and inhibits DENV infection in vitro.[132] Mice defective in TRAIL also have a much greater mortality rate following subcutaneous infection with WNV. In a few surviving animals, viral load is higher in the brain and spinal cord, but not in peripheral tissues, indicating that the TRAIL produced by CD8[+] T killer cells also helps in the clearance of WNV infection in the CNS.[133]

In order to target WNV in the CNS, CD8[+] T killer cells first must pass through the BBB. This barrier normally prevents the entry of most immune cells, including T lymphocytes, into the CNS parenchyma. This is necessary in order to prevent the development of pathogenic inflammation in the CNS, such as that occurring in multiple sclerosis. However, the BBB also inhibits the elimination of viruses that are already present in that location. The chemokine CXCL12 and its receptor, CXCR4, are present on T cells at the BBB. Normally, the interaction between these molecules serves to localize T cells to the perivascular spaces of the CNS microvasculature and restricts their entry into the brain parenchyma, thus limiting their access to the virus. Inhibition of CXCR4 binding to its ligand enhances T cell entry into the CNS and increases viral clearance by 1000-fold. This improves the survival of experimentally infected mice by 10%–50%, while reducing the development of a local pathologic immune response by activated astrocytes or microglia. CXCR4 antagonists are thus potentially beneficial in treating WNV infection.[134]

The binding of the proinflammatory TNF-α cytokine to its receptor, TNF-R1, enhances the migration of antiviral CD8[+] T killer cells and macrophages into the brain during the acute phase of WNV infection. Meningeal and perivascular inflammation occurs in infected mice lacking the TNF-R1 and increases the viral titer to 70-fold higher than that found in infected wild-type animals. The influx of inflammatory cells into the brain of these mice is associated with decreased viral titers in the CNS in the absence of any direct anti-WNS activity by TNF-α.[135] By contrast, only small changes in viral load occur in the peripheral tissues of these mice. Once CD8[+] T killer cells enter the CNS, CD4[+] T helper cells help in the maintenance of antiviral CD8[+] T killer cell numbers in that location.[134]

The number of a minor T cell population, the γ/δ T cells, increases during WNV infection. These cells help in viral elimination by producing high levels of IFN-γ.[136] γδ T cells additionally help in the maturation of professional antigen-presenting cells, including B cells, splenic DCs, and macrophages.[137] These macrophages then stimulate the activity of WNV-specific CD4[+] T helper cells. The addition of WNV-specific antibodies increases the efficiency of antigen presentation by macrophages, perhaps via opsonization. The loss of macrophages decreases the time required to produce encephalitis. Mortality rates increase from 50% in mice with normal macrophage numbers to 100% in mice deficient in macrophages following infection with a virulent WNV strain. Furthermore, the mortality rate of infected with an attenuated WNV strain rises from almost 0% to 70%–79% mortality in mice with or without normal macrophage numbers, respectively.[138]

WNV Evasion of the Immune Response

Some of the host immune responses discussed earlier may be subverted by viruses. When inoculated with WNV via the peritoneal route, the endosomal virus sensors TLR3 and TLR7 and the inflammatory cytokine TNF-α may alter the permeability of the endothelial cells of the CNS, allowing the virus to cross the BBB and, accordingly, to increase the risk of developing lethal encephalitis. By contrast, deficiency in TLR3 decreases the viral load and inflammatory responses in the CNS.[90] Within 2 h of viral infection, WNV also induces the expression of cell adhesion molecules in cultured endothelial cells, including intracellular adhesion molecule-1 (ICAM-1), VCAM-1, and E-selectin. These molecules help in the entry of leukocytes into the brain parenchyma. P-selectin levels, however, are unchanged by WNV infection.[60,139]

In vitro, WNV increases the expression of MHC-I and MHC-II molecules at 24 and 72h, respectively. The proinflammatory Th1 cytokines IFN-γ and TNF-α, as well as IL-1, act synergistically with WNV and cause greater increases in MHC-I expression than those caused by WNV or the cytokines alone.[139] By contrast, the Th2 cytokine IL-4 completely abrogates WNV-induced increases in E-selectin.

PREVENTION
Vaccines
No effective vaccines against WNV are currently licensed for use in humans. Four vaccines are approved for use in horses, but may not be safe for use in humans.[38] Two of these vaccines use inactivated whole viruses, one uses a nonreplicating live recombinant canarypox vector, and the fourth is an inactivated flavivirus chimeric vaccine. These vaccines are quite effective and disease incidence in horses fell soon after the first vaccine became available.

Several human vaccine candidates are in clinical trials, including some chimeric viruses in which WNV genes are inserted into live, attenuated YFV or a DENV-4 backbone. Vaccination of humans against other flaviviruses (DENV, JEV, and yellow fever virus) does not lead to the production of protective, cross-reactive neutralizing antibody responses to WNV.[28]

Education
Education of the general population is considered to be a vital part of disease prevention. During the 1999 WNV outbreak in New York City, a massive educational program was developed to inform city residents of protective strategies. This program included a door-to-door campaign, a telephone hotline, and a website. Media also communicated valuable information to those people in the affected area.[5] Nevertheless, despite an excellent educational program, WNV spread across the country to California in less than 10 years. The disease outcomes would likely have been even worse in developing regions of the world where large sections of the public are illiterate and may not have access to television or radios. In tropical regions, it is very difficult and expensive to escape contact with mosquito vectors.

Even though contact with live or dead infected birds has not been shown to transmit WNV, dead birds should not be handled with bare hands, especially in regions with ongoing WNV activity. If dead birds are found in a region, especially crows or blue jays that

have died for no apparent reason, they should be reported to the local health department. If the proper authorities wish for individuals to dispose of a dead bird, disposable gloves or an inverted plastic bag should be used to handle the bird, which should be sealed in double plastic bags before being placed in the garbage container.

Since, on very rare occasions, WNV transmission has been shown to occur by contact with contaminated blood or organs, the American Red Cross asks potential blood donors whether they know that they have ever been infected by WNV and whether they have been at high risk for infection. The blood supply in the United States and Canada has additionally been screened for the presence of WNV since 2003 using a nucleic acid amplification test in order to discard contaminated blood units. This is very important since the majority of human infections are asymptomatic.

TREATMENT
No specific and effective treatment measures are currently licensed for those people who develop neuro-invasive West Nile diseases. Individuals with serious illness should be hospitalized since they may require supportive care, such as intravenous fluids or mechanical respiration. Care should be taken to prevent the development of secondary infections. Since the vast majority of infections are asymptomatic or produce only mild manifestations, such as West Nile fever, they resolve spontaneously. Medications may, however, reduce the symptoms of West Nile fever, such as head and body aches.

The general antiviral compound ribavirin has in vitro activity against WNV but has not been shown to be effective in experimentally infected animals or in people. Indeed, it perhaps even increases pathology in humans with neuroinvasive disease. IFN, but not ribavirin, reduces disease in Syrian golden hamsters. Case reports in humans indicate potential clinical improvement in people treated with IFN-α2b. High-titer virus-specific gamma globulin (containing anti-WNV antibodies) appears to be beneficial in animal models. Another general antiviral compound, 6-azauridine, also inhibits flavivirus replication.[140] A broad-spectrum antiviral derivative of N-methylisatin-beta-thiosemicarbazone completely inhibits WNV replication in kidney cell lines in vitro at concentrations much lower than those required for ribavirin activity.[141] This compound has similar efficacy against JEV.

Several NS3 protease inhibitors decrease WNV numbers. For some of these compounds, interaction with the viral NS3 anchor region is important in inhibitor binding and efficacy.[142] Aprotinin and D-arginine-based 9–12-mer peptides potently inhibit the WNV NS3 protease with K_i values of 26 and 1 nM, respectively. Additionally, D-arginine-based peptides decrease WNV infection in primary neuron cultures.[143]

Lycorine is an alkaloid compound present in plants, such as daffodils and bush lilies. It functions as a potent inhibitor of WNV, DENV, and yellow fever virus RNA synthesis in kidney cell cultures, decreasing viral load by 2–4 orders of magnitude.[144] It does so without affecting WNV protease, nucleotide phosphatase, methyltransferase, or RNA-dependent RNA polymerase activities.

Some iminocyclitol derivatives that inhibit the glycan-processing enzyme endoplasmicreticular glucosidase also inhibit morphogenesis of WNV and other viruses that bud from the ER[145]. Flaviviruses are unusual in that they require calnexin-mediated folding in the ER. Calnexin recognizes the nascent viral glycoproteins only after modification by cellular glucosidases, thus making these ER enzymes attractive therapeutic targets.

The adenosine analog imino-C-nucleoside strongly inhibits the replication of WNV in kidney cell lines in vitro. It also decreases the replication of some tick-borne species of flaviviruses, including TBE, louping ill, and Kyasanur Forest disease viruses, although the effective dose varies greatly among viruses.[146] Another adenosine analog, the polymerase inhibitor NITD008, also blocks WNV replication in kidney cells in vitro. It also decreases viremia and prevents neuroinvasion in a mouse model system in vivo, completely protecting the animals from mortality and morbidity. However, it is ineffective when administered during the chronic phase of infection. The combination of NITD008 with the antiinflammatory histone deacetylase inhibitor vorinostat, however, decreases WNV disease by reducing both inflammation and neuronal cell death, even when administered during the chronic phase.[147] Other drug combinations that target different viral pathways simultaneously may also be effective in preventing disease if given during the chronic phase of WNV infection. For example, the combination of inhibitors of MMP-9 and COX-2 act together with neutralizing antibodies against cytokines decreases BBB disruption and neuronal injury.[54,55]

Isoforms of the cellular enzyme protein kinase C (PKC) regulate many cellular processes, including apoptosis, differentiation, and proliferation. The broad-base PKC inhibitor chelerythrine targets conventional, novel, and atypical PKCs and significantly decreases WNV replication in kidney cells in vitro.[148] Two other

PKC inhibitors, staurosporine and enzastaurin, that are specific for conventional and novel PKC isoforms, however, are not effective against WNV. This suggests that atypical PKCs also take part in WNV replication and provide a new host cell target for anti-WNV drugs.

Atypical PKC isoforms are unusual in that they do not require Ca^{2+} or diacylglycerol for activation. The WNV NS5 polymerase contains three potential PKC phosphorylation sites that modulate viral replication. The WNV NS5 RNA polymerase is phosphorylated at least in one of these sites during infection.[118,149,150] The activation of atypical PKC activity requires lipids that are enriched in the plasma membrane of normal nervous system cells, including ceramides and sphingomyelin. WNV infection stimulates the synthesis and accumulation of several lipids in cellular membranes, including fatty acids, cholesterol, glycerophospholipids, lyso-phospholipids, and sphingolipids. Sphingomyelin, but not phosphatidylcholine, is enriched in the lipid envelope of WNV and takes part in virus assembly.[149,151,152] Cells from humans with Niemann–Pick disease type A and mice have increased levels of sphingomyelin due to a genetic deficiency in acid sphingomyelinase activity. This enzyme normally converts sphingomyelin into ceramide. Ceramide helps to promote membrane bending and budding processes. Cells without functional sphingomyelinase are more susceptible to WNV multiplication.[153] Taken together, these findings provide further evidence of the importance of specific lipids and atypical PKC isoforms in WNV pathogenicity.

Other molecules also alter lipid types and levels in WNV-infected cells. The ISG viperin regulates cholesterol and isoprenoid biosynthesis, lipid raft formation, and the composition and localization of lipid droplets. Ectopic expression of viperin changes the ER membrane morphology. This decreases viral protein secretion and perhaps alters the assembly and secretion of WNV virions.[110]

Several drugs that are FDA-approved for use against JEV replication also decrease WNV replication. Three of these drugs, manidipine, cilnidipine, and benidipine hydrochloride, are voltage-gated Ca^{2+} channel antagonists. Another drug, pimecrolimus, inhibits the secretion of inflammatory cytokines.[154] Nelfinavir mesylate, an HIV-1 protease blocker, also reduces WNV replication.

Imidazo[4,5-d]pyridazine nucleosides are purine nucleoside analogs, in which a pyridazine is substituted for a pyrimidine fused to an imidazole ring. In a kinetic study of one such purified compound, the unwinding activities of purified WNV NS3 NTPases and helicases were enhanced in a time-dependent manner.[155] In cell culture, however, these analogs also uncouple the viral ATPase and helicase activities, thus decreasing the unwinding of the genome and reducing viral replication. Indeed, the analog that most efficiently enhances enzyme-mediated ATP hydrolysis also inhibits WNV helicase activity. Which of these two antagonistic actions occurs is dependent upon the nucleoside analogs' concentration in a given area.[155]

The viral capping enzyme is another potential target of antiflavivirus drugs. Several members of the 2-thioxothiazolidin-4-ones family of drugs potently inhibit the capping enzyme's GTP binding and guanylyltransferase functions. It reduces the replication of several flaviviruses, including the Kunjin type of WNV, in kidney cell cultures by almost 3 orders of magnitude and is a promising candidate for further in vivo testing in animal model systems.[156]

SUMMARY OVERVIEW

Diseases: West Nile fever, West Nile encephalitis, West Nile meningitis, West Nile meningoencephalitis, West Nile poliomyelitis, inflammation of peripheral nerves

Causative agent: WNV

Type of agent: flavivirus, Japanese encephalitis virus serocomplex

Vector: mosquitoes, primarily *Culex* species

Common reservoir: wild birds

Mode of transmission: bite of infected mosquitoes; blood transfusion or organ donation; rarely, transplacentally or by breastfeeding

Geographical distribution: Africa; the Middle East; Europe; South Asia; Australia; and North, Central, and South America

Year of emergence: 1937 in Uganda; 1999 in the Western Hemisphere (in the United States)

REFERENCES

1. Smithburn C, Hughes TP, Burke AW, Paul JH. A neurotropic virus isolated from the blood of a native of Uganda. *Am J Trop Med Hyg.* 1940;20:471–492.
2. Weaver SC, Reisen WK. Present and future arboviral threats. *Antiviral Res.* 2010;85(2):328.
3. Blitvich BJ. Transmission dynamics and changing epidemiology of West Nile virus. *Anim Health Res Rev.* 2008;9:71–86.
4. Centers for Disease Control and Prevention. *West Nile Virus Statistics and Maps. West Nile Virus Homepage;* 2017. Accessed, https://www.cwc.gov/westnile/statsmaps/index.html.
5. Beltz LA. *Emerging Infectious Diseases: A Guide to Diseases, Causative Agents, and Surveillance.* Jossey-Bass; 2011.
6. Lanciotti RS, Roehrig JT, Deubel V, et al. Origin of the West Nile virus responsible for an outbreak of encephalitis in the Northeastern United States. *Science.* 1991;286(5448):2333–2337.
7. Donadieu E, Bahuon C, Lowenski S, Zientara S, Coulpier M, Lecollinet S. Differential virulence and pathogenesis of West Nile viruses. *Viruses.* 2013;5:2856–2880.
8. Zeller HG, Schuffenecker I. West Nile virus: an overview of its spread in Europe and the Mediterranean Basin in contrast to its spread in the Americas. *Eur J Clin Microbiol Infect Dis.* 2004;23:147–156.
9. Bin H, Grossman Z, Pokamunski S, et al. West Nile fever in Israel 1999–2000: from geese to humans. *Ann NY Acad Sci.* 2001;951:127–142.
10. Davis LE, DeBiasi R, Goade DE, et al. West Nile virus neuroinvasive disease. *Ann Neurol.* 2006;60:286–300.
11. Rappole JH, Derrickson SR, Hubalek Z. Migratory birds and spread of West Nile virus in the Western Hemisphere. *Emerg Infect Dis.* 2000;6:319–327.
12. Komar N, Panella NA, Burns JE, Dusza SW, Mascarenhas TM, Talbot TO. Serologic evidence for West Nile virus infection in birds in the New York City vicinity during an outbreak in 1999. *Emerg Infect Dis.* 2001;7:621–625.
13. Brault AC, Huang CY, Langevin SA, et al. A single positively selected West Nile viral mutation confers increased virogenesis in American crows. *Nat Genet.* 2007;39:1162–1166.
14. Hamer GL, Kitron UD, Goldberg TL, et al. Host selection by *Culex pipiens* mosquitoes and West Nile virus amplification. *Am J Trop Med Hyg.* 2009;80:268–278.
15. Kilpatrick AM, Meola MA, Moudy RM, Kramer LD. Temperature, viral genetics, and the transmission of West Nile virus by *Culex pipiens* mosquitoes. *PLoS Pathol.* 2008;4, e1000092.
16. Moudy RM, Meola MA, Morin LL, Ebel GD, Kramer LD. A newly emergent genotype of West Nile virus is transmitted earlier and more efficiently by *Culex* mosquitoes. *Am J Trop Med Hyg.* 2007;77:365–370.
17. Centers for Disease Control and Prevention. *West Nile Virus Homepage;* 2020. Accessed June 22, 2020, https://www.cdc.gov/westnile/statsmaps/finalmapsdata/ioindex.html.
18. Estrada-Franco JG, Navarro-Lopez R, Beasley DWC, et al. West Nile virus in Mexico: evidence of widespread circulation since July 2002. *Emerg Infect Dis.* 2003;9:1604–1607.
19. Dupuis II AP, Marra PP, Kramer LD. Serologic evidence of West Nile virus transmission, Jamaica, West Indies. *Emerg Infect Dis.* 2003;9:860–863.
20. Samuel MA, Diamond MS. Pathogenesis of WNV infection: a balance between virulence, innate and adaptive immunity, and viral evasion. *J Virol.* 2006;80:9349–9360.
21. Samuel MA, Morrey JD, Diamond MS. Caspase 3-dependent cell death of neurons contributes to the pathogenesis of WNV encephalitis. *J Virol.* 2007;81:2614–2623.
22. Hayes EB, Gubler DJ. West Nile virus: epidemiology and clinical features of an emerging epidemic in the United States. *Annu Rev Med.* 2006;57:181–194.

23. Leis AA, Fratkin J, Stokic DS, Harrington T, Webb RM, Slavinski SA. West Nile poliomyelitis. *Lancet Infect Dis.* 2003;3:9–10.

24. Klee AL, Maidin B, Edwin B. Long-term prognosis for clinical West Nile virus infection. *Emerg Infect Dis.* 2004;10:1405–1411.

25. Sejvar JJ. The long-term outcomes of human West Nile virus infection. *Clin Infect Dis.* 2007;44:1617–1624.

26. Kleinschmidt-DeMasters BK, Marder BA, Levi ME, et al. Naturally acquired West Nile virus encephalomyelitis in transplant recipients: clinical, laboratory, diagnostic, and neuropathological features. *Arch Neurol.* 2004;61:1210–1220.

27. Sejvar JJ, Haddad MB, Tierney BC, et al. Neurologic manifestations and outcome of West Nile virus infection. *JAMA.* 2003;290:511–515.

28. DeBiasi RL, Tyler KL. West Nile virus meningoencephalitis. *Nat Clin Pract Neurol.* 2006;2(5):264–275.

29. Hershkovitz O, Rosental B, Rosenberg LA, et al. NKp44 receptor mediates interaction of the envelope glycoproteins from the West-Nile and dengue viruses with natural killer cells. *J Immunol.* 2009;183(4):2610–2621.

30. Lopez-Denman AJ, Russo A, Wagstaff KM, White PA, Jans DA, Mackenzie JM. Nucleocytoplasmic shuttling of the West Nile virus RNA-dependent RNA polymerase NS5 is critical to infection. *Cell Microbiol.* 2018;20(8):e12848.

31. Shrestha B, Gottlieb D, Diamond M. Infection and injury of neurons by West Nile encephalitis virus. *J Virol.* 2003;77:13203–13213.

32. Green AM, Beatty PB, Hadjilaou A, Harris E. Innate immunity to dengue virus infection and subversion of antiviral responses. *J Mol Biol.* 2014;426(6):1148–1160.

33. Beloor J, Maes N, Ullah I, et al. Small interfering RNA-mediated control of virus replication in the CNS is therapeutic and enables natural immunity to West Nile virus. *Cell Host Microbe.* 2018;23:549–556.

34. Smith JL, Jeng S, McWeeney SK, Hirsch AJ. A microRNA screen identifies the Wnt signaling pathway as a regulator of the interferon response during flavivirus infection. *J Virol.* 2017;91(8). e02388-16.

35. Slonchak A, Shannon RP, Pali G, Khromykh AA. Human microRNA miR-532-5p exhibits antiviral activity against West Nile virus via suppression of host genes SESTD1 and TAB3 required for virus replication. *J Virol.* 2016;90(5):2388–2402.

36. Kanayama A, Seth RB, Sun L, et al. TAB2 and TAB3 activate the NF-κB pathway through binding to polyubiquitin chains. *Mol Cell.* 2004;15:535–548.

37. Smith JL, Grey FE, Uhrlaub JL, Nikolich-Zugich J, Hirsch AJ. Induction of the cellular microRNA, Hs-154, by West Nile virus contributes to virus-mediated apoptosis through repression of antiapoptotic factors. *J Virol.* 2012;86:5278–5287.

38. Ahlers LRH, Goodman AG. The immune responses of the animal hosts of West Nile virus: a comparison of insects, birds, and mammals. *Front Cell Infect Microbiol.* 2018;81:96.

39. Slonchak A, Hussain M, Torres S, Asgari S, Khromykh AA. Expression of mosquito microRNA Aae-Mir-2940-5p is downregulated in response to West Nile virus infection to restrict viral replication. *J Virol.* 2014;88:8457–8467.

40. Lim P-Y, Behr MJ, Chadwick CM, Shi P-Y, Bernard KA. Keratinocytes are cell targets of West Nile virus *in vivo. J Virol.* 2011;85(10):5197–5201.

41. Bai F, Kong K-F, Dai J, et al. A paradoxical role for neutrophils in the pathogenesis of West Nile virus. *J Infect Dis.* 2010;202(12):1804–1812.

42. Byrne SN, Halliday GM, Johnston LJ, King NJ. Interleukin-1 beta but not tumor necrosis factor is involved in West Nile virus-induced Langerhans cell migration from the skin in C57BL/6 mice. *J Invest Dermatol.* 2001;117:702–709.

43. Chu JJ, Ng ML. Interaction of West Nile virus with alpha V beta 3 integrin mediates viral entry into cells. *J Biol Chem.* 2004;279:54533–54541.

44. Scherbik SV, Brinton MA. Virus-induced Ca^{2+} influx extends survival of West Nile virus-infected cells. *J Virol.* 2010;84:8721–8731.

45. Beatman E, Oyer R, Shives KD, et al. West Nile virus growth is independent of autophagy activation. *Virology.* 2015;433:262–272.

46. Bryan MA, Giordano D, Draves KE, Green R, Gale Jr M, Clark EA. Splenic macrophages are required for protective innate immunity against West Nile virus. *PLoS One.* 2018;13(2), e0191690.

47. Brown AN, Kent KA, Bennett CJ, Bernard KA. Tissue tropism and neuroinvasion of West Nile virus do not differ for two mouse strains with different survival rates. *Virology.* 2007;368(2):422.

48. Samuel MA, Diamond MS. Alpha/beta interferon protects against lethal West Nile virus infection by restricting cellular tropism and enhancing neuronal survival. *J Virol.* 2005;79(21):13350–13361.

49. Suthar MS, Brassil MM, Blahnik G, et al. A systems biology approach reveals that tissue tropism to West Nile virus is regulated by antiviral genes and innate immune cellular processes. *PLoS Pathol.* 2013;9(2), e1003168.

50. Samuel MA, Wang H, Siddharthan V, Morrey JD, Diamond MS. Axonal transport mediates West Nile virus entry into the central nervous system and induces acute flaccid paralysis. *Proc Natl Acad Sci USA.* 2007;104(43):17140–17145.

51. Arjona A, Foellmer HG, Town T, et al. Abrogation of macrophage migration inhibitory factor decreases West Nile virus lethality by limiting viral neuroinvasion. *J Clin Invest.* 2007;117(10):3059–3066.

52. Sampey AV, Hall PH, Mitchell RA, Metz CN, Morand EF. Regulation of synoviocyte phospholipase a2 and cyclooxygenase 2 by macrophage migration inhibitory factor. *Arthritis Rheumatol.* 2001;44:1273–1280.

53. van Marle G, Antony J, Ostermann H, et al. West Nile virus-induced neuroinflammation: glial infection and capsid protein-mediated neurovirulence. *J Virol.* 2007;81:10933–10949.

54. Verma S, Kumar M, Nerurkar VR. Cyclooxygenase-2 inhibitor blocks the production of West Nile virus-induced neuroinflammatory markers in astrocytes. *J Gen Virol.* 2011;92:507–515.

55. Verma S, Kumar M, Gurjav U, Lum S, Nerurkar VR. Reversal of West Nile virus-induced blood-brain barrier disruption and tight junction proteins degradation by matrix metalloproteinases inhibitor. *Virology.* 2010;397(1):130–138.

56. Cheeran MC, Hu S, Sheng WS, Rashid A, Peterson PK, Lokensgard JR. Differential responses of human brain cells to West Nile virus infection. *J Neurovirol.* 2005;11:512–524.

57. Bazan NG. COX-2 as a multifunctional neuronal modulator. *Nat Med.* 2001;7:414–415.

58. Palus M, Vancov M, Sirmarova J, Elsterova J, Perner J, Ruzek D. Tick-borne encephalitis virus infects human brain microvascular endothelial cells without compromising blood-brain barrier integrity. *Virology.* 2017;507:110–122.

59. Roe K, Kumar M, Lum S, Orillo B, Nerurkar VR, Verma S. West Nile virus-induced disruption of the blood-brain barrier in mice is characterized by the degradation of the junctional complex proteins and increase in multiple matrix metalloproteinases. *J Gen Virol.* 2012;93:1193–1203.

60. Roe K, Orillo B, Verma S. West Nile virus-induced cell adhesion molecules on human brain microvascular endothelial cells regulate leukocyte adhesion and modulate permeability of the *in vitro* blood-brain barrier model. *PLoS One.* 2014;9(7), e102598.

61. Ambrose RL, Mackenzie JM. West Nile virus differentially modulates the unfolded protein response to facilitate replication and immune evasion. *J Virol.* 2011;85(6):2723–2732.

62. Medigeshi GR, Lancaster AM, Hirsch AJ, et al. West Nile virus infection activates the unfolded protein response, leading to CHOP induction and apoptosis. *J Virol.* 2007;81(20):10849–10860.

63. Klein RS, Lin E, Zhang B, et al. Neuronal CXCL10 directs CD8 T-cell recruitment and control of West Nile virus encephalitis. *J Virol.* 2005;79(17):11457–11466.

64. Glass WG, McDermott DH, Lim JK, et al. CCR5 deficiency increases risk of symptomatic West Nile virus infection. *J Exp Med.* 2006;203:35–40.

65. Beasley DWC, Li L, Suderman MT, Barret ADT. Mouse neuroinvasive phenotype of West Nile virus strains varies depending upon virus genotype. *Virology.* 2002;296:17–23.

66. Pérez-Ramírez E, Llorente F, del Amo J, et al. Pathogenicity evaluation of twelve West Nile virus strains belonging to four lineages from five continents in a mouse model: discrimination between three pathogenicity categories. *J Gen Virol.* 2017;98:662–670.

67. McMullen AR, May FJ, Guzman LLH, et al. Evolution of new genotype of West Nile virus in North America. *Emerg Infect Dis.* 2011;17(5):785–793.

68. Szentpáli-Gavallér K, Lim SM, Dencső L. *In vitro* and *in vivo* evaluation of mutations in the NS region of lineage 2 West Nile virus associated with neuroinvasiveness in a mammalian model. *Viruses.* 2016;8:49.

69. Beasley DW, Barrett AD. Identification of neutralizing epitopes within structural domain II of the West Nile virus envelope protein. *J Virol.* 2002;76:13097–13100.

70. Hussmann KL, Samuel MA, Kim KS, Diamond MS, Fredericksen BL. Differential replication of pathogenic and nonpathogenic strains of West Nile virus within astrocytes. *J Virol.* 2013;87(5):2814–2822.

71. Beasley DWC, Whiteman MC, Zhang S. Envelope protein glycosylation status influences mouse neuroinvasion phenotype of genetic lineage 1 West Nile virus strains. *J Virol.* 2005;79(13):8339–8347.

72. Keller BC, Fredericksen BL, Samuel MA, et al. Resistance to alpha/beta interferon is a determinant of West Nile virus replication fitness and virulence. *J Virol.* 2016;80(19):9424–9434.

73. Botha EM, Markotter W, Wolfaardt M, et al. Genetic determinants of virulence in pathogenic lineage 2 West Nile virus strains. *Emerg Infect Dis.* 2008;14(2):222–230.

74. Davis CT, Galbraith SE, Zhang S, et al. A combination of naturally occurring mutations in North American West Nile virus nonstructural protein genes and in the 3′ untranslated region alters virus phenotype. *J Virol.* 2007;81:6111–6116.

75. Moudy RM, Zhang B, Shi P-Y, Kramer LD. West Nile virus envelope protein glycosylation is required for efficient viral transmission by *Culex* vectors. *Virology.* 2009;387(1):222–228.

76. Glaser RL, Meola MA. The native *Wolbachia* endosymbionts of *Drosophila melanogaster* and *Culex quinquefasciatus* increase host resistance to West Nile virus infection. *PLoS One.* 2010;5:e11977.

77. Dodson BL, Hughes GL, Paul O, Matacchiero AC, Kramer LD, Rasgo JL. *Wolbachia* enhances West Nile virus (WNV) infection in the mosquito *Culex tarsalis.* *PLoS Negl Trop Dis.* 2014;8, e2965.

78. Liu WJ, Chen HB, Khromykh AA. Molecular and functional analyses of Kunjin virus infectious cDNA clones demonstrate the essential roles for NS2a in virus assembly and for a nonconservative residue in NS3 in RNA replication. *J Virol.* 2003;77:7804–7813.

79. Audsley M, Edmonds J, Liu W, et al. Virulence determinants between New York 99 and Kunjin strains of West Nile virus. *Virology.* 2011;414:63–73.

80. Puig-Basagoiti F, Tilgner M, Bennett CJ, et al. A mouse cell-adapted NS4B mutation attenuates West Nile virus RNA synthesis. *Virology.* 2007;361:229–241.

81. Wicker JA, Whiteman MC, Beasley DWC, et al. A single amino acid substitution in the central portion of the West Nile virus NS4b protein confers a highly attenuated phenotype in mice. *Virology.* 2006;349:245–253.

82. Kinney RM, Huang CY-H, Whiteman MC, et al. Avian virulence and thermostable replication of the North American strain of West Nile virus. *J Gen Virol.* 2006;87:3611–3622.

83. Schuler LA, Khaitsa ML, Dyer NW, Stoltenow CL. Evaluation of an outbreak of West Nile virus infection in horses: 569 cases (2002). *J Am Vet Med Assoc.* 2004;225:1084–1089.

84. McIntosh B. Mosquito-borne virus disease of man in southern Africa. *Suppl S Afr Med J.* 1986;1986:69–72.

85. Venter M. Assessing the zoonotic potential of arboviruses of African origin. *Currt Opin Virol.* 2018;28:74–84.

86. Colmant AMG, Hall-Mendelin S, Ritchie SA, et al. The recently identified flavivirus Bamaga virus is transmitted horizontally by *Culex* mosquitoes and interferes with West Nile virus replication in vitro and transmission in vivo. *PLoS Negl Trop Dis.* 2018;12(10), e0006886.

87. Daniels BP, Holman DW, Cruz-Orengo L, Jujjavarapu H, Durrant DM, Klein RS. Viral pathogen-associated molecular patterns regulate blood brain barrier integrity via competing innate cytokine signals. *mBio.* 2014;5, e01476-14.

88. Ramos HJ, Gale Jr M. RIG-I-like receptors and their signaling crosstalk in the regulation of antiviral immunity. *Curr Opin Virol.* 2011;1:167–176.

89. Daffis S, Samuel MA, Suthar MS, Gale Jr M, Diamond MS. Toll-like receptor 3 has a protective role against West Nile virus infection. *J Virol.* 2008;82(21):10349–10358.

90. Wang T, Town T, Alexopoulou L, Anderson JF, Fikrig E, Flavell RA. Toll-like receptor 3 mediates West Nile virus entry into the brain causing lethal encephalitis. *Nat Med.* 2004;10(12):1366–1373.

91. Daffis S, Samuel MA, Keller BC, Gale Jr M, Diamond MS. Cell-specific IRF-3 responses protect against West Nile virus infection by interferon-dependent and -independent mechanisms. *PLoS Pathog.* 2007;3(7):e106.

92. Daffis S, Samuel MA, Suthar MS, Keller BC, Gale Jr M, Diamond MS. Interferon regulatory factor IRF-7 induces the antiviral alpha interferon response and protects against lethal West Nile virus infection. *J Virol.* 2008;82(17):8465–8475.

93. Daffis S, Suthar MS, Szretter KJ, Gale Jr M, Diamond MS. Induction of IFN-β and the innate antiviral response in myeloid cells occurs through an IPS-1-dependent signal that does not require IRF-3 and IRF-7. *PLoS Pathog.* 2009;5(10), e1000607.

94. Samuel MA, Whitby K, Keller BC, et al. PKR and RNase L contribute to protection against lethal West Nile virus infection by controlling early viral spread in the periphery and replication in neurons. *J Virol.* 2006;80(14):7009–7019.

95. Lazear HM, Daniels BP, Pinto AK, et al. Interferon-λ restricts West Nile virus neuroinvasion by tightening the blood-brain barrier. *Sci Transl Med.* 2015;7(284):284ra59.

96. Shrestha B, Wang T, Samuel MA, et al. Gamma interferon plays a crucial early antiviral role in protection against West Nile virus infection. *J Virol.* 2006;80(11):5338–5348.

97. Liu WJ, Chen HB, Wang XJ, Huang H, Khromykh AA. Analysis of adaptive mutations in Kunjin virus replicon RNA reveals a novel role for the flavivirus nonstructural protein NS2a in inhibition of beta interferon promoter-driven transcription. *J Virol.* 2004;78:12225–12235.

98. Guo JT, Hayashi J, Seeger C. West Nile virus inhibits the signal transduction pathway of alpha interferon. *J Virol.* 2005;79:1343–1350.

99. Muñoz-Jordán JL, Laurent-Rolle M, Ashour J, et al. Inhibition of alpha/beta interferon signaling by the NS4b protein of flaviviruses. *J Virol.* 2005;79(13):8004–8013.

100. Liu WJ, Wang XJ, Mokhonov VV, Shi P-Y, Randall R, Khromykh AA. Inhibition of interferon signaling by the New York 99 strain and Kunjin subtype of West Nile virus involves blockage of STAT1 and STAT2 activation by nonstructural proteins. *J Virol.* 2005;79(3):1934–1942.

101. Lazear HM, Pinto A, Ramos HJ. Pattern recognition receptor MDA5 modulates CD8+ T cell-dependent clearance of West Nile virus from the central nervous system. *J Virol.* 2013;87(21):11401–11415.

102. Fredericksen BL, Keller BC, Fornek J, Katze MG, Gale Jr M. Establishment and maintenance of the innate antiviral response to West Nile virus involves both RIG-I and MDA5 signaling through IPS-1. *J Virol.* 2008;82(2):609–616.

103. Errett JS, Suthar MS, McMillan A, Diamond MA, Gale Jr M. The essential, nonredundant roles of RIG-I and MDA5 in detecting and controlling West Nile virus infection. *J Virol.* 2013;87(21):11416–11425.

104. Cho H, Proll SC, Szretter KJ, Katze MG, Gale Jr M, Diamond MS. Differential innate immune response programs in neuronal subtypes determine susceptibility to infection in the brain by positive-stranded RNA viruses. *Nat Med.* 2013;19:458–464.

105. Suthar MS, Ma DY, Thomas S, et al. IPS-1 is essential for the control of West Nile virus infection and immunity. *PLoS Pathog.* 2010;6(2), e1000757.

106. Lanteri MC, O'Brien KM, Purtha WE, et al. Tregs control the development of symptomatic West Nile virus infection in humans and mice. *J Clin Invest.* 2009;119(11):3266–3277.

107. Bai F, Town T, Qian F, et al. IL-10 signaling blockade controls murine West Nile virus infection. *PLoS Pathog.* 2009;5(10), e1000610.

108. Wacher C, Muller M, Hofer MJ, et al. Coordinated regulation and widespread cellular expression of interferon-stimulated genes (ISG) ISG-49, ISG-54, and ISG-56 in the central nervous system after infection with distinct viruses. *J Virol.* 2007;81:860–871.

109. Calistri P, Giovannini A, Hubalek Z, et al. Epidemiology of West Nile in Europe and in the Mediterranean Basin. *Open Virol J.* 2010;4:29–37.

110. Szretter KJ, Brien JD, Thackray LB, Virgin HW, Cresswell P, Diamond MS. The interferon-inducible gene *viperin* restricts West Nile virus pathogenesis. *J Virol.* 2011;85(22):11557–11566.

111. Lindqvist R, Kurhade C, Gilthorpe JD, Överby AK. Cell-type- and region-specific restriction of neurotropic flavivirus infection by viperin. *J Neuroinflammation.* 2018;15:80.

112. Perwitasari O, Cho H, Diamond MS, Gale Jr M. Inhibitor of κB kinase ε (IKKε), STAT1, and IFIT2 proteins define novel innate immune effector pathway against West Nile virus infection. *J Biol Chem.* 2011;286(52):44412–44423.

113. Jiang D, Weidner JM, Qing M, et al. Identification of five interferon-induced cellular proteins that inhibit West Nile virus and dengue virus infections. *J Virol.* 2010;84:8332–8341.

114. Szretter KJ, Samuel MA, Gilfillan S, Fuchs A, Colonna M, Diamond MS. The immune adaptor molecule SARM modulates tumor necrosis factor alpha production and microglia activation in the brainstem and restricts West Nile virus pathogenesis. *J Virol.* 2009;83(18):9329–9338.

115. Ramos HJ, Lanteri MC, Blahnik G, et al. IL-1β signaling promotes CNS-intrinsic immune control of West Nile virus infection. *PLoS Pathog.* 2012;8(11), e1003039.

116. Das S, Mishra MK, Ghosh J, Basu A. Japanese encephalitis virus infection induces IL-18 and IL-1beta in microglia and astrocytes: correlation with *in vitro* cytokine responsiveness of glial cells and subsequent neuronal death. *J Neuroimmunol.* 2008;195:60–72.

117. Daffis S, Szretter KJ, Schriewer J, et al. 2'-O methylation of the viral mRNA cap evades host restriction by IFIT family members. *Nature.* 2010;468:452–456.

118. Keating JA, Bhattacharya D, Lim P-Y, et al. West Nile virus methyltransferase domain interacts with protein kinase G. *Virol J.* 2013;10:242.

119. Mehlhop E, Whitby K, Oliphant T, Marri A, Engle M, Diamond MS. Complement activation is required for induction of a protective antibody response against West Nile virus infection. *J Virol.* 2005;79(12):7466–7477.

120. Silva MC, Guerrero-Plata A, Gilfoy FD, Garofalo PD, Mason PW. Differential activation of human monocyte-derived and plasmacytoid dendritic cells by West Nile virus generated in different host cells. *J Virol.* 2007;81(24):13640–13648.

121. Tyler KL, Pape J, Goody RJ, Corkill M, Kleinschmidt-DeMasters BK. CSF findings in 250 patients with serologically confirmed West Nile virus meningitis and encephalitis. *Neurology.* 2006;66:361–365.

122. Halevy M, Akov Y, Ben-Nathan D, Kobiler D, Lachmi B, Lustig S. Loss of active neuroinvasiveness in attenuated strains of West Nile virus: pathogenicity in immunocompetent and SCID mice. *Arch Virol.* 1994;137:355–370.

123. Diamond MS, Sitati E, Friend L, Shrestha B, Higgs S, Engle M. Induced IgM protects against lethal West Nile virus infection. *J Exp Med.* 2003;198:1–11.

124. Cardosa MJ, Gordon S, Hirsch S, Springer TA, Porterfield JS. Interaction of West Nile virus with primary murine macrophages: role of cell activation and receptors for antibody and complement. *J Virol.* 1986;57:952–959.

125. Shrestha B, Diamond MS. Role of CD8+ T cells in control of West Nile virus infection. *J Virol.* 2004;78:8312–8321.

126. Town T, Bai F, Wang T, et al. Toll-like receptor 7 mitigates lethal West Nile encephalitis via interleukin 23-dependent immune cell infiltration and homing. *Immunity.* 2009;30:242–253.

127. Acharya D, Wang P, Paul AM, et al. Interleukin-17A promotes CD8+ T cell cytotoxicity to facilitate West Nile virus clearance. *J Virol.* 2017;91(1), e01529-16.

128. Wang T, Gao Y, Scully E, et al. Gamma delta T cells facilitate adaptive immunity against West Nile virus infection in mice. *J Immunol.* 2006;177(3):1825–1832.

129. Wang P, Bai F, Zenewicz LA, et al. IL-22 signaling contributes to West Nile encephalitis pathogenesis. *PLoS One.* 2012;7:1–10.

130. Shrestha B, Samuel M, Diamond MS. CD8+ T cells require perforin to clear WNV from infected neurons. *J Virol.* 2006;80:119–129.

131. Shrestha B, Diamond MS. Ligand interactions contribute to CD8+ T cell-mediated control of West Nile virus infection in the central nervous system. *J Virol.* 2007;81:11749–11757.

132. Warke RV, Martin KJ, Giaya K, Shaw SK, Rothman AL, Bosch I. TRAIL is a novel antiviral protein against dengue virus. *J Virol.* 2008;82:555–564.

133. Shrestha B, Pinto AK, Green S, Bosch I, Diamond MS. CD8+ T cells use TRAIL to restrict West Nile virus pathogenesis by controlling infection in neurons. *J Virol.* 2012;86(17):8937–8948.

134. McCandless EE, Zhang B, Diamond MS, Klein RS. CXCR4 antagonism increases T cell trafficking in the central nervous system and improves survival from WNV encephalitis. *Proc Natl Acad Sci USA.* 2008;105:11270–11275.

135. Shrestha B, Zhang B, Purtha WE, Klein RS, Diamond MS. Tumor necrosis factor alpha protects against lethal West Nile virus infection by promoting trafficking of mononuclear leukocytes into the central nervous system. *J Virol.* 2008;82(18):8956–8964.

136. Wang T, Scully E, Yin Z, et al. IFN-gamma-producing gamma delta T cells help control murine West Nile virus infection. *J Immunol.* 2003;171(5):2524–2531.

137. Kulkarni AB, Müllbacher A, Blanden RV. Functional analysis of macrophages, B cells and splenic dendritic cells as antigen-presenting cells in West Nile virus-specific murine T lymphocyte proliferation. *Immunol Cell Biol.* 1991;69(2):71–80.

138. Ben-Nathan D, Huitinga I, Lustig S, van Rooijen N, Kobiler D. Macrophage depletion in mice. *Arch Virol.* 1996;141(3–4):459–469.

139. Shen J, T-To SS, Schrieber L, King NJ. Early E-selectin, VCAM-1, ICAM-1, and late major histocompatibility complex antigen induction on human endothelial cells by flavivirus and comodulation of adhesion molecule expression by immune cytokines. *J Virol.* 1997;71(12):9323–9332.

140. Crance JM, Scaramozzino N, Jouan A, Garin D. Interferon, ribavirin, 6-azauridine and glycyrrhizin: antiviral compounds active against pathogenic flaviviruses. *Antiviral Res.* 2003;58:73–79.

141. Sebastian L, Desai A, Shampur MN, Perumal Y, Sriram D, Vasanthapuram RN. Methylisatin-beta-thiosemicarbazone derivative (SCH 16) is an inhibitor of Japanese encephalitis virus infection *in vitro* and *in vivo*. *Virol J.* 2008;5:64.

142. Pathak N, Lai M-L, Chen W-Y, Hsieh BW, Yu G-Y, Yang J-M. Pharmacophore anchor models of flaviviral NS3

proteases lead to drug repurposing for DENV infection. *BMC Bioinformatics.* 2017;18(suppl. 16):548.

143. Shiryaev SA, Ratnikov BI, Chekanov AV, et al. Cleavage targets and the D-arginine-based inhibitors of the West Nile virus NS3 processing proteinase. *Biochem J.* 2006;393:503–511.

144. Zou G, Puig-Basagoiti F, Zhang B, et al. A single-amino acid substitution in West Nile virus 2K peptide between NS4a and NS4b confers resistance to lycorine, a flavivirus inhibitor. *Virology.* 2009;84(1):242–252.

145. Gu B, Mason P, Wang L, et al. Antiviral profiles of novel iminocyclitol compounds against bovine viral diarrhea virus, West Nile virus, dengue virus and hepatitis B virus. *Antivir Chem Chemother.* 2007;18:49–59.

146. Eyer L, Zouharová D, Sirmarová J. Antiviral activity of the adenosine analogue BCX4430 against West Nile virus and tick-borne flaviviruses. *Antiviral Res.* 2017;142:63–67.

147. Nelson J, Roe K, Orillo B, Shi P-Y, Verma S. Combined treatment of adenosine nucleoside inhibitor NITD008 and histone deacetylase inhibitor vorinostat represents an immunotherapy strategy to ameliorate West Nile virus infection. *Antiviral Res.* 2015;122:39–45.

148. Blázquez AB, Vázquez-Calvo A, Martín-Acebes MA, Saiz J-C. Pharmacological inhibition of protein kinase C reduces West Nile virus replication. *Viruses.* 2018;10:91.

149. Mackenzie JM, Khromykh AA, Parton RG. Cholesterol manipulation by West Nile virus perturbs the cellular immune response. *Cell Host Microbe.* 2007;2:229–239.

150. Reed KE, Gorbalenya AE, Rice CM. The NS5A/NS5 proteins of viruses from three genera of the family Flaviviridae are phosphorylated by associated serine/threonine kinases. *J Virol.* 1998;72(7):6199–6206.

151. Martín-Acebes MA, Merino-Ramos T, Blázquez A-B, et al. The composition of West Nile virus lipid envelope unveils a role of sphingolipid metabolism in flavivirus biogenesis. *J Virol.* 2014;88(20):12041–12054.

152. Aktepe TE, Pham H, Mackenzie JM. Differential utilisation of ceramide during replication of the flaviviruses West Nile and dengue virus. *Virology.* 2015;484:241–250.

153. Martín-Acebes MA, Gabandé-Rodríguez E, García-Cabrero AM, et al. Host sphingomyelin increases West Nile virus infection *in vivo. J Lipid Res.* 2017;57:422–432.

154. Wang S, Liu Y, Guo J, et al. Screening of FDA-approved drugs for inhibitors of Japanese encephalitis virus infection. *J Virol.* 2017;91(21), e01055-17.

155. Borowski P, Lang M, Haag A, et al. Characterization of imidazo[4,5-*d*]pyridazine nucleosides as modulators of unwinding reaction mediated by West Nile virus nucleoside triphosphatase/helicase: evidence for activity on the level of substrate and/or enzyme. *Antimicrob Agents Chemother.* 2002;46(5):1231–1239.

156. Stahla-Beek HJ, April DG, Saeedi BJ, Hannah AM, Keenan SM, Geiss BJ. Identification of a novel antiviral inhibitor of the flavivirus guanylyltransferase enzyme. *J Virol.* 2012;86(16):8730–8739.

CHAPTER 5

Kunjin Virus

INTRODUCTION

Australia hosts at least 75 species of arboviruses, several of which are associated with mild to life-threatening human disease.[1] Among these are encephalitic flaviviruses, such as the Kunjin strain of WNV (KUNV), Japanese encephalitis virus (JEV), and Murray Valley encephalitis virus (MVEV).[2] Australia is also home to Ross River and Barmah Forest alphaviruses, which cause severe, and sometimes chronic, polyarthritis.[3] The numbers of locally acquired dengue virus (DENV) infections have been increasing as well, resulting in fever, intense bone pain, and hemorrhagic manifestations.[1] Alfuy virus, a close relative of MVEV, has been isolated from mosquitoes in northern Australia and may also cause mild disease in humans.[4,5] Kokobera and Stratford viruses are other flaviviruses that infect humans in Australia[2] and are discussed in Chapter 8. Other flaviviruses that have recently emerged in Oceania and Southeast Asia include Edge Hill and New Mapoon viruses in Australia, Sitiawan virus in Malaysia, and ThCAr virus in Thailand.[6] Though infection with these viruses may currently be asymptomatic in humans or cause mild disease, there is always the threat that they may undergo minor mutations that lead to large changes in virulence, as it was the case in the 2011 KUNV outbreak in horses (discussed in the following section). These viruses may also expand their geographical range by genetic adaptation to climatic conditions, human modification of the environment, or carriage by migratory birds. The latter is believed to have been the case for KUNV spread to new regions of Australia east of the Great Dividing Range.

Although WNV and KUNV were originally categorized as separate but related viruses, on the basis of genetic and antigenic studies, KUNV is now considered to be an Australian cluster of lineage 1 WNV.[7,8] Members of the KUNV cluster share 94% identity in the E protein gene and 90% in NS5/3'UTR nucleosides. Since WNV is the subject of a separate chapter in this book, this chapter will focus primarily on KUNV, and how it differs from other lineage 1 WNVs. KUNV is present primarily in the northwestern portions of Australia[9] and, rarely, in the temperate regions of central and southern Australia during periods of heavy rainfall.[10]

Instances of KUNV-associated disease typically appear as isolated, sporadic cases or as occasional small outbreaks in humans.[11] However, KUNV is present in a large proportion of people in some regions of the continent. In a study of indigenous populations in rural endemic regions in the top end of the Northern Territory in 1988 and 1989, KUNV seroprevalance increased with age and was 30% overall in adults ($n=834$).[12] Serological data suggest that KUNV may also be present from New Guinea to parts of the eastern Indonesian archipelago, Borneo, and Cambodia.[6] It is not known whether this seropositivity is associated with KUNV infection or merely reflects exposure to a similar antigen on another flavivirus. A virus that is genetically very closely related to KUNV has been isolated in Iran[13] and another close relative is found in Malaysia, although the latter has been placed into a separate WNV lineage.[14]

HISTORY

Infection with WNV primarily led to occasional cases of mild febrile illness at the time of its discovery in 1937 in the West Nile district of Uganda.[15] For several decades, infections were generally mild and infrequent. In 1957, however, an outbreak produced severe neurological symptoms in residents of Israeli nursing homes. Such serious disease manifestations remained uncommon until the mid-1990s, when large outbreaks of severe disease became increasingly common and widespread in Africa, Europe, and the Middle East.[16] Cases of mild to severe infection were first seen in the Americas in New York City in 1999 and spread across the continent to the Pacific Coast during the next several years. WNV is now endemic throughout much of North, South, and Central America.[17]

In 1960, KUNV was detected in *Culex annulirostris* mosquitoes from northern Queensland, Australia.[18] It became enzootic across the northern parts of the Northern Territory and the Kimberly region of Western Australia[19] and has since extended its range southward. While a 2019 report by the Australian National Arbovirus and Malaria Advisory Committee found no reports of KUNV infection in Australia in 2014–15,[20] the epidemiology of KUNV has recently changed. The virus has now spread into new areas of Australia in a manner that is not linked to floods.[21] Using high-throughput sequencing together with bioinformatics to study archival KUNV genomic material, Huang et al.[22] traced the evolution of KUNV over 50 years and found the presence of only a single long-term lineage in affected regions of the continent. At most six fixed substitutions are present in individual proteins. Most of the changes are in variable regions, indicative of stochastic drift. The substitutions in functional domains are conservative and lead to minor changes at most.

In 2011, a major change in KUNV virulence occurred as a strain with far greater pathogenicity sickened almost 1000 horses. A study of KUNV isolates from a variety of locations in Australia from 1960 to 2012 found additional isolates in 1984, 2000, and 2012 that were of similar virulence in mice as the highly pathogenic 2011 outbreak strain, despite the fact that no disease in animals was reported in 2000 or 2012.[21,22] Potentially virulent strains of KUNV have, therefore, been present in Australia for at least 30 years and neuroinvasive strains may be circulating in the absence of associated disease outbreaks,[21] thus having the potential to severely infect horses or cause zoonotic infection in humans without warning.

THE DISEASE

Disease Caused by Virulent WNV Lineage 1 Strains in the Americas

Approximately 80% of infected individuals remain asymptomatic. About 20% of those infected by WNV develop West Nile fever, a mild illness that is found in all age groups. It is characterized by fever and chills, severe frontal headache, ache in the eyes upon movement, pain in the chest and lumbar regions, tiredness, nausea and vomiting, lymphadenopathy, or a nonitching skin rash. This condition may last from several days to several weeks. No permanent ill effects are associated with West Nile fever.[23,24]

Serious disease symptoms occur in 0.75% of those infected with WNV. The fatality rate is 3%–15% and over half of those with neuroinvasive illness develop long-term nervous system disorders. Most of the damage occurs in the brainstem, hippocampus, cerebellum, and anterior horn of the spinal cord.[25] Following a 3–4-day incubation period, a small percentage of infected individuals develop at least one of the following symptoms: severe headache, high fever, stiff neck, stupor, disorientation, confusion, coma, tremors, convulsions, muscle weakness, parkinsonism, loss of vision, numbness, or paralysis.[26,27] These symptoms may persist for several weeks. The CSF contains WNV-specific IgM antibodies in the presence of pleocytosis, composed primarily of neutrophils, in approximately half of the patients.[28] Frequently, long-term sequelae, such

as weakness, myalgia, persistent movement disorders, and cognitive deficits, follow recovery from the acute West Nile neuroinvasive disease.[16,29–31] Neuroinvasive disease may be manifested in several forms: West Nile encephalitis, meningitis, poliomyelitis, or a Guillain–Barré-like syndrome.[24]

Disease Caused by KUNV in Australia

Symptoms of KUNV infection in humans, though rare, range from mild to severe, including mild fever, lymphadenopathy, headache, rash, photophobia, myalgia, arthralgia, and potentially encephalomyelitis.[11,32] In a 1992–2010 study of human KUNV cases in the Northern Territory ($n = 10$), all symptomatic patients developed fever, 30% presented with encephalitis, 30% presented with meningitis, 30% presented with arthralgia, myalgia, or rash, and 10% of the patients presented with fever alone.[33] Morbidity is limited, but some patients develop persisting mild neurological disorders, such as vertigo, left facial weakness, and unsteady gait.[34] In one study, MRIs of the brain found increased T2 signal in the right thalamus and, to a lesser degree, in the cerebellum and brainstem. The cerebral spinal fluid (CSF) contained protein and 10^6 leukocytes/mL, almost all of which were lymphocytes. All of the patients with encephalitis in this study survived.[33] By comparison, fatality rates of 5%–15% are seen in encephalitis from the WNV_{NY99} strain in the United States that is associated with severe neurological disease in about 50% of the encephalitis survivors.[33] During the severe outbreak of KUNV-induced disease in horses in 2011, the animals developed symptoms similar to those seen in WNV-related disease in the United States, including incoordination, ataxia, weakness, muscle paralysis, and tremors.[35]

THE VIRUS

WNV Lineages

KUNV is a mosquito-borne subtype of WNV in the JEV antigenic complex of flaviviruses. WNV has been divided into seven to nine lineages, several of which cause disease in humans. Lineages 1 and 2 are the best studied groups. Lineage 1 WNVs are present in North Africa, the Middle East, Europe, India, Asia, the Americas, and Australia. WNV lineage 2 viruses are present predominately in Africa. Lineage 3 is composed of the Rabensburg strain from *Culex pipiens* mosquitoes in the Czech Republic. Lineage 4 is composed of the LEIVKrnd88–190 strain isolated from *Dermacentor marginatus* ticks in Russia. Lineage 5 is formed of isolates from *Culex* and *Anopheles* mosquitoes and humans in

India. Lineages 6, 7, and 8 are composed of Sarawak virus in Malaysia, Koutango virus in Senegal, and a Spanish virus from *Cx. pipiens*, respectively.[16]

Lineage 1 viruses are typically more pathogenic than those from lineage 2,[36] but highly virulent neuroinvasive and less virulent strains exist in both the lineages.[37] KUNV belongs to clade 1B and is confined to Australia. A recent report examined relative pathogenicity in various lineage 1 viral strains in mice, based on LD_{50} (the dose at which 50% of the subjects die), median survival times, ID_{50} (the dose at which 50% of subjects are infected), ability to replicate in neural and extraneural tissues, and ability to stimulate antibody production. Using these criteria, KUNV isolates in general, as well as lineage 6 (Malaysian) viruses, are categorized as being of low virulence. KUNV normally has limited ability to invade the human central nervous system (CNS).[37,38] For the most part, KUNV infections are infrequent and less severe than infection with MVEV,[19] although KUNV is present in the brains and hearts, but not the livers, of artificially infected young mice.[38]

Factors Involved in Differing Virulence Among WNV Strains

Virulence is at least partially associated with the process of protein production. When virulent WNV strains are compared to the relatively attenuated KUNV strains, WNV prompts phosphorylation of elongation initiation factor 2α (eIF2α) and induces activating transcription factor 4 (ATF4) production. KUNV strains, however, are associated with only minimal eIF2α phosphorylation and ATF4 induction.[39] Both strains induce the unfolded protein response. KUNV preferentially activates ATF6, while this activation may be nonessential for other, more pathogenic, WNV functioning.[39,40]

A 2002 study suggested that the differences in WNV neuroinvasiveness are not linked to the isolate source (mosquito, mammal, or bird), in vitro passage history of virus strains, or age of the infected person.[36] The pathogenic 2011 strain contains E protein glycosylation and a substitution in the polymerase portion of the NS5 gene, which are not present in the original 1960 $KUNV_{MRM61C}$ strain.[22] A 1982 study found that 19 of 33 KUNV isolates derived from mosquitoes, horses, humans, and chickens possessed a glycosylated E protein.[10] With the exception of the 1960 prototype strain, the changes in the E protein and NS5 are present in all of the strains isolated since the 1980s. A highly conserved 8-base deletion in the 3'UTR is also found in all KUNV isolates collected after 2000, regardless of their virulence.[21]

Replacing KUNV prM residues 22 and 72 with the corresponding WNV_{NY99} residues increases the secretion of prM/E and virus particles and also increases virulence in weanling mice.[41] This is due to increased prM/E heterodimerization and nucleocapsid incorporation into virions. These effects occur in the presence or absence of KUNV E protein glycosylation.[42] Both prM residues 20 and 31 play an important role in prM/E particle secretion as well due to increased prM/E accumulation in the interfaces between the endoplasmic reticulum (ER) and Golgi apparatus.[43]

Bingham[44] compared pathogenicity of several WNV strains to each other in a mouse model system using the highly pathogenic American WNV_{NY99}, the prototypical $KUNV_{MRM16}$ strain, two KUNV isolates from the 2011 Australian horse outbreak, and a more typical KUNV horse isolate.[44] Following intraperitoneal inoculation of weanling mice, all WNV isolates induced meningoencephalitis in at least three of the tested inoculum doses, which ranged from 1 to 10,000 $TCID_{50}$ (the dose at which 50% of the tissue culture cells are infected). The $TCID_{50}$ for WNV_{NY99} was 3.16 and increased to 19.9 for both 2011 pathogenic horse isolates, 79.4 for the typical horse isolate, and the $TCID_{50}$ was too high to be determined for WNV_{MRM16} strain. In vivo, WNV_{NY99} caused disease in all infected mice, the horse isolates caused disease in 85%–94%, which $KUNV_{MRM16}$ only caused disease in 29% of the mice. As expected, WNV_{NY99} infection resulted in the most severe neurological symptoms followed by intermediate disease by the horse isolates, and, while seroconversion was seen after inoculation with $KUNV_{MRM16}$, infection was typically asymptomatic. A viral antigen was detected in the cell bodies of neurons in the CNS and ganglia, including those of the enteric nervous system. The antigen was also seen in the connective tissues, including those of the bone marrow, kidney tubules, and pancreas, as well as all three muscle types. While all WNV_{NY99}-infected mice had extra-neural antigens, they were only occasionally present in the KUNV horse or human strains.[44] WNV_{NY99}, but not KUNV, is also neuroinvasive in adult mice infected by the intraperitoneal route.[45] Mouse model systems may therefore be useful in determining pathogenicity of new WNV strains as well as in examining factors influencing pathogenicity.

Using a different approach, chimeric KUNVs expressing 5'UTR from the WNV_{NY99} are more virulent in mice than wild-type KUNV in spite of the lack of significant changes in replication kinetics and in vitro virus spread through mammalian and mosquito cell lines.[45] Four nucleoside differences exist in this region between the 5'UTR of KUNV and WNV_{NY99}. The presence of four nucleoside differences between these two viruses in the 3'UTR, however, does not affect viral virulence. Chimeric KUNV expressing WNV_{NY99} NS2A or NS5 proteins produces intermediate replication, cell-to-cell spread, and virulence in mice. Similarly, chimeric WNV_{NY99} containing the KUNV NS2A protein with a point mutation in residue 30 causes less cytopathic effect in cell culture and are less virulent in mice.[45] Differences in the NS4B, NS5, and the 3'UTR of WNV_{NY99} and another, attenuated, American isolate also alter virulence in mice.[46]

The highly virulent lineage 1 American WNV_{NY99} and the avirulent lineage 2 African WNV_{MAD78} strains are both able to effectively replicate in neurons and transverse brain microvascular endothelial cells. The WNV_{MAD78} strain replication is delayed and reduced in astrocytes, however.[47] This delay is due at least in part due to a type I IFN-independent reduction in viral spread between cells. This information may aid in determining factors involved in the reduced virulence characteristic of the early KUNV strains as well as the increased virulence of the horse strain in 2011.[47] It should be noted, however, that the WNV_{MAD78} strain is from lineage 2, while KUNV is from lineage 1. Also, WNV_{MAD78} induces less IFN than does WNV_{NY99}, while KUNV infection is associated with higher levels of IFN-β, as discussed later. Nevertheless, studies of WNV_{MAD78} as well as other less virulent strains of WNV may yield clues to the ways in which KUNV is rendered less virulent than many other lineage 1 strains.

Microarray technology also reveals differences in gene expression among WNV strains with high and low neuroinvasiveness.[37] KUNV belongs to the latter category. The highly neuroinvasive WNV strains upregulate those brain, liver, and spleen genes that are involved in IFN pathways, protein degradation, acute phase and inflammatory responses, and hematopoietic cell surface molecules involved in signal transduction and cell activation, T lymphocyte proliferation, and apoptosis. Expression of these genes is generally not increased or increased to a lesser degree in KUNV and other low virulence WNV types. For a complete list of genes specifically upregulated in highly neuroinvasive KUNV strains, see Venter et al.[37]

Factors Involved in Differing Virulence Between KUNV and MVEV

MVEV and KUNV are two of the mosquito-borne encephalitis viruses found in Australia. They share several key traits and differ in others. While most wild mice are resistant to intracranial infection with many flaviviruses, including KUNV and MVEV, only a few strains

of laboratory mice are resistant.[48] A laboratory mouse strain has been developed, however, that is highly resistant to flaviviruses due to the presence of an intact oligoadenylate synthetase 1b (OAS1b) gene. A defect in this gene leads to susceptibility to flavivirus pathogenicity, while natural flavivirus resistance was shown to be consistent with the presence of an intact OAS1b gene.[49–51]

KUNV is typically attenuated in adult mice[36] and is only usually virulent in weanling animals that lack a fully developed immune response.[52] Following intracranial inoculation of laboratory mouse strains, however, KUNV persists in mice that are normally resistant to flaviviruses, including those resistant to the generally more pathogenic MVEV.[16,53] The failure of these mice to completely clear KUNV infection appears to be the major factor contributing to the late-stage pathogenesis associated with death.[54] KUNV-induced pathogenicity in these mice may be due to the induction of suboptimal immune responses, which fail to eliminate KUNV, but not WVEV. KUNV-infected mice have a lesser degree of gross brain tissue immunopathology and lower levels of type I IFNs and TNF-α in the brain when compared to those seen in MVEV-infected mice. Continued low stimulation of the host immune system may lead to the late-term disease and death in these mice.[53]

KUNV Insect Vectors and Avian Reservoir Hosts

In addition to *Cx. annulirostris*, KUNV has been isolated from *Culex australicus*, *Culex squamosus*, *Culex quinquefasciatus*, *Aedes tremulus*, *Aedes alternans*, *Aedes nomanensis*, *Aedes vigilax*, and *Anopheles amictus* mosquitoes.[14,55] *Cx. annulirostris* is the primary KUNV vector.[2] *Culex gelidus*, an important vector for JEV, is also competent to transmit both KUNV and MVEV. These mosquitoes are potentially problematic in Australia since they are resistant to the insecticides DDT and malathion, breed in fresh and dirty waters, demonstrate high anthropophily, and are rapidly increasing in numbers.[56] It should be noted that since most *Aedes* species feed primarily on mammals and not typically on birds, *Aedes* mosquitoes are unlikely to maintain endemic KUNV transmission in Australia.[57,58]

By comparison, the vectors for other strains of WNV include the following: *Cx. univittatus* in Africa; *Cx. pipiens*, *Cx. modestus* and *Coquillettidia richiardii* in Europe; *Cx. quinquefasciatus*, *Cx. tritaeniorhynchus*, and *Cx. vishnui* in Asia; *Cx. pipiens* and *Cx. restuans* in the northeastern and north central United States; *Cx. tarsalis* in the Great Plains and western United States; and *Cx. nigripalpus* and *Cx. quinquefasciatus* in the southeastern

United States.[58] *Culex* species are considered to be the primary vectors throughout their geographical ranges.

Of these mosquito species, only *Cx. quinquefasciatus* is present in Australia. This species is highly ornithophilic in urban areas of Australia, although it does feed on humans and other mammals as well. Unlike some other WNV strains, however, KUNV is rarely reported in urban areas.[58] In the Americas, *Cx. quinquefasciatus* effectively transmits WNV_{NY99} and, of note, it was also abundant at some of the outbreak sites in Australia in 2011; thus, it may have also had an important role in the eastern portion of the 2011 KUNV outbreak.[59,60]

KUNV's primary vector, *Cx. annulirostris*, and another, lesser vector, *Cx. australicus*, were experimentally exposed to infectious blood meals containing low pathogenic KUNV or the 2011 horse outbreak strain.[61] Few significant differences exist in the susceptibility of *Cx. annulirostris* between these two KUNV strains, including the kinetics of virus replication and transmission. On days 12–14 postexposure, however, significantly more of the pathogenic KUNV 2011 strain was expectorated by the insects. The rate of transmission and levels of virus expectorated were higher in *Cx. annulirostris* than in *Cx. australicus*.[61]

KUNV is maintained and amplified in mosquito–bird cycles. It is undergoing an epizootic spread from northwestern into central and southern areas of Australia as infected wading birds and mosquito numbers increase during times of greater than normal rainfall.[62] Wading birds, especially the rufous night heron (*Nycticorax caledonicus*) and egrets, are the most important reservoir hosts of KUNV. Both of these bird species develop high-level viremia.[63,64] These birds also serve as an important reservoir of Australian MVEV, but not American WNV strains.[64,65] American crows (*Corvus brachyrhynchos*) are important amplifying hosts of American WNV strains. All crows experimentally infected with the WNV_{NY99} strain die; however, inoculation with KUNV does not sicken or kill infected birds.[19,66] Inoculation of crows with KUNV produces lower levels of viremia than that caused by the WNV_{NY99}.[66] Other birds and mammals, including feral pigs and feral rabbits, horses, and cattle, have also been found to be seropositive for KUNV and may act as a reservoir or amplifying hosts as well.[63,67]

WNV in Humans, Horses, and Rabbits

Few cases of KUNV-related encephalitis have been reported in humans: five in 1978, 1991, 1995, 1998, and 1999 in Western Australia; four in the Northern Territory in 1997 and 2000; two in 1984 and 1991 in Victoria; and four in 1991 and 1999 in New South Wales. None of these cases were fatal.[11] The known numbers of human KUNV infection were larger in 2003 and 2004 (18 and 12 cases, respectively).[1] The virus has also been isolated from mosquitoes in Western Australia in the regions where seropositive humans and sentinel chickens are present.[11] Sentinel chicken surveillance programs provide an early warning of the presence of KUNV and other flaviviruses in a region.[20]

Horses are susceptible to WNV, particularly to viral strains found in the United States. In Australia, KUNV infection is found intermittently in horses in the Southeast, but rarely has been known to cause encephalitis in these animals.[19] In New South Wales, the seroprevalance of KUNV in horses is usually less than 5%[68] and is found in flooded inland areas that support large mosquito populations. Waterbirds act as both a reservoir and an amplifying host in those areas.

While KUNV infection is typically mild in horses, an unusually large and severe outbreak of encephalitis involving almost 1000 Australian horses occurred in New South Wales in 2011. This epidemic was due to infection with either or both MVEV and KUNV. The responsible KUNV variant has greatly enhanced neuroinvasiveness when compared to typical KUNV strains.[68,69] The 2011 KUNV had a case fatality rate of 10%–15%.[68] An epidemic involving 119 horses also occurred in Victoria. Full genome sequences determined by epigenomics revealed that KUNV isolates are highly homogenous and only three amino acid differences separated KUNV from the 2011 epidemics in New South Wales and Victoria.[69] One difference is that the New South Wales E protein is glycosylated at residue 154. Glycosylation of this amino acid was previously shown to increase virus dissemination by enhancing the efficiency of viral assembly and virion release.[70] A substitution at residue 653 of NS5 is also present, which may permit NS5 to antagonize type I IFN-mediated Janus kinase-signal transducer and activator of transcription (JAK–STAT) signaling, as described later. While a change was also present in residue 249 of NS2A, a key alteration in NS3 was not present. An alteration in the NS2 gene also leads to increased virulence in birds.[69]

The abnormally high rainfall and flood prior to the 2011 outbreak is believed to have been a major factor in the high number of horse infections since the mosquito vector numbers increased sixfold.[67] It should be noted, however, that many horses were also infected east of the Great Dividing Range, near the major coastal centers of Sydney, Newcastle, and Wollongong. It is noteworthy because this area is much drier, did not experience floods, and its mosquito numbers remained low.[68,71]

This change in KUNV disease in horses, especially its appearance in drier regions of the continent, emphasizes the need for continued monitoring of disease in birds and humans over large and somewhat unsuspected areas. Monitoring should also include watching for genetic changes in KUNV that might lead to a severe outbreak in humans.

No bird or human encephalitis was recorded during the 2011 outbreak in horses, although a mild case of disease was seen in one person.[68] KUNV seroprevalence in humans prior to the 2011 horse outbreak ($n = 148$) was only 0.7% and was 0.6% afterward ($n = 169$),[67] suggesting a very low rate of human infection with this highly virulent horse strain of the virus. Serological testing of feral rabbits (*Oryctolagus cuniculus*), however, revealed a 12.7% seropositivity rate between April 2011 and November 2012 ($n = 675$), with the rate peaking in February 2012 (19.3% seropositive; $n = 145$). Feral rabbits are abundant throughout the outbreak region and are a potential KUNV reservoir host since they can be infected with the KUNV 2011 horse strain and remain asymptomatic.[67] In the Americas, the Eastern cottontails (*Sylvilagus floridanus*) experimentally infected with WNV_{NY99} produce a high enough viremia to allow viral transmission to mosquitoes.[72] While it is not known whether wild Australian rabbits also produce a sufficient level of viremia to play a role in the viral life cycle, they may, nevertheless, be a valuable sentinel species for monitoring KUNV incidence in a given region,[67] especially since detection of infection in these rabbits could provide a longer interval of time for the implementation of preventative strategies than would be seen using only domestic chickens, which most likely would warn of a potential outbreak only once the disease was already in close proximity to humans. Since feral rabbits are an imported pest species, testing could easily be performed during their culling.[67]

WNV in Reptiles

KUNV infects some economically valuable reptiles. It is present in the belly skin lesions in farmed juvenile saltwater crocodiles (*Crocodylus porosus*) just as WNV has been found in the lesions in American alligators (*Alligator mississippiensis*). While KUNV does not appear to lead to morbidity or mortality in crocodiles, up to 60% of WNV-infected alligators die after exhibiting neurological disease.[73] As seen in other vertebrates, KUNV also appears to be less virulent than American WNV strains in these reptiles. Alligators appear to become infected by consumption of WNV-contaminated horsemeat.

Replication of KUNV and Other Flaviviruses

Flavivirus replication, including that of WNV, occurs within the intracellular membranous structures in the cytoplasm, which is ideal for efficient replication and avoidance of the immune response.[74,75] Replication of these viruses' RNA is performed by their RNA-dependent RNA polymerase, a part of the viral NS5 protein. Despite the cytoplasmic location for replication, flaviviruses also need NS5 to enter the nucleus. Some NS5 proteins of JEV, YFV, DENV-2, and ZIKV have, accordingly, been visualized in the nucleus.[75] A more recent report found that NS5 trafficking between the cytoplasm and the nucleus is essential for Kunjin replication.[75] Blocking nuclear import, but not export, of NS5 inhibits KUNV replication, apparently indirectly, and decreases the production of infectious virus. Kinetic studies show that trafficking of NS5 between the cytoplasm and the nucleus occurs very rapidly and may explain why nuclear KUNV NS5 was not previously observed. Since specific inhibitors of NS5 nuclear import decrease the KUNV production, targeting this process may be useful in anti-KUNV drug development.[75]

KUNV and RNAi

The microRNA (miRNA), miR-532-5p, is upregulated by KUNV infection in vitro and in vivo in the brains of infected mice. This small inhibitory RNA (siRNA) downregulates the production of the cellular proteins SEC14, spectrin domain 1 (SESTD1), and TAK1-binding protein (TAB3) in a human kidney cell line as well as in infected mouse brains.[76] Both SESTD1 and TAB3 are required for efficient Kunjin replication. SESTD1 inhibits Ca^{2+}-mediated signals, while TAB3 influences activation of transforming growth factor-β-activated kinase 1 (TAK1). The latter phosphorylates c-Jun N-terminal kinases and the IkBα/β subunit of NF-κB, allowing nuclear translocation of the transcription factors AP-1 and NF-κB. This nuclear translocation is required for the survival of the virus' target cell.[77]

RNA interference (RNAi) also plays a protective role in mosquito immune responses to KUNV. Both *Cx. quinquefasciatus*-infected cells in vitro and orally-infected *Cx. quinquefasciatus* mosquitoes in vivo circumvent RNAi pathways by producing viral noncoding subgenomic flavivirus RNAs (sfRNAs) that interact with the RNAi-processing enzymes Dicer and Argonaute 2.[78] Additionally, in KUNV-infected mosquito cells, the miRNA aae-miR-2940-5p is downregulated. This miRNA suppresses production of a host metalloprotease that is required for virus replication.[79]

THE IMMUNE RESPONSE

A large amount of information is available that describes the immune response to WNV; however, since KUNV differs in virulence from many of the WNV strains used in these studies, much of this information may not be pertinent to KUNV. The following subsections describe relationships that are known to be true for the KUNV strain of WNV.

KUNV and Cytokines

The bite of an infected mosquito inserts KUNV into the skin, the site of initial viral infection and replication of keratinocytes and skin-resident dendritic cells (DCs) such as Langerhans cells, before migrating to cutaneous lymph nodes.[80] KUNV-infected human monocyte-derived DCs permit synthesis of viral mRNA and proteins without undergoing apoptosis. Expression of the T cell costimulatory molecules CD86 and CD40 is upregulated and infected DCs secrete, at best, small amounts of the cytokines IL-12, IL-23, IL-18, or IL-10.[81] KUNV infection stimulates the production of significant amounts of type I IFN, however, with greater amounts of IFN-α than IFN-β. Expression of the IFN-γ receptor is decreased.[81]

KUNV and IFNs

Type I IFNs, but not IFN-γ, play a vital role in clearance of WNV from the CNS and in controlling virus in the periphery.[16] The attenuated phenotype of KUNV in humans can at least partially be explained by its higher degree of sensitivity to type I IFNs, since it is not able to suppress the IFN-signaling JAK–STAT pathway that controls type I IFN production. Pretreatment of cultured cells with 1–10,000 IU/mL of IFN-α decreases KUNV infectivity by 5–1000-fold, while such pretreatment only decreases WNV$_{NY99}$ by up to 50-fold.[52] When IFN-α is added 3 h after infection, both titers of KUNV and WNV are also decreased although KUNV production was decreased to a greater extent than that of WNV$_{NY99}$. Taken together, the low virulent KUNV is more susceptible to type I IFN than the highly virulent WNV$_{NY99}$ strain.

Even though both KUNV and WNV$_{NY99}$ decrease IFN responses by reducing phosphorylation of STAT1 and STAT2, downstream mediators of type I IFN activation, the percentage of infected cells containing nuclear, phosphorylated STAT1 is greater in KUNV-infected cells than that found in WNV$_{NY99}$-infected cells after IFN-α treatment, with the latter cells lacking detectable nuclear STAT1, as determined by immunofluorescence assays.[52,82] Additionally, infection of mice lacking an intact IFN response system resulted in a 100% mortality

rate in mice, compared to no deaths in wild-type mice infected with KUNV. KUNV virulence is increased, however, in cultured cells and mice that lack a combination of interferon regulatory factor-3 and -7 (IRF-3; IRF-7) or the common type I IFN receptor.[52] Together, these findings emphasize the role of IFN sensitivity to WNV strain virulence.

Type I IFNs act by stimulating the cytoplasmic IFN-induced MxA protein that sequesters the KUNV capsid protein in cytoplasmic tubular structures, thus decreasing levels of secreted, infectious, KUNV particles.[83] When MxA expression is retargeted from the cytoplasmic inclusions to the ER, the formation and spread of infectious KUNV is decreased.

Changes in several KUNV nonstructural proteins are involved in its high susceptibility to type I IFN. Even though a virulent American WNV and the relatively nonpathogenic KUNV are very similar at the protein level a point mutation can greatly affect virulence. KUNV and WNV$_{NY99}$ differ at the NS5 residue 653. When this amino acid in KUNV is changed to that present in WNV$_{NY99}$, the resulting virus has greatly decreased sensitivity to IFN and increased virulence.[84] NS2A also plays a role in IFN-β production by host cells. A change in residue 30 of the wild-type KUNV NS2A gene promotes a 15- to 50-fold increase in establishing noncytopathic, persistent infection in hamster and human cell lines without decreasing viral replication or virion formation and secretion. Infection of IFN-β-deficient cultured kidney cells with this point mutation reduced DNA degradation, suggesting that the NS2A protein plays a role in IFN-independent apoptosis. Introduction of several other amino acids into the NS2A gene also affect KUNV virulence in different manners, depending on the nature of the substituted amino acid.[85] Mutation of NS2A residue 30, nevertheless, increases IFN-β promoter activity as seen in a KUNV replicon, a luciferase reporting system.[86] A second change in the KUNV NS2A protein, in residue 101, also increases persistence of the virus in cell lines, although to a lesser extent than that seen in KUNV residue 30 alterations. Wild-type NS2A may therefore be useful as a new target for attenuation of a KUNV-based vaccine active against the pathogenic strains of West Nile virus,[86] especially since attenuated KUNV is also protective against WNV$_{NY99}$ infection in mice and crows.[58,66,87]

Using chimeric WNV$_{NY99}$ and KUNV 2011 strains, NS3 was found to increase WNV replication in cells having normal type I IFN responses, leading to increased virulence in mice.[88] Using a similar approach, placing the viral protease and helicase domains of

WNV_{NY99} NS3 on the background of the KUNV 2011 strain, the viral helicase, but not viral protease, domain of NS3 was found to inhibit type I IFN signaling via decreased STAT1 phosphorylation. Additionally, the activity of the WNV_{NY99} helicase is more efficient than that of the 2011 KUNV strain.[89]

Structural genes, however, are also important to the viral response to type I IFN. A typically nonpathogenic KUNV engineered to express prM/E genes from Rocio virus (another mosquito-borne flavivirus) inhibits IFN-α, IFN-β, and JAK–STAT signaling and enhances viral replication and virulence in young mice when compared to the parent KUNV.[90]

PREVENTION AND TREATMENT
Prevention of KUNV Infection
Wolbachia pipientis is an intracellular endosymbiotic bacterium of arthropods, including mosquitoes. In cultured *Ae. aegypti* mosquito cells infected with *Wolbachia*, accumulation of genomic RNA from several strains of WNV (WNV_{NY99}, KUNV, and the 2011 KUNV strain) are increased. By contrast, the amount of secreted KUNV was decreased. *Wolbachia* completely blocked in vivo WNV replication in *Ae. aegypti* mosquitoes as well as viral infection, transmission, and dissemination rates.[91] It should be noted that this mosquito species is a poor vector for WNV. Other studies have shown an inhibition of WNV replication in *Cx. quinquefasciatus* mosquitoes harboring *Wolbachia* as well.[92] Further in vivo testing using other *Culex* species mosquitoes need to be pursued in order to evaluate the usefulness of *Wolbachia* reducing KUNV transmission to mosquitoes, birds, horses, and humans in natural settings.

Vaccines could play a major role in preventing infection. One vaccine approach uses a strain of KUNV that contains large deletions in the C protein gene. These replication-competent RNAs secrete highly immunogenic subviral particles. The particles are noninfectious since they cannot be packaged into virions, making them safe while still able to generate strong immune responses, similar to live vaccines.[93,94] One potential vaccine construct uses a cytomegalovirus promoter-driven KUNV cDNA with specific deletions of alphahelices 1, 2, and 4 in the C protein. When these deletions are combined with the addition of a glycosylation motif in the E protein gene, viral secretion is enhanced. This construct produces many subviral particles and may prove to be an effective vaccine candidate.[95]

Treatment of KUNV Infection
No effective means of treatment is currently licensed for use in humans with neuroinvasive WNV diseases. Individuals with serious illness should be hospitalized. They may require supportive care, such as intravenous fluids and mechanical respiration. Care should be taken to prevent the development of secondary infections.

Several drugs are being developed to combat severe WNV-induced diseases in general. These include ribavirin, nucleoside analogs, a broad-spectrum antiviral derivative of N-methylisatin-beta-thiosemicarbazone, the proteinase inhibitors aprotinin and D-arginine-based peptides, lycorine, iminocyclitol derivatives, and protein kinase C inhibitors.[96–103] Given the differences in KUNV and other more neuroinvasive WNV strains, these drugs may or may not be active against KUNV.

The efficacy of several drugs against KUNV-related disease is, however, being tested. One potential target of antiflavivirus drugs is the capping enzyme. Several members of the 2-thioxothiazolidin-4-ones family of drugs potently inhibit the capping enzyme's GTP binding and guanylyltransferase functions. These drugs reduced replication of several flaviviruses, including the Kunjin type of WNV, in in vitro kidney cell cultures by almost three orders of magnitude.[10]

Another drug, lactimidomycin, targets the cellular translation elongation process. Since viruses lack a translational apparatus, they are forced to use the host cell's protein synthesis machinery. Lactimidomycin has antiviral activity against KUNV in in vitro cell cultures at concentrations that do not affect cell viability.[104] Since it has higher potency and selectivity than other antiviral agents, it may be found to be very useful in treating KUNV-infected vertebrates after undergoing in vivo testing.

SUMMARY OVERVIEW
Diseases: usually asymptomatic but may cause mild to severe neurological disease in humans
Causative agent: Kunjin strain, West Nile virus lineage 1b
Vector: primarily *Culex*, but occasionally *Aedes*, mosquitoes
Common reservoir: wading birds, especially night herons and egrets
Mode of transmission: mosquito bite
Geographical distribution: Australia, primarily northwestern regions
Year of emergence: 1960

REFERENCES

1. Gyawali N, Bradbury RS, Aaskov JG, Taylor-Robinson AW. Neglected Australian arboviruses: quam gravis? *Microbes Infect.* 2017;19:388–401.
2. Russell RC. Arboviruses and their vectors in Australia: an update on the ecology and epidemiology of some mosquito-borne arboviruses. *Rev Med Vet Entomol.* 1995;83:141–158.
3. Tesh RB. Arthritis caused by mosquito-borne viruses. *Annu Rev Med.* 1982;33:31–40.
4. May FJ, Lobigs M, Lee E, et al. Biological, antigenic and phylogenetic characterization of the flavivirus Alfuy. *J Gen Virol.* 2006;87:329–337.
5. Whitehead RH, Doherty RL, Domrow R, Standfast HA, Wetters EJ. Studies of the epidemiology of arthropod-borne virus infections at Mitchell River Mission, Cape York Peninsula, North Queensland. *Trans R Soc Trop Med Hyg.* 1968;62:439–445.
6. Mackenzie JS, Williams DT. The zoonotic flaviviruses of Southern, South-Eastern and Eastern Asia, and Australasia: the potential for emergent viruses. *Zoonoses Public Health.* 2009;56:338–356.
7. Scherret H, Poidinger M, Mackenzie JS, et al. The relationships between West Nile and Kunjin viruses. *Emerg Infect Dis.* 2001;7:697–705.
8. Felsenstein J. PHYLIP—phylogeny inference package (version 3.2). *Cladistics.* 1989;5:164–166.
9. Hall RA, Scherret JH, Mackenzie JS. Kunjin virus: an Australian variant of West Nile? *Ann N Y Acad Sci.* 2001;951:153–160.
10. Adams SC, Broom AK, Sammels LM, et al. Glycosylation and antigenic variation among Kunjin virus isolates. *Virology.* 1995;206:49–56.
11. Russell RC, Dwyer DE. Arboviruses associated with human disease in Australia. *Microbes Infect.* 2000;2:1693–1704.
12. Holland J, Smith DW, Broom AK, Currie B. A comparison of seroprevalence of arboviral infections between three northern territory regions. *Microbiol Aust.* 1994;15:A105.
13. Shahhosseini N, Chinikar S. Genetic evidence for circulation of Kunjin-related West Nile virus strain in Iran. *J Vector Borne Dis.* 2016;53:384–386.
14. Prow NA. The changing epidemiology of Kunjin virus in Australia. *Int J Environ Res Public Health.* 2013;10(12):6255–6272.
15. Smithburn KC, Hughes TP, Burke AW, Paul JH. A neurotropic virus isolated from the blood of a native of Uganda. *Am J Trop Med Hyg.* 1940;20:471–492.
16. Donadieu E, Bahuo C, Lowenski S, Zientara S, Coulpier M, Lecollinet S. Differential virulence and pathogenesis of West Nile viruses. *Viruses.* 2013;5:2856–2880.
17. Blitvich BJ. Transmission dynamics and changing epidemiology of West Nile virus. *Anim Health Res Rev.* 2008;9:71–86.
18. Doherty RL, Carley JG, Mackerras MJ, Marks EN. Studies of arthropod-borne virus infections in Queensland. III. Isolation and characterization of virus strains from wild-caught mosquitoes in North Queensland. *Aust J Exp Biol Med Sci.* 1963;41:17–39.
19. Hall RA, Broom AK, Smith DW, Mackenzie JS. The ecology and epidemiology of Kunjin virus. *Curr Top Microbiol Immunol.* 2002;267:253–269.
20. Knope K, Doggett SL, Jansen CC, et al. Arboviral diseases and malaria in Australia, 2014-15: annual report of the National Arbovirus and Malaria Advisory Committee. *Commun Dis Intell.* 2019;29:43.
21. Prow N, Edmonds J, Williams D, et al. Virulence and evolution of West Nile virus, Australia, 1960-2012. *Emerg Infect Dis.* 2016;22(8):1353–1362.
22. Huang B, Prow NA, van den Hurk AF, et al. Archival isolates confirm a single topotype of West Nile virus in Australia. *PLoS Negl Trop Dis.* 2016;10(12):e0005159.
23. Samuel MA, Diamond MS. Pathogenesis of WNV infection: a balance between virulence, innate and adaptive immunity, and viral evasion. *J Virol.* 2006;80:9349–9360.
24. Beltz LA. West Nile disease in the United States. In: *Emerging Infectious Diseases: A Guide to Diseases, Causative Agents, and Surveillance.* Jossey-Bass; 2011:475–497.
25. Samuel MA, Morrey JD, Diamond MS. Caspase 3-dependent cell death of neurons contributes to the pathogenesis of WNV encephalitis. *J Virol.* 2007;81:2614–2623.
26. Hayes EB, Gubler DJ. West Nile virus: epidemiology and clinical features of an emerging epidemic in the United States. *Annu Rev Med.* 2006;57:181–194.
27. Leis AA, Fratkin J, Stokic DS, Harrington T, Webb RM, Slavinski SA. West Nile poliomyelitis. *Lancet Infect Dis.* 2003;3:9–10.
28. Davis LE, DeBiasi R, Goade DE, et al. West Nile virus neuroinvasive disease. *Ann Neurol.* 2006;60:286–300.
29. Klee AL, Maidin B, Edwin B, et al. Long-term prognosis for clinical West Nile virus infection. *Emerg Infect Dis.* 2016;10:1405–1411.
30. Sejvar JJ, Bode AV, Marfin AA, et al. West Nile virus-associated flaccid paralysis outcome. *Emerg Infect Dis.* 2006;12:514–516.
31. Sejvar JJ. The long-term outcomes of human West Nile virus infection. *Clin Infect Dis.* 2007;44:1617–1624.
32. Naim H, Wild J, Boughton CR, Hawkes RA. Arbovirus surveillance in the Murray-Riverina region, New South Wales (1981-82). *Commun Dis Intell Q Rep.* 1982;82:5–6.
33. Gray TJ, Burrow JN, Markey PG, et al. Case report: West Nile virus (Kunjin subtype) disease in the Northern Territory of Australia—a case of encephalitis and review of all reported cases. *Am J Trop Med Hyg.* 2011;85(5):952–956.
34. Mackenzie JS, Smith DW, Broom AK, Bucens MR. Australian encephalitis in Western Australia, 1978-1991. *Med J Aust.* 1993;158:591–595.
35. Ostlund EN, Crom RL, Pedersen DD, Johnson DJ, Williams WO, Schmitt BJ. Equine West Nile encephalitis, United States. *Emerg Infect Dis.* 2001;7:665–669.
36. Beasley DWC, Li L, Suderman MT, Barrett ADT. Mouse neuroinvasive phenotype of West Nile virus strains varies depending upon virus genotype. *Virology.* 2002;296:17–23.

37. Venter M, Myers TG, Wilson MA, et al. Gene expression in mice infected with West Nile virus strains of different neurovirulence. *Virology*. 2005;342:119–140.

38. Pérez-Ramírez E, Llorente F, del Amo J, et al. Pathogenicity evaluation of twelve West Nile virus strains belonging to four lineages from five continents in a mouse model: discrimination between three pathogenicity categories. *J Gen Virol*. 2017;98:662–670.

39. Lewy TG, Grabowski JM, Bloom ME. BiP: master regulator of the unfolded protein response and crucial factor in flavivirus biology. *Yale J Biol Med*. 2017;90:291–300.

40. Ambrose RL, Mackenzie JM. ATF6 signaling is required for efficient West Nile virus replication by promoting cell survival and inhibition of innate immune responses. *J Virol*. 2013;87:2206–2214.

41. Setoh YX, Prow NA, Hobson-Peters J, et al. Identification of residues in West Nile virus pre-membrane protein that influence viral particle secretion and virulence. *J Gen Virol*. 2012;93(9):1965–1975.

42. Setoh YX, Tan CSE, Prow NA, et al. The I22V and L72S substitutions in West Nile virus prM protein promote enhanced prM/E heterodimerisation and nucleocapsid incorporation. *Virol J*. 2015;12:72.

43. Calvert AE, Huang CY, Blair CD, Roehrig JT. Mutations in the West Nile prM protein affect VLP and virion secretion in vitro. *Virology*. 2012;433(1):35–44.

44. Bingham J, Payne J, Harper J, et al. Evaluation of a mouse model for the West Nile virus group for the purpose of determining viral pathotypes. *J Gen Virol*. 2014;95:1221–1232.

45. Audsley M, Edmonds J, Liu W, et al. Virulence determinants between New York 99 and Kunjin strains of West Nile virus. *Virology*. 2011;414(1):63–73.

46. Davis CT, Galbraith SE, Zhang S, et al. A combination of naturally occurring mutations in North American West Nile virus nonstructural protein genes and in the 3′ untranslated region alters virus phenotype. *J Virol*. 2007;81:6111–6116.

47. Hussmann KL, Samuel MA, Kim KS, Diamond MS, Fredericksen BL. Differential replication of pathogenic and nonpathogenic strains of West Nile virus within astrocytes. *J Virol*. 2013;87:2814–2822.

48. Sangster MY, Heliams DB, MacKenzie JS, Shellam GR. Genetic studies of flavivirus resistance in inbred strains derived from wild mice: evidence for a new resistance allele at the flavivirus resistance locus (*Flv*). *J Virol*. 1993;6(1):340–347.

49. Urosevic N, Silvia OJ, Sangster MY, Mansfield JP, Hodgetts SI, Shellam GR. Development and characterization of new flavivirus-resistant mouse strains bearing *Flv(r)*-like and *Flv(mr)* alleles from wild or wild-derived mice. *J Gen Virol*. 1999;80(pt. 4):897–906.

50. Mashimo T, Lucas M, Simon-Chazottes D, et al. A nonsense mutation in the gene encoding 2′-5′-oligoadenylate synthetase/L1 isoform is associated with West Nile virus susceptibility in laboratory mice. *PNAS*. 2002;99(17):11311–11316.

51. Perelygin AA, Scherbik SV, Zhulin IB, Stockman BM, Li Y, Brinton MA. Positional cloning of the murine flavivirus resistance gene. *PNAS*. 2002;99(14):9322–9327.

52. Daffis S, Lazear HM, Liu WJ, et al. The naturally attenuated Kunjin strain of West Nile virus shows enhanced sensitivity to the host type I interferon response. *J Virol*. 2011;85:5664–5668.

53. Shueb RH, Papadimitriou J, Urosevic N. Fatal persistence of West Nile virus subtype Kunjin in the brains of flavivirus resistant mice. *Virus Res*. 2013;155(2011):455–461.

54. Shueb RH, Pantelic L, Urosevic N. A delayed morbidity in genetically resistant mice triggered by some flaviviruses. *Arbovirus Res Aust*. 2013;9:344–351.

55. Kay BH, Standfast HA. Ecology of arboviruses and their vectors in Australia. *Curr Top Vector Res*. 1978;3:1–36.

56. Sudeep AB. *Culex gelidus*: an emerging mosquito vector with potential to transmit multiple virus infections. *J Vector Borne Dis*. 2014;51:251–258.

57. Jansen CC, Web CE, Graham GC, et al. Blood sources of mosquitoes collected from urban and periurban environments in eastern Australia with species-specific molecular analysis of avian blood meals. *Am J Trop Med Hyg*. 2013;81:849–857.

58. Jansen CC, Ritchie SA, van den Hurk AF. The role of Australian mosquito species in the transmission of endemic and exotic West Nile Virus strains. *Int J Environ Res Public Health*. 2013;10:3735–3752.

59. Jansen CC, Webb CE, Northill JA, Ritchie SA, Russell RC, van den Hurk AF. Vector competence of Australian mosquito species for a North American strain of West Nile virus. *Vector Borne Zoonotic Dis*. 2008;8(6):805–811.

60. Doggett S, Clancy J, Haniotis J, et al. *The New South Wales Arbovirus Surveillance and Mosquito Monitoring Program 2010–2011 Annual Report*. Westmead, Australia: Department of Medical Entomology; 2011.

61. van den Hurk AF, Hall-Mendelin S, Webb CE, et al. Role of enhanced vector transmission of a new West Nile virus strain in an outbreak of equine disease in Australia in 2011. *Parasit Vectors*. 2011;7:586.

62. Broom A, Whelan P, Smith D, et al. An outbreak of Australian encephalitis in Western Australia and Central Australia (Northern Territory and South Australia) during the 2000 wet season. *Arbovirus Res Aust*. 2001;8:37–42.

63. Marshall ID. Kunjin virus isolates of Australia are genetically homogeneous. In: Monath T, ed. *The Arboviruses: Epidemiology and Ecology*. vol. III. CRC Press; 1988:151–190.

64. Boyle DB, Dickerman RW, Marshall ID. Primary viraemia responses of herons to experimental infection with Murray Valley encephalitis, Kunjin and Japanese encephalitis viruses. *Aust J Exp Biol Med Sci*. 2001;61:655–664.

65. Reisen WK, Wheeler SS, Yamamoto S, Fang Y, Garcia S. Nesting *Ardeid* colonies are not a focus of elevated West Nile virus activity in southern California. *Vector Borne Zoonotic Dis*. 2005;5:258–266.

66. Braul AC, Langevin SA, Bowen RA, et al. Differential virulence of West Nile strains for American crows. *Emerg Infect Dis*. 2004;5:2161–2168.

67. Prow NA, Hewlett EK, Faddy HM, et al. The Australian public is still vulnerable to emerging virulent strains of West Nile virus. *Front Public Health.* 2014;2:146.

68. Frost MJ, Zhang J, Edmonds JH, et al. Characterization of virulent West Nile Virus Kunjin strain, Australia, 2011. *Emerg Infect Dis.* 2012;18:792–800.

69. Mann RA, Fegan M, O'Riley K, Motha J, Warner S. Molecular characterization and phylogenetic analysis of Murray Valley encephalitis virus and West Nile virus (Kunjin subtype) from an arbovirus disease outbreak in horses in Victoria, Australia, in 2011. *J Vet Diagn Invest.* 2013;25(1):35–44.

70. Hanna SL, Pierson TC, Sanchez MD, Ahmed AA, Murtadha MM, Doms RW. N-linked glycosylation of West Nile virus envelope proteins influences particle assembly and infectivity. *J Virol.* 2005;79:13262–13674.

71. Roche SE, Wicks R, Garner MG, et al. Descriptive overview of the 2011 epidemic of arboviral disease in horses in Australia. *Aust Vet J.* 2013;91:5–13.

72. Tiawsirisup S, Platt KB, Tucker BJ, Rowley WA. Eastern cottontail rabbits (*Sylvilagus floridanus*) develop West Nile virus viremias sufficient for infecting select mosquito species. *Vector Borne Zoonotic Dis.* 2005;5:342–350.

73. Isberg SR, Moran JL, De Araujo R, Elliott N, Davisb SS, Melville L. First evidence of Kunjin strain of West Nile virus associated with saltwater crocodile (*Crocodylus porosus*) skin lesions. *Aust Vet J.* 2019;97:390–393.

74. Gillespie LK, Hoenen A, Morgan G, Mackenzie JM. The endoplasmic reticulum provides the membrane platform for biogenesis of the flavivirus replication complex. *J Virol.* 2010;84(20):10438–10447.

75. Lopez-Denman AJ, Russo A, Wagstaff KM, White PA, Jans DA, Mackenzie JM. Nucleocytoplasmic shuttling of the West Nile virus RNA-dependent RNA polymerase NS5 is critical to infection. *Cell Microbiol.* 2018;20(8):12848.

76. Slonchak A, Shannon RP, Pali G, Khromykh AA. Human microRNA miR-532-5p exhibits antiviral activity against West Nile virus via suppression of host genes SESTD1 and TAB3 required for virus replication. *J Virol.* 2016;90(5):2388–2402.

77. Kanayama A, Seth RB, Sun L, et al. TAB2 and TAB3 activate the NF-κB pathway through binding to polyubiquitin chains. *Mol Cell.* 2004;15:535–548.

78. Ahlers LRH, Goodman AG. The immune responses of the animal hosts of West Nile virus: a comparison of insects, birds, and mammals. *Front Cell Infect Microbiol.* 2018;81:96.

79. Slonchak A, Hussain M, Torres S, Asgari S, Khromykh AA. Expression of mosquito microRNA Aae-Mir-2940-5p is downregulated in response to West Nile virus infection to restrict viral replication. *J Virol.* 2014;88:8457–8467.

80. Suthar MS, Diamond MS, Gale MJ. West Nile virus infection and immunity. *Nat Rev Microbiol.* 2013;11:115–128.

81. Kovats S, Turner S, Simmons A, Powe T, Chakravarty E, Alberola-Ila J. West Nile virus-infected human dendritic cells fail to fully activate invariant natural killer T cells. *Clin Exp Immunol.* 2016;186:214–226.

82. Liu WJ, Wang XJ, Mokhonov VV, Shi P-Y, Randall R, Khromykh AA. Inhibition of interferon signaling by the New York 99 strain and Kunjin subtype of West Nile virus involves blockage of STAT1 and STAT2 activation by nonstructural proteins. *J Virol.* 2005;79:1934–1942.

83. Hoenen A, Gillespie L, Morgan G, van der Heide P, Khromykh A, Mackenzie J. The West Nile virus assembly process evades the conserved antiviral mechanism of the interferon-induced MxA protein. *Virology.* 2014;448:104–116.

84. Laurent-Rolle M, Boer EF, Lubick KJ, et al. The NS5 protein of the virulent West Nile virus NY99 strain is a potent antagonist of type I interferon-mediated JAK-STAT signaling. *J Virol.* 2010;84:3503–3515.

85. Melian EB, Edmonds JH, Nagasaki TK, Hinzman E, Floden N, Khromykh AA. West Nile virus NS2A protein facilitates virus-induced apoptosis independently of interferon response. *J Gen Virol.* 2013;94:308–313.

86. Liu WJ, Chen HB, Wang XJ, Huang H, Khromykh AA. Analysis of adaptive mutations in Kunjin virus replicon RNA reveals a novel role for the flavivirus nonstructural protein NS2A in inhibition of beta interferon promoter-driven transcription. *J Virol.* 2004;78:12225–12235.

87. Hall RA, Nisbet DJ, Pham KB, Pyke AT, Smith GA, Khromykh AA. DNA vaccine coding for the full-length infectious Kunjin virus RNA protects mice against the New York strain of West Nile virus. *PNAS.* 2003;100:10460–10464.

88. Setoh YX, Prow NA, Rawle DJ, et al. Systematic analysis of viral genes responsible for differential virulence between American and Australian West Nile virus strains. *J Gen Virol.* 2015;96:1297–1308.

89. Setoh YX, Periasamy P, Peng NYG, Amarilla AA, Slonchak A, Khromykh AA. Helicase domain of West Nile virus NS3 protein plays a role in inhibition of type I interferon signaling. *Viruses.* 2017;9:326.

90. Amarill AA, Fumagalli MJ, Figueiredo ML, et al. Ilheus and Saint Louis encephalitis viruses elicit cross-protection against a lethal Rocio virus challenge in mice. *PLoS One.* 2018;13(6):e0199071.

91. Hussain M, Lu G, Torres S, et al. Effect of *Wolbachia* on replication of West Nile virus in a mosquito cell line and adult mosquitoes. *J Virol.* 2013;87(2):851–858.

92. Glaser RL, Meola MA. The native Wolbachia endosymbionts of *Drosophila melanogaster* and *Culex quinquefasciatus* increase host resistance to West Nile virus infection. *PLoS One.* 2010;5:e11977.

93. Mandl CW. Flavivirus immunization with capsid-deletion mutants: basics, benefits, and barriers. *Viral Immunol.* 2004;17:461–472.

94. Roby JA, Hall RA, Khromykh AA. Nucleic acid-based infectious and pseudo-infectious flavivirus vaccines. In: Dormitzer PR, Mandl CW, Rapuoli R, eds. *Replicating Vaccines: A New Generation.* Birkhauser Verlag AG; 2011:299–320.

95. Roby JA, Hall RA, Khromykh AA. West Nile virus genome with glycosylated envelope protein and deletion of

alpha helices 1, 2, and 4 in the capsid protein is noninfectious and efficiently secretes subviral particles. *J Virol.* 2013;87(23):13063–13069.

96. Crance JM, Scaramozzino N, Jouan A, Garin D. Interferon, ribavirin, 6-azauridine and glycyrrhizin: antiviral compounds active against pathogenic flaviviruses. *Antiviral Res.* 2003;58:73–79.

97. Pathak N, Lai M-L, Chen W-Y, Hsieh BW, Yu G-Y, Yang J-M. Pharmacophore anchor models of flaviviral NS3 proteases lead to drug repurposing for DENV infection. *BMC Bioinformatics.* 2017;18(suppl. 16):548.

98. Shiryaev SA, Ratnikov BI, Chekanov AV, et al. Cleavage targets and the D-arginine-based inhibitors of the West Nile virus NS3 processing proteinase. *Biochem J.* 2006;393:503–511.

99. Zou G, Puig-Basagoiti F, Zhang B, et al. A single-amino acid substitution in West Nile virus 2K peptide between NS4a and NS4b confers resistance to lycorine, a flavivirus inhibitor. *Virology.* 2009;84(1):242–252.

100. Gu B, Mason P, Wang L, et al. Antiviral profiles of novel iminocyclitol compounds against bovine viral diarrhea virus, West Nile virus, dengue virus and hepatitis B virus. *Antivir Chem Chemother.* 2007;8:49–59.

101. Sebastian L, Desai A, Shampur MN, Perumal Y, Sriram D, Vasanthapuram RN. Methylisatin-beta-thiosemicarbazone derivative (SCH 16) is an inhibitor of Japanese encephalitis virus infection *in vitro* and *in vivo. Virol J.* 2008;5:64.

102. Eyer L, Zouharová D, Sirmarová J, et al. Antiviral activity of the adenosine analogue BCX4430 against West Nile virus and tick-borne flaviviruses. *Antiviral Res.* 2017;142:63–67.

103. Blázquez AB, Vázquez-Calvo A, Martín-Acebes MA, Saiz J-C. Pharmacological inhibition of protein kinase C reduces West Nile virus replication. *Viruses.* 2018;10:91.

104. Carocci M, Yang PL. Lactimidomycin is a broad-spectrum inhibitor of dengue and other RNA viruses. *Antiviral Res.* 2016;128:57–62.

CHAPTER 6

Usutu Virus

INTRODUCTION AND HISTORY

USUV was first identified in South Africa in *Culex naevei* mosquitoes in 1959 and subsequently spread to regions thousands of kilometers apart, such as Senegal, Central African Republic, Nigeria, Uganda, Burkina Faso, Cote d'Ivoire, and Morocco.[1,2] At that time, it was not associated with clinical disease in birds or mammals. Recently, these and other flaviviruses have spread and are now found in Tunisian oases, where 10% of the tested anthropophilic mosquitoes as well as the abundant population of loving doves were seropositive for WNV and 4% were seropositive for USUV. Occurrence of such antiflavivirus antibodies increases with dove age and proximity to the coast, rather than vegetation type.[3] Although surrounded by dry, barren desert, oases are wet and densely vegetated areas that support rich local bird populations as well as providing climatic conditions appropriate for mosquitoes. Oases also have concentrated human populations, many of whom are farmers with a high rate of exposure to mosquitoes.

Outside of Africa, USUV was first documented in Central European birds in 2001 and the following years. Retrospective studies, however, suggest that this virus was present in 6% of those tested in Italy in 1996[4] and may have arrived in Europe in the early 1990s.[5] In 2001, USUV was first detected near or in Vienna and elsewhere in Austria and later in Switzerland, where it caused avian deaths, especially among wild blackbirds, captive great gray owls, and barn swallows.[6,7] In the following years, this viral strain continued to kill birds in Austria,[8,9] suggesting that the virus is able to overwinter and establish a local bird–mosquito transmission cycle in that region.

Between 2006 and 2009, USUV caused outbreaks in free and captive wild birds in Budapest, Hungary[10] and Italy (2008–2009), in which over 1000 birds died.[11,12] In a Zurich zoo, USUV was particularly deadly for wild members of Passeriformes (particularly blackbirds and house sparrows), and, to a lesser extent, Strigiformes species.[13] Based upon the 99.9% identity of the nearly complete genomes of the Austrian and Hungarian viruses, it is most likely that the USUV strains from wild birds in Austria spread to Hungarian wild birds rather than from a separate introduction from Africa.[10] Despite winter temperatures as low as −20°C in Central Europe, USUV has adapted to local mosquito species

and is endemic in several European countries, with different viral genetic lineages emerging and undergoing multiple dispersal events.[6,14] In Italy alone from 2008 to 2009, at least 11 viral strains were found in sentinel horses, dead blackbirds, and a very small number of magpies.[2,11] It should be noted that almost half of the blackbirds examined were coinfected by hemosporidia (blood protozoans), perhaps weakening the hosts and contributing to disease severity of *Plasmodium* species. This is similar to the situation occurring in a large disease outbreak in the Netherlands in 2016, in which many blackbirds and great gray owls were coinfected with USUV and *Plasmodium*, the hemosporidian causative agent of malaria.[15] It was suggested that the coinfections may be partially explained by the fact that mosquitoes are vectors for both pathogens; however, *Culex* species mosquitoes are the primary vectors for USUV in Europe, while *Anopheles* mosquito species primarily transmit *Plasmodium*. Alternatively, coinfection may lead to increased severity of USUV-related disease.[15] Notably, USUV-infected *Aedes albopictus* mosquitoes have been found in Italy[16] and are also vectors for DENV and Zika virus (ZIKV).

USUV has been found in a variety of mosquitoes, birds, and bats in Europe, including Hungary, Switzerland, Spain, Italy, the Czech Republic, Germany, Belgium, and France.[17] Moreover, antibodies to the virus in birds are present in Poland and Greece and in a horse in Serbia.[17] USUV infection is also recurrent in Austria (2001–2006), Hungary (2005–2006), Italy (2009–2016), Spain (2006, 2009, 2012), and Germany (2010–2015). A large European outbreak in humans occurred in 2016 in Belgium, Germany, France, and the Netherlands.[18] The complete genome of the responsible USUV strain is closely related to isolates from Germany (Europe 3 lineage, described later). The North Eastern Italian strain nucleosides are identical to an USUV strain later detected in an immunocompromised human patient's brain and are highly similar to viruses isolated from birds in Vienna and Budapest. Interestingly, the Italian isolates from birds as well as those from Spanish *Cx. pipiens* mosquitoes were 97%–99% identical to the 1959 South African reference strain.[12,19] In the 2009 USUV outbreak in Spain, the virus was detected in *Cx. perexiguus* mosquitoes and, later,

Zika and Other Neglected and Emerging Flaviviruses. https://doi.org/10.1016/B978-0-323-82501-6.00011-6

in two ill song thrushes in 2012. Comparisons of these Spanish strains, however, found differences between the mosquito and bird isolates.[20]

The first report of human infection was in the early 1980s in Africa.[17] In 2009, the first two human cases of USUV infection were reported in Europe after isolating the virus from patients' blood and detecting viral RNA in the cerebrospinal fluid (CSF) in immunocompromised patients in Italy. One of the patients who developed severely impaired cerebral functions had very recently undergone orthotropic liver transplantation as a treatment for thrombotic thrombocytopenic purpura.[21]

At least 21 human cases of USUV infection have been reported as of 2017 with moderate (rash, fever, and headache) to severe (neurological disorders) illness. Two human cases from the Central African Republic (1980s) and Burkina Faso (2004) presented with moderate symptoms, such as fever, rash, and jaundice.[17] The first cases of meningoencephalitis due to USUV were reported in 2009 in two immunocompromised subjects in Italy. USUV was also present in the CSF from three patients with acute meningoencephalitis in 2008–2009.[17] A retrospective study in Italy detected USUV infection in patients with suspected viral encephalitis or meningoencephalitis and comorbidities during the same time period. Intriguingly, in a retrospective study of CSF and serum, not only was USUV infection first detected in Italy in 2008, but also the first case of WNV neuroinvasive disease in humans was found in Italy in that year.[22,23] The number of human USUV-related neurological disease cases in 2009 was fivefold higher than the corresponding number of WNV cases in that area.[22,24] Additionally, 6.6% of well, ill, or hospital inpatients and outpatients tested ($n = 609$) had anti-USUV antibodies, while 3.0% had anti-WNV antibodies.[22] From 2008 to 2009, in the tested region of Italy, therefore, incidence of USUV infection and neurological disease in humans was much higher than those of WNV. Prevalence of USUV-specific antibodies in healthy blood donors, however, ranged from 0.02% to 1.1% in Italy and Germany from 2010 to 2011.[25,26] The prevalence of USUV may be underestimated due to its high serological cross-reactivity and cocirculation with the closely related WNV and tickborne encephalitis virus (TBEV). In 2013, neuroinvasive infection was found in three patients from Croatia as well.[17]

THE DISEASE

Symptomatic infection of wild birds may be either mild or lead to serious infection or death. Multiorgan failure, especially brain lesions, seems to be the most likely cause of death.[7] Symptoms involve depression, ruffled plumage, half-closed eyes, anorexia, inability to fly, jerky movements, torticollis, nystagmus, incoordination, and seizures, as well as loss of mistrust of humans. These symptoms are associated with brainstem and cortical neuron necrosis.[18,27] Upon necropsy, most birds have marked splenomegaly, mild hepatomegaly, and pulmonary hyperemia. Lesions are very discrete and are composed primarily of neuronal necrosis, leukocytolysis in and around brain blood vessels, myocardial degeneration, coagulative necrosis of the liver and spleen, hyperemia and edema of the lungs, perivascular infiltration of the kidneys, and intestinal inflammation.[7,8,13] USUV infection of domestic chickens and domestic geese, however, leads to minimal pathology.[28,29]

In humans, infection is typically mild. USUV was found in an African patient with fever and rash, and viral RNA was present in an Austrian patient with rash.[13] In a small number of cases, however, infection leads to neurological disease or death.[30,31] In a retrospective survey of over 650 CSF samples collected in 2016 from patients with infectious or neurologic syndromes in France, only 1 CSF sample contained USUV RNA.[31]

In addition to meningitis or meningoencephalitis, symptoms in severe human cases include persistent high fever, headache, hepatitis, or idiopathic facial paralysis (one patient each for the latter two symptoms).[21,31,32] Only one case of neurological disease is known to have occurred in an infected immunocompetent person: a 29-year-old female from Croatia in 2013.[30] The two other cases reported in this outbreak both had comorbidities and were middle-aged (56 and 61 years of age), indicating that disease is not confined to the young and elderly. The immunocompetent woman displayed disorientation and somnolence preceding an elongated period of memory and speech dysfunction. She and the two other patients in this outbreak had nuchal rigidity, hand tremor, and hyperreflexia. Their electroencephalography showed diffusely slow activity. Since USUV neurological signs may be very similar to those of WNV neuroinvasive disease, it is important to consider USUV infection in areas in which both viruses are present.[16,30] Unfortunately, no USUV-specific treatment or vaccines are currently available.[33]

Both African and European strains of USUV upregulate the cellular autophagic pathway by inducing the unfolded protein response. During this pathway, cytoplasmic components are sequestered into double-membrane vesicles where they are degraded and which, under normal circumstances, help to maintain cellular homeostasis as well as limiting the extent of apoptosis. Rapamycin, an inductor of autophagy, increased the virus yield of both USUV strains, while two inhibitors of autophagy decreased virus yield.[34] Rapamycin activates type I IFN production that protects normal adult mice, but not in those animals lacking the IFN receptor or in suckling mice,[35-37] the latter of which develop depression, disorientation, paraplegia, paralysis, and coma.[38] Moderate neuron cell death was also seen in the spinal cords of very young mice, especially in the ventral horns, in addition to multifocal demyelination, while apoptosis was spread throughout the brain, particularly the brain stem, but also in white matter of the cerebellum and medulla, most likely in oligodendrites. This was often in conjunction with primary demyelination.[38] Skeletal muscle appears to be the only location of peripheral USUV replication.

USUV-induced mortality in suckling mice is dose-dependent, with 60% dying after infection with 10^4 plaque-forming units of virus, while all tested adult mice survived at all doses tested.[37,39] Accordingly, while the brains of suckling mice were positive for USUV RNA on day 7 postinfection, no such RNA was detected in the brains of adults. In contrast, suckling and adult mice had higher mortality rates when infected by WNV.[37] USUV infection does not lead to cross-protection against WNV infection in adult mice; however, almost all USUV-infected mice survive infection with a neuro-invasive strain of WNV. Sera from WNV-infected mice also cross-react with USUV, neutralizing both flaviviruses and, upon challenge, protect animals from disease and death.[37] Additionally, immunization with WNV lineage 1 recombinant subviral particles, which share antigenic features with infectious virions, stimulates the production of low levels of USUV-specific antibodies, which are active during subsequent USUV infection.[39] Comparison of multiple USUV strains to WNV defines residues of the E protein that are important or critical to the observed serological cross-reactivity.[40]

THE VIRUS

Most USUV characteristics are typical of other members of the JEV complex of flaviviruses, especially WNV, with which it may interact at the population level. USUV and WNV are antigenically cross-reactive and infect human and animal populations throughout Europe, where they cocirculate in 10 countries. USUV and WNV both infect 34 bird species from 11 orders, including carrion crows, Eurasian blackbirds, Eurasian blackcaps, European robins, and magpies. At least four mosquito species are potential vectors for both flaviviruses, most importantly, *Cx. pipiens* with a feeding preference for blackbirds and Eurasian magpies. USUV-infected *Ae. albopictus* has an expanding geographical range and is also another important vector in urban transmission cycles of DENV.[41] Such cocirculation may alter the epidemiology of these viruses, such as occurred with the displacement of St. Louis encephalitis virus by WNV in the United States and may also increase disease severity, such as the increase in DENV pathology in individuals previously infected by JEV in Thailand.[41]

USUV does not display tropism to any specific cell, tissue, or organ. One study of dead birds in Austria detected viral nucleic acid in brain neurons (100%; $n=40$ birds), proventricular glands (86%; $n=22$), myocardial fibers (73%; $n=33$), renal tubular cells (53%; $n=36$), intestinal tunica muscularis (41%; $n=32$), splenic macrophages (35%; $n=34$), hepatic Kupffer cells (32%; $n=38$), and lungs (21%, $n=34$). USUV is able to grow in cultured cells from a wide range of vertebrates, including humans, monkeys, horses, pigs, rabbits, cattle, dogs, cats, hamsters, rats, and turtles, as well as primary goose embryo fibroblasts. USUV causes cytopathic effect in Vero (monkey), PK-15 (pig), and goose embryo fibroblast cells in vitro.[42] USUV also infects astrocytes, microglia, and neuronal stem cells.[43] The infection rate of human astrocytes and the amount of viral production is greater than that caused by Zika virus, while astrocyte proliferation is decreased. USUV also induces massive amounts of caspase-dependent cell death in neural stem cells ex vivo and a strong anti-USUV immune response that may lead to inflammation.[43]

The USUV reference strain (SAAR-1776; from South African mosquitoes in 1958) is not associated with avian deaths, while European strains have caused massive bird deaths. Austrian and South African isolates, nevertheless, have 97% nucleoside and 99% amino acid identities.[44] Among tested members of the JEV serogroup, USUV is most closely related to Murray Valley encephalitis virus (73% nucleoside and 82% amino acid identities), followed by JEV (71% and 81%), and is furthest from West Nile virus (68% and 75%).

Sequence analysis indicates the existence of at least seven USUV strains with nucleoside and amino acid identities of 96%–99% and 99%, respectively. USUV also shares nucleoside and amino acid identities of 81% and 94%, with an outlier USUV subtype strain, respectively.[45] The first USUV strain isolated from an immunocompromised patient with neuroinvasive disease has overall genome identities of 99% and 96%, respectively, with those of isolates from Europe and Africa. Comparison of the complete human USUV polyprotein sequence to those of bird-derived strains revealed two unique amino acid substitutions, one that is believed to be in the receptor-binding domain of the

E protein. In WNV, substitutions within this domain alter virus infectivity, virulence, antigenicity, and escape from neutralizing antibodies.[46] The other substitution is in a residue in the viral RNA polymerase domain of the NS5 protein. This domain is highly conserved among USUV isolates that are not associated with human infection.[47]

USUV in Birds

At least 62 species of birds are infected by USUV in Europe.[17] Most African viral isolates were derived from mosquitoes or a small number of nonmigratory African birds: hornbills, little greenbuls, and Kurrichane thrushes.[48] Increased African bird deaths due to USUV infection have not been reported.[33] Some European bird species, however, develop life-threatening disease. Several migratory birds, including the common kestrel, Eurasian reed warbler, lesser and common whitethroats, and European pied flycatcher are believed to have introduced USUV into Europe, while other bird species, such as the Eurasian magpie, house sparrow, red junglefowl, and common blackbirds, may have disseminated the virus throughout Europe. USUV causes high mortality rates among several bird species, particularly in blackbirds in most of Europe, but not in Africa or Spain.[17] In a study of dead birds collected in Germany from 2011 to 2013, almost one-third carried USUV and greater than 88% of them were blackbirds. During the same time period, none of more than 900 live migratory and resident birds in the area carried USUV RNA.[49]

Several raptor species, such as the Spanish imperial eagle and the golden eagle, are infected in Spain, putting additional stress on the populations of these already critically endangered birds.[50] Coinfection with both USUV and WNV or other bird flaviviruses is found in several European countries and might result in beneficial or pathogenic antigenic cross-reactivity. USUV is also present in and pathogenic to other European raptor species, including long-eared owls, Egyptian vultures, snowy owls, and Ural owls.[51] Alarmingly, sentinel chickens and some wild, nonmigratory birds in the United Kingdom are seropositive for USUV,[52,53] indicating spread of the virus beyond Africa and continental Europe.

USUV in Mosquitoes

USUV has been detected in a wide range of mosquito species in the genera *Aedes, Anopheles, Culex, Culiseta, Ochlerotatus, Coquillettidia,* and *Mansonia.*[17] While *Cx. naevei* is believed to be the major viral vector in Africa, *Cx. pipiens* is the most common USUV vector in

Europe.[54] The ability of *Cx. pipiens* to act as a vector for USUV was compared to its well-characterized ability to act as a vector for WNV. These northwestern European mosquitoes are highly effective vectors for USUV, with infection rates of 11% at 18°C and an impressive 53% at 23°C, comparable to their infection values for WNV. At the even higher temperature of 28°C, the infection rate of *Cx. pipiens* for USUV was much higher than that for WNV (90% vs 58%, respectively). Furthermore, in 2010, USUV was found to be much more prevalent in birds and mosquitoes in one region of Italy than WNV. *Cx. pipiens* is by far the major USUV vector species in that area. Interestingly, no evidence of human infection was found in over 1000 blood donors.[55] A defined 21-nucleoside small interfering RNA (siRNA) is the major small RNA pathway, which targets both USUV and WNV infections in *Cx. pipiens* mosquitoes.[56] From February–March, 2009–2011, Italian *Cx. pipiens* mosquitoes were not found to be infected with WNV, while USUV-infected mosquitoes were detected during that time period. Both viruses were present in these mosquitoes between May and October. USUV and a smaller number of WNV, however, were found in birds, with USUV being present continuously during this time period.[57] Additionally, year-to-year USUV sequence identity was high. These data suggest that these USUVs are not reintroduced yearly, but overwinter in the region, primarily in birds.

A German study of almost 100,000 mosquitoes from 2011 to 2016 found USUV RNA in *Cx. pipiens* in only 2 of 4144 mosquito pools.[58] These pools contained different USUV lineages. USUV present in one of the mosquito pools belonged to Europe lineage 3, and the other pool belonged to African lineage 3, previously known to be present in northwestern Germany, the Netherlands, Belgium, and France. Members of the Africa 2 strain are also present in Germany and are restricted to the area around Berlin. Multiple USUV strains may also cocirculate in a region. A WNV surveillance program in Northern Italy during 2010–2014 detected USUV nucleoside sequences belonging to two distinct groups, apparently resulting from two different routes of introduction—over the Alps and from Eastern Europe.[5] Europe 3, Africa 2, and Africa 3-like lineages were simultaneously present in Eastern Germany during a large, fatal outbreak in birds. Interestingly, infected *Cx. pipiens* were also present in regions without reports of dead birds.[59] Incidental, dead-end USUV hosts include several mammal species, especially the insectivorous common pipistrelle bats, horses, dogs, and wild boars, although fruit-eating African bats could not be experimentally infected.[17,60]

USUV Groups and Lineages

USUV has been divided into African and European groups that are based upon their geographical origin of isolation.[17] Phylogenetic analysis of the NS5 gene revealed three distinct African lineages in birds or humans.[19,61] African 1 lineage (Africa 1) is composed of only one strain that was isolated in the Central African Republic in 1969. African lineage 2 (Africa 2) originated in South Africa in mid-1940s and contains strains from Senegal, Spain, Germany, and France. African lineage 3 (Africa 3) includes strains from Senegal, Germany, the Netherlands, and Belgium as well as a human isolate from the Central African Republic in 1981.

The European USUV group is also subdivided into several lineages, the majority of which may have resulted from autochthonous evolution of a single common ancestor.[5] European 1 lineage (Europe 1) in birds and human isolates from Italy consists of viral strains from Austria, Hungary, Switzerland, and Senegal. European 2 lineage (Europe 2) strains are present in Italy and the Czech Republic, including the Bologna 2009 strain from a patient with meningoencephalitis. Europe 3 lineage is present in Germany, Belgium, and France; Europe 4 lineage is found in Italy and includes human isolates; and Europe 5 lineage isolates are present in Germany.

Most of the above lineages are highly conserved (genomic identity of 94%). Nevertheless, specific nucleoside mutations do appear, at least in parts of Germany, to arise rapidly, especially in the NS3 region.[59] Mutations are also present in the 5′ UTR of African and European lineages, while highly variable size heterogeneity among the 3′ UTR is found in different USUV lineages. The Bologna/09 strains contain specific mutations that alter tropism to human neurological cells and neuroinvasive capacity.[47] Based upon complete genomic sequencing, a virulent USUV strain isolated in southern Spain in *Cx. perexiguus* mosquitoes in 2009 differs from that isolated from song thrushes in 2012. The latter has not been shown to cause wild bird mortality. This indicates that USUV strains from the same region may vary in their virulence, at least in birds, and suggests that the geographical range and distribution of USUV strains may be much wider than currently known because of possible covert viral cycles in bird hosts and mosquito vectors.[19]

USUV RNA from European birds has high homology to the original South African isolate, but several adaptive mutations were present as well. An examination of RNA from more than 25,000 female mosquitoes (753 pools) from urbanized, human-inhabited areas in Serbia in 2014 detected USUV RNA in 3 pools of *Cx. pipiens* mosquitoes. Due to the sequence identity in a partial NS5 gene, complete genome sequencing was performed on one of these strains. This Serbian sequence is most closely related to USUV Europe 1 strains that emerged in Austria in 2001, in Hungary in 2005, and in Austria in 2006. This strain circulated in Hungary until 2015.[14] This suggests that these USUV strains were introduced once from Africa to Vienna and then spread across Central Europe.[13] Spanish strains of USUV differ genetically from those of Central Europe, suggesting independent introductions from Africa.[13]

THE IMMUNE RESPONSE

Cytokines and Chemokines

Various cytokine and chemokine genes are upregulated during infection of CNS cells by USUV. Some of the genes have a 100-fold greater induction than that caused by ZIKV infection. CNS genes that are induced by USUV infection include those for the cytokines interferon-β (IFN-β) (> 7000 times upregulated), tumor necrosis factor-α, interleukin-12A (IL-12A), IL-15, and IL-6; the chemokines CCL3, CCL5, CXCL8, CXCL10, and CXCL11; CD40, and cathepsin B; and the transcription factors Fos and interferon response factor 7 (IRF7) in USUV-infected astrocytes, as well as the genes producing the pattern recognition receptors retinoic acid-inducible gene-I (RIG-1), laboratory of genetics and physiology 2 (LGP2), and toll-like receptor 3 (TLR3).[43] In contrast, the ZIKV inflammatory profile is more centered on the specific induction of several mitogen-activated protein kinase (MAPK) genes. USUV induction of IFN-β expression is particularly noteworthy since pretreating the cells with type I or III IFN decreases USUV replication in liver cells and kidney cell lines. Decreased viral replication is not seen, however, when IFN is added after infection of these cell lines.[36] In addition to CNS cells, the activity of mature and immature monocyte-derived dendritic cells of the innate immune response is linked to IFN levels during USUV infection. USUV infects these cells and induces IFN-α production and the IFN-stimulated gene 15 pathway to a greater extent than that found in WNV lineages 1 and 2. USUV is also more sensitive to type I and III IFNs than these WNV lineages.[35]

Antibodies

The arrival of USUV in Central Europe in 2001 led, at first, to an increase in avian mortality that lasted until the end of the 2003 transmission cycle. This was followed rapidly by a decrease in USUV-associated deaths from 2004 to 2006, which corresponded to an increased proportion of infected birds having only low levels of virus in their tissues.[9,62] In order to determine the production and protective role of antibodies against USUV, the proportion of 442 primarily juvenile wild birds dying or undergoing seroconversion was studied from 2003 to 2006 in eastern Austria.[62] USUV antibody prevalence was 10% in 2003–2004 and significantly increased in 2005–2006 to greater than 50%. This suggests that humoral immunity plays an important role in decreasing USUV-related avian disease. However, the summers of 2004 and 2005 also had low average temperatures in Austria, which might have played a role in decreased USUV-induced bird deaths (5% or less), in addition to a decrease in virulence of the circulating USUV strain.[62] The rise and fall of disease incidence in wild birds, therefore, is complex and multifactorial.

The above study also examined seropositivity at three time points per year in two highly susceptible species of captive owls, which were housed in open environments at a rehabilitation center. Interestingly, some of the owls had a pronounced drop in antibody titer between subsequent assays in a single year, suggesting that even after natural infection, the antibody response is not long-lasting.[62] Additionally, since USUV and WNV have high amino acid sequence similarity in their E proteins, the main target of flavivirus antibody responses, the presence of both flaviviruses in the same region may cause immunological cross-reactions within their vertebrate hosts, producing either beneficial neutralizing antibodies or a pathogenic antibody-dependent enhancement.[40]

The reduction in pathology of birds in Central Europe in 2004–2006 described earlier could be due to the development of "flock immunity" in susceptible bird groups in which a sufficient number of animals are partially or completely immune to that particular viral strain to inhibit transmission to the few remaining nonimmune birds. Pathology is much less likely to occur in previously infected individuals, as is also the case with JEV and WNV infections.[52,63] Thus, the significant decline of USUV-associated avian mortality parallels increased the numbers of seropositive birds in the region, despite the continuing presence of the virus. While indoor housing of captive birds appears to provide them with protection; it might, however, interfere with the development of flock immunity in wild birds.[13] Additionally, a large number of bird species are infected, produce anti-USUV antibodies, and remain asymptomatic.[33] As mentioned previously, domestic geese and chickens suffer little ill effects from USUV infection.

SURVEILLANCE AND PREVENTION

In some incidences, the presence of USUV in an area has been detected via WNV surveillance programs using mosquitoes, wild birds, and, sometimes, horses. Such programs have been used to examine the temporal and geographical spread of USUV across Europe since USUV and WNV share many serological, biological, and ecoepidemiological characteristics.[5,61] Additionally, the common blackbird is the most important bird reservoir in Europe, while the suspected WNV reservoir in the United States is the American robin.[56,64] Unfortunately, misdiagnosis may occur often in many locales in which differentiation between WNV and USUV is not routinely assessed.[65] It may be advisable to adapt WNV surveillance programs to intentionally screen for USUV in samples from birds, horses, mosquitoes, and humans. Interestingly, long-term surveillance of infected mosquitoes indicates that USUV prevalence in these vectors increases during drought conditions.[55] This knowledge may aid in predicting the areas that need to implement prevention strategies at any given time.

Zoological facilities are important in detecting and monitoring the spread of USUV infection and, possibly, the emergence of new zoonotic infection into a region, using the One Health approach. The Austrian, Italian, and Swiss avian USUV outbreaks were first found in zoos. These facilities have intensive health surveillance programs and trained personnel who can detect early symptoms in captive birds from a wide variety of species with different habitats.[13] Information about the health of individual birds and avian carcasses are also more readily available in captive birds, allowing a more complete understanding of pathology over the course of the disease. The facilities also allow the birds to readily receive supportive care and, when developed, treatment specifically for USUV or for a related flavivirus, such as WNV. Restricting captive birds to indoor areas and treatment against ectoparasites also reduces risk of viral introduction to that population. This may prove to be critical in the case of endangered, susceptible, species of birds.

In light of the modest increase in USUV prevalence in birds and humans in Europe as well as the possibility of further adaptation for survival in the humans, USUV may be one of a growing list of emerging infections of public health concern, especially among the expanding population of immunocompromised people. USUV may also spread to the Americas, as recently occurred for ZIKV.[66,67] Additionally, anticipated increases in temperature could expand the established USUV European foci and initiate large outbreaks in regions currently containing immunologically näive birds.[61] Unfortunately, incentives for preventative measures, such as vaccination development, may be limited due to the small numbers of human cases and the mild symptoms seen in the limited species of domestic fowls tested. This, however, may change rapidly if, as in the case of Zika virus, the virus increases its geographical range or mutates in such a manner as to become more pathogenic.

SUMMARY OVERVIEW

Diseases: asymptomatic to severe neurological disease that is similar to neuroinvasive WNV encephalitis

Causative agent: Usutu virus

Type of agent: member of the Japanese encephalitis virus complex

Vectors: Culex naevei mosquitoes in Africa and *Culex pipiens* mosquitoes in Europe

Common reservoirs: birds (blackbirds in Europe and possibly hornbills, little greenbuls, and Kurrichane thrushes in Africa)

Mode of transmission: mosquito bite

Geographical distribution: Africa and Europe

Year of emergence: 1959 in Africa and 2001 in Europe

REFERENCES

1. Woodall JP. The viruses isolated from arthropods at the East African Virus Research Institute in the 26 years ending December. *Proc E Afr Acad II.* 1964;2:141–146.
2. Nikolay B, Diallo M, Boye CS, Sall AA. Usutu virus in Africa. *Vector Borne Zoonotic Dis.* 2011;11(11):1417–1423.
3. Ayadi T, Hammouda A, Poux A, Boulinier T, Lecollinet S, Selmi S. Evidence of exposure of laughing doves (*Spilopelia senegalensis*) to West Nile and Usutu viruses in Southern Tunisian oases. *Epidemiol Infect.* 2017;145:2808–2816.
4. Weissenböck H, Bakonyi T, Rossi G, Mani P, Nowotny N. Usutu virus, Italy, 1996. *Emerg Infect Dis.* 2013;19:274–277.
5. Calzolari M, Chiapponi C, Bonilauri P, et al. Co-circulation of two Usutu virus strains in Northern Italy between 2009 and 2014. *Infect Genet Evol.* 2017;51:255–262.
6. Weissenböck H, Kolodziejek J, Url A, Lussy H, Rebel-Bauder B, Nowotny N. Emergence of Usutu virus, an African mosquito-borne flavivirus of the Japanese encephalitis virus group, Central Europe. *Emerg Infect Dis.* 2002;8:652–656.
7. Chvala S, Kolodziejek J, Nowotny N, Weissenböck H. Pathology and viral distribution in fatal Usutu virus infections of birds from the 2001 and 2002 outbreaks in Austria. *J Comp Pathol.* 2004;131:176–185.
8. Weissenböck H, Kolodziejek J, Fragner K, Kuhn R, Pfeffer M, Nowotny N. Usutu virus activity in Austria, 2001-2002. *Microbes Infect.* 2003;5:1132–1136.
9. Chvala S, Bakonyi T, Bukovsky C, et al. Monitoring of Usutu virus activity and spread by using dead bird surveillance in Austria, 2003-2005. *Vet Microbiol.* 2007;122:237–245.
10. Bakonyi T, Erdélyi K, Ursu K, et al. Emergence of Usutu virus in Hungary. *J Clin Microbiol.* 2007;45(12):3870–3874.
11. Manarolla G, Bakonyi T, Gallazzi D, et al. Usutu virus in wild birds in Northern Italy. *Vet Microbiol.* 2010;141:159–163.
12. Savini G, Monaco F, Terregino C, et al. Usutu virus in Italy: an emergence or a silent infection? *Vet Microbiol.* 2011;151:264–274.
13. Steinmetz HW, Bakonyi T, Weissenböck H, et al. Emergence and establishment of Usutu virus infection in wild and captive avian species in and around Zurich, Switzerland—genomic and pathologic comparison to other Central European outbreaks. *Vet Microbiol.* 2011;148:207–212.
14. Kemenesi G, Buzás D, Zana B, et al. First genetic characterization of Usutu virus from *Culex pipiens* mosquitoes, Serbia, 2014. *Infect Genet Evol.* 2018;63:58–61.
15. Rijks J, Kik M, Slaterus R, et al. Widespread Usutu virus outbreak in birds in the Netherlands, 2016. *Euro Surveill.* 2016;21:30–39.
16. Tamba M, Bonilauri P, Bellini R, et al. Detection of Usutu virus within a West Nile virus surveillance program in Northern Italy. *Vector Borne Zoonotic Dis.* 2011;11(5):551–557.
17. Gaibani P, Rossini G. An overview of Usutu virus. *Microbes Infect.* 2017;19:382–387.
18. Garigliany M, Linden A, Gilliau G, et al. Usutu virus, Belgium, 2016. *Infect Genet Evol.* 2017;48:116–119.
19. Bakonyi T, Busquets N, Nowotny N. Comparison of complete genome sequences of Usutu virus strains detected in Spain, Central Europe, and Africa. *Vector Borne Zoonotic Dis.* 2014;14(5):324–329.
20. Höfle U, Gamino V, de Mera IG, Mangold AJ, Ortíz JA, de la Fuente J. Usutu virus in migratory song thrushes, Spain. *Emerg Infect Dis.* 2013;19:1173–1175.
21. Cavrini F, Gaibani P, Longo G, et al. Usutu virus infection in a patient who underwent orthotropic liver transplantation, Italy, August-September 2009. *Euro Surveill.* 2009;14(50):9448.
22. Grottola A, Marcacci M, Tagliazucchi S, et al. Usutu virus infections in humans: a retrospective analysis in the municipality of Modena, Italy. *Clin Microbiol Infect.* 2017;23:3337.
23. Rossini G, Cavrini F, Pierro A, et al. First human case of West Nile virus neuroinvasive infection in Italy, September 2008—case report. *Euro Surveill.* 2008;13:19002.
24. Rizzo C, Salcuni P, Nicoletti L, et al. Epidemiological surveillance of West Nile neuroinvasive diseases in Italy, 2008 to 2011. *Euro Surveill.* 2012;17:20172.
25. Pierro A, Gaibani P, Spadafora C, et al. Detection of specific antibodies against West Nile and Usutu viruses in healthy blood donors in Northern Italy, 2010-2011. *Clin Microbiol Infect.* 2013;19:451–453.

26. Allering L, Jöst H, Emmerich P, et al. Detection of Usutu virus infection in a healthy blood donor from south-west Germany, 2012. *Euro Surveill.* 2012;17:20341.

27. Garigliany M-M, Marlier D, Tenner-Racz K, et al. Detection of Usutu virus in a bullfinch (*Pyrrhula pyrrhula*) and a great spotted woodpecker (*Dendrocopos major*) in Northwest Europe. *Vet J.* 2014;199:191–193.

28. Chvala S, Bakonyi T, Hackl R, Hess M, Nowotny N, Weissenböck H. Limited pathogenicity of Usutu virus for the domestic chicken (*Gallus domesticus*). *Avian Pathol.* 2005;34:392–395.

29. Chvala S, Bakonyi T, Hackl R, Hess M, Nowotny N, Weissenböck H. Limited pathogenicity of Usutu virus for the domestic goose (*Anser anser f. domestica*) following experimental inoculation. *J Vet Med B Infect Dis Vet Public Health.* 2006;53:171–175.

30. Santini M, Vilibic-Cavlek T, Barsic B, et al. First cases of human Usutu virus neuroinvasive infection in Croatia, August-September 2013: clinical and laboratory features. *J Neurovirol.* 2015;21(1):92–97.

31. Simonin Y, Sillam O, Carles MJ, et al. Human Usutu virus infection with atypical neurologic presentation, Montpellier, France, 2016. *Emerg Infect Dis.* 2018;24:875–878.

32. Pecorari M, Longo G, Gennari W, et al. First human case of Usutu virus neuroinvasive infection, Italy, August-September 2009. *Euro Surveill.* 2009;14(50):15–16.

33. Pauli G, Bauerfeind U, Blumel J, et al. Usutu virus. *Transfus Med Hemother.* 2014;41(1):73–82.

34. Blázquez A-B, Escribano-Romero E, Merino-Ramos T, Saiz J-C, Martín-Acebes MA. Infection with Usutu virus induces an autophagic response in mammalian cells. *PLoS Negl Trop Dis.* 2013;7(10):e2509.

35. Cacciotti G, Caputo B, Selvaggi C, et al. Variation in interferon sensitivity and induction between Usutu and West Nile (lineages 1 and 2) viruses. *Virology.* 2015;485:189–198.

36. Scagnolari C, Caputo B, Trombetti S, et al. Usutu virus growth in human cell lines: induction of and sensitivity to type I and III interferons. *J Gen Virol.* 2013;94:789–795.

37. Blázquez A-B, Escribano-Romero E, Martín-Acebes MA, Petrovic T, Saiz J-C. Limited susceptibility of mice to Usutu virus (USUV) infection and induction of flavivirus cross-protective immunity. *Virology.* 2015;482:67–71.

38. Weissenböck H, Bakonyi T, Chvala S, Nowotny N. Experimental Usutu virus infection of suckling mice causes neuronal and glial cell apoptosis and demyelination. *Acta Neuropathol.* 2014;108:453–460.

39. Merino-Ramos T, Blazquez AB, Escribano-Romero E, et al. Protection of a single dose West Nile virus recombinant subviral particle vaccine against lineage 1 or 2 strains and analysis of the cross-reactivity with Usutu virus. *PLoS One.* 2014;9(9):e108056.

40. Nikolay B, Fall G, Boye CSB, Sall AA, Skern T. Validation of a structural comparison of the antigenic characteristics of Usutu virus and West Nile virus envelope proteins. *Virus Res.* 2014;189:87–91.

41. Nikolay B. A review of West Nile and Usutu virus co-circulation in Europe: how much do transmission cycles overlap? *Trans R Soc Trop Med Hyg.* 2015;109:609–618.

42. Ashraf U, Ye J, Ruan X, Wan S, Zhu B, Cao S. Usutu virus: an emerging flavivirus in Europe. *Viruses.* 2015;7:219–238.

43. Salinas S, Constant O, Desmetz C, et al. Deleterious effect of Usutu virus on human neural cells. *PLoS Negl Trop Dis.* 2017;11(9), e0005913.

44. Bakonyi T, Gould EI, Kolodziejek J, Weissenbock H, Nowotny N. Complete genome analysis and molecular characterization of Usutu virus that emerged in Austria in 2001: comparison with the South African strain SAAR-1776 and other flaviviruses. *Virology.* 2004;328:301–310.

45. Nikolay B, Dupressoir A, Firth C, et al. Comparative full length genome sequence analysis of Usutu virus isolates from Africa. *Virol J.* 2013;10:217.

46. Chu JJ, Rajamanonmani R, Li J, Bhuvanakantham R, Lescar J, Ng ML. Inhibition of West Nile virus entry by using a recombinant domain III from the envelope glycoprotein. *J Gen Virol.* 2005;86:405–412.

47. Gaibani P, Cavrini F, Gould EA, et al. Comparative genomic and phylogenetic analysis of the first Usutu virus isolate from a human patient presenting with neurological symptoms. *PLoS One.* 2013;8(5):e64761.

48. CDC Arbocat. *USUV;* 2012. www.cdc.gov/arbocat/catalog-listing.asp?VirusID=503&SI=1. Accessed September 19, 2012.

49. Ziegler U, Jöst H, Müller K, et al. Epidemic spread of Usutu virus in Southwest Germany in 2011 to 2013 and monitoring of wild birds for Usutu and West Nile viruses. *Vector Borne Zoonotic Dis.* 2015;15(8):481–488.

50. Jiménez-Clavero MA, Sotelo E, Fernandez-Pinero J, et al. West Nile virus in golden eagles, Spain, 2007. *Emerg Infect Dis.* 2008;14:1489–1491.

51. Jurado-Tarifa E, Napp S, Lecollinet S, et al. Monitoring of West Nile virus, Usutu virus and Meaban virus in waterfowl used as decoys and wild raptors in Southern Spain. *Comp Immunol Microbiol Infect Dis.* 2016;49:58–64.

52. Buckley A, Dawson A, Moss SR, Hinsley SA, Bellamy PE, Gould EA. Serological evidence of West Nile virus, Usutu virus and Sindbis virus infection of birds in the UK. *J Gen Virol.* 2003;84:2807–2817.

53. Buckley A, Dawson A, Gould EA. Detection of seroconversion to West Nile virus, Usutu virus and Sindbis virus in UK sentinel chickens. *Virol J.* 2006;3:71.

54. Mancini G, Montarsi F, Calzolari M, et al. Mosquito species involved in the circulation of West Nile and Usutu viruses in Italy. *Vet Ital.* 2017;53(2):97–110.

55. Calzolari M, Gaibani P, Bellini R, et al. Mosquito, bird and human surveillance of West Nile and Usutu viruses in Emilia-Romagna region (Italy) in 2010. *PLoS One.* 2012;7(5):e38058.

56. Fros JJ, Miesen P, Vogels CB, et al. Comparative Usutu and West Nile virus transmission potential by local *Culex pipiens* mosquitoes in North-Western Europe. *One Health.* 2015;1:31–36.

57. Calzolari M, Bonilauri P, Bellini R, et al. Usutu virus persistence and West Nile virus inactivity in the Emilia-Romagna region (Italy) in 2011. *PLoS One.* 2013;8(5), e63978.

58. Scheuch DE, Schäfer M, Eiden M, et al. Detection of Usutu, Sindbis, and Batai viruses in mosquitoes (Diptera: Culicidae) collected in Germany, 2011-2016. *Viruses.* 2018;10:389.

59. Sieg M, Schmidt V, Ziegler U, et al. Outbreak and cocirculation of three different Usutu virus strains in Eastern Germany. *Vector Borne Zoonotic Dis.* 2017;17:662–664.

60. Simpson DIH, O'Sullivan JP. Studies on arboviruses and bats (Chiroptera) in East Africa. I. Experimental infection of bats and virus transmission attempts in *Aedes (Stegomyia) aegypti. Ann Trop Med Parasitol.* 1968;62:422–431.

61. Cadar D, Lühken R, van der Jeugd H, et al. Widespread activity of multiple lineages of Usutu virus, Western Europe, 2016. *Euro Surveill.* 2017;22:30452.

62. Meiste T, Lussy H, Bakonyi T, et al. Serological evidence of continuing high Usutu virus (Flaviviridae) activity and establishment of herd immunity in wild birds in Austria. *Vet Microbiol.* 2008;127:237–248.

63. Endy TP, Nisalak A. Japanese encephalitis virus: ecology and epidemiology. *Curr Top Microbiol Immunol.* 2002;267:11–48.

64. Kilpatrick AM, Daszak P, Jones MJ, Marra PP, Kramer AD. Host heterogeneity dominates West Nile virus transmission. *Proc Biol Sci.* 2006;273:2327–2333.

65. Beck C, Jimenez-Claverom MA, Leblond A, et al. Flaviviruses in Europe: complex circulation patterns and their consequences for the diagnosis and control of West Nile disease. *Int J Environ Res Public Health.* 2013;10:6049–6083.

66. Tetr A. Is Usutu virus ready for prime time? *Microbes Infect.* 2017;19:380–381.

67. Paniz-Mondolfi AE, Villamil-Gómez WE, Rodríguez-Morales AJ. Usutu virus infection in Latin America: a new emerging threat. *Travel Med Infect Dis.* 2017;4:641–643.

CHAPTER 7

Murray Valley Encephalitis Virus

INTRODUCTION

Murray Valley encephalitis virus (MVEV) is one of several mosquito-borne flaviviruses of the Japanese encephalitis virus complex that causes severe disease in humans. It is restricted to a small region of Oceania and, with the exception of travel-related cases, has been exclusively reported in Australia and Papua New Guinea. It is endemic in tropical portions of the Northern Territory and Kimberley region of Western Australia, found periodically in Central Australia and occasionally in southeastern regions of the continent. Kunjin virus is another mosquito-borne encephalitic flavivirus found in Australia and is a subset of West Nile virus (WNV). WNV and Kunjin virus are the subject of separate chapters.

Although relatively rarely reported, Murray Valley encephalitis (MVE) has a high mortality rate and almost half of the survivors have long-term or permanent neurological disease. Disease occurs primarily during times of mosquito activity during the wet season (December–June), especially in years with above-average amounts of rainfall or flooding.

Given the remoteness of some of the areas in which MVE is found and its presence among Aboriginal populations, disease incidence is most likely underreported. MVE may also be misdiagnosed as infection with Kunjin virus. Due to its high morbidity and mortality rates and its propensity to cause outbreaks, MVEV is a potential threat to not only Australia and Papua New Guinea, but also other, surrounding regions of Oceania. Fortunately, infections in sentinel chickens often are detected prior to human cases and may provide important warning of impending outbreaks, especially if these affected regions experience increased rainfall. These factors suggest that MVEV is an excellent candidate for study by the One Health Initiative.

HISTORY

During the summers of 1917–18, 1922, and 1950–51, outbreaks of severe, highly lethal encephalitis were reported in eastern Australia. The first case of this disease, originally named Australian X disease, was reported in October 1916 in New South Wales. Over the next 17 months, 184 additional cases were reported, most of which were from the Murray Valley region or in Queensland. During the 1922 outbreak, at least 75 cases were reported throughout Queensland. Fatality rates for these epidemics averaged 68% and were most frequent in children under the age of 15 years. Infections in males were more common than in females. Another major epidemic of 45 encephalitis cases occurred in the Murray Valley region during the summers of 1950–51 with similar characteristics. This disease was subsequently named Murray Valley encephalitis and is believed to be identical to Australian X encephalitis.[1]

MVEV was first isolated during the 1951 epidemic in southeast Australia. Previously, MVE cases were present in large outbreaks in eastern Australia. The disease was first reported in Papua New Guinea in 1956. The next major epidemic of 58 cases occurred in 1974, with early cases widely scattered along the Murray Valley.[1] This outbreak was preceded by the detection of antibodies against MVEV in domestic fowl in the beginning of February 1974, prior to the first human case being reported in Queensland. Antibodies to MVEV in sentinel chickens were also found prior to human cases in a 1993 outbreak, suggesting the potential usefulness of sentinel chickens to warn about potential outbreaks in both endemic and nonendemic regions, and appear to have a greater predictive value in rural than in urban areas.[2,3] Since 1974, most symptomatic human infections moved across the continent and are being reported in Western Australia, primarily as outbreaks after heavy rainfall events, notably in 2011. The correlation between heavy rainfall or flooding and the seroconversion of sentinel chickens may be the most useful predictive model of subsequent human infections in a region; however, this model is not absolute.[3] Another factor that may play an important role in human infections by MVEV is the ability of virus to survive the dry season, due to the desiccation-resistance of *Aedes* mosquito species eggs.[4] While *Culex* species remain the major MVEV vectors, several *Aedes* species serve as MVEV vectors.

MVEV and the Kunjin type of WNV underwent a 26-year absence from Central Australia between 1976 and March and April of 2000, when five laboratory-confirmed cases of flavivirus-associated encephalitis were reported in Aboriginal populations from remote

Zika and Other Neglected and Emerging Flaviviruses. https://doi.org/10.1016/B978-0-323-82501-6.00003-7

communities in the normally dry inland region near Alice Springs, the largest township in Central Australia and a major tourist center. This was preceded or accompanied by seroconversion of sentinel chickens in northern Western Australia in early January, in the Northern Territory in late February, in Tennant Creek in early March, and in Alice Springs in late March. The appearance of these cases followed unusually high amounts of rainfall from a tropical cyclone. These conditions led to a sharp rise in the numbers of the common banded mosquito (*Culex annulirostris*), another MVEV vector, at multiple rural sites in Central Australia, beginning in January 2000 and remaining high to very high until early April.[5] More MVE cases were reported during the following wet season in both Aboriginals and Caucasians in the urban Alice Springs.[6] Interestingly, most of the Aboriginal cases were among children. The low incidence of disease in Aboriginal adults may result from high infection rates during childhood, rendering the adults resistant to WNV infection.[5] After the year 2000, disease incidence has shifted more toward non-Aboriginal populations, perhaps due to increased mining, agriculture, and tourism in northern Australia.[7]

In 2011, after record high levels of rainfall, MVEV activity was present in all mainland states of Australia and caused 17 human encephalitis and numerous equine disease cases.[8] In the 2011 epidemic, unlike earlier outbreaks, the majority of cases were non-Aboriginal adults. This may be indicative of a change in the demographics of MVE cases and suggests a risk of the virus expanding its range to include the heavily populated areas of southeastern Australia.[9]

The first reported case of MVE in Europe was in a young German male who had visited the Northern Territory of Australia prior to his return to Europe in May of 2001.[9] Despite severe illness, he fully recovered after 2 months. The 2011 epidemic in Australia caused at least one travel-associated case, in a healthy 19-year-old Canadian woman who visited, among other places, Darwin, in the tropical region of Top End in the Northern Territory, and Alice Springs in Central Australia.[10] Upon her return to Canada, she was drowsy, confused, and febrile. Despite administration of high-dose intravenous ceftriaxone, vancomycin, and acyclovir, she continued to experience progressive neurological deterioration. Despite the absence of MVEV in cultures of blood, urine, cerebrospinal fluid (CSF), and respiratory secretions, her condition continued to decline and she became deeply comatose with progressively worsening seizures that were refractory to treatment prior to her death. Upon autopsy, she was found to have had lymphocytic myocarditis, pulmonary

edema, and acute tubular necrosis of the kidney as well as congestion of the liver and spleen.[10] These two travel-related cases demonstrate the possibility of acquiring severe or fatal MVE when visiting endemic areas of Australia, even though both patients were young and previously healthy. It is imperative, therefore, to include recent travel in the diagnosis of patients with encephalitis. It should also be noted that travel-related infections may be much more common than realized, since MVEV infections are typically asymptomatic, as discussed below.

THE DISEASES

Human infections with MVEV are usually asymptomatic, with only a small number of those infected developing clinical disease, including fever with headache, irritability, seizures, altered state of consciousness, or encephalitis. The latter is associated with high mortality and morbidity. Outcomes have included cognitive impairment, hypotonia, and quadriplegia.[6] The CSF often contains proteins, as well as neutrophils and monocytes. Other symptoms of infection include respiratory failure resulting from brain stem involvement and respiratory muscle paralysis, requiring supportive ventilation. Seizures are the predominant manifestations in children, while adults usually present with more typical encephalitic symptoms.[11] Cranial nerve palsies, especially those involving the seventh nerve, are found in 50% of cases. Movement disorders are significant in 40% of patients and include choreiform movements, Parkinsonism and other tremors, as well as flaccid paralysis.[11] Necrosis of white matter, the thalamus, and the cerebellar cortex can occur later in the course of the disease.[12]

Only 0.1%–0.2% of MVEV infections result in encephalitis; however, approximately 20% of those cases are fatal and permanent neurological sequelae are seen in about half of the survivors.[5] Encephalitis is reported primarily among Aboriginal children, tourists, and newcomers to the region.[13] Disease clusters have been present sporadically in Australia for the past 100 years. These outbreaks are reported every few years and are seasonal, occurring during or following the wet season of February to May.[9] Approximately one-third of MVE patients completely recover. Fatalities are most common in infants less than 2 years of age and those over the age of 60.[5]

In the CNS, MVEV only infects neurons and has not been found in glial cells, the ependyma, the choroid plexus, or meninges.[14] Microscopic analysis of the brains of MVEV-infected mice reveals necrosis in the olfactory bulb and hippocampus neurons by 5 days postinfection, proliferation of the endoplasmic reticulum (ER) and Golgi apparatus membranes, and abnormal membrane-bound tubular and spherical vesicles structures in the ER cisternae similar to those present in other flaviviruses. After 7–8 days, apoptotic neurons are seen, particularly in the hippocampus and, late in the course of infection, apoptotic immune cells are also prominent.[15] Mortality rate in these infected mice correlates with the presence of inflammatory cells, especially neutrophils, but also includes some lymphocytes and macrophages.

In a 2007–2011 study of nine encephalitis patients with altered mental state and seizures, tremor, weakness, or paralysis, all of the patients had elevated levels of C-reactive protein in the blood and most patients developed peripheral neutrophilia and thrombocytosis, as well as acute liver injury with raised ALT and creatine kinase levels. Bilateral cerebral peduncle involvement was also detected by early magnetic resonance imaging (MRI); however, only one patient had an abnormal CT scan early during the illness.[16] T1-weighted MRIs reveal bilateral, symmetrical, thalamic hypointensity with prominence of the ventricles. Thalamic hyperintensity may also be seen with involvement of the red nucleus, substantia nigra, and cervical cord; however, T2-weighted MRIs of patients with MVE are similar to those present during infection with JEV, while other related flaviviruses have a lower propensity to involve the thalamus.[17] Patients without MRI hyperintensity during acute illness had better neurological outcomes, whether or not they had leptomeningeal enhancement. In contrast, patients with widespread abnormalities involving the thalamus, midbrain, and cerebral cortex or cerebellum typically had severe neurological outcomes.[16] Of note: in a 2005 case report, a man living in the Northwest Territory who had recently camped in northeastern Kimberley presented with symptoms clinically and radiologically characteristic of herpes simplex encephalitis, with MRI temporal lobe changes indicative of herpes infection, rather than MVEV.[18] Serological findings demonstrated the presence of anti-MVEV IgM, however, as well as a hemagglutination inhibition antibody titer of 1:1280.

In a 2016 report of 39 survivors of MVEV infection, the long-term sequelae include paralysis or paresis in nine patients, which was more common and severe in those under the age of 5 years, requiring lengthy hospitalization. This differs from WNV encephalitis in which children typically have less severe disease.[19] Two of these patients died due to complications of quadriplegia. Two patients who were discharged with neurological sequelae required no further hospitalizations but reported ongoing cognitive dysfunction and inability to work.[20] This is similar to findings in long-term survivors of WNV infection, who also report cognitive dysfunction, memory loss, and poor physical health lasting up to 8 years, especially in those people initially presenting with neuroinvasive disease.[21,22]

Inborn resistance to flaviviruses in wild mice and in some laboratory strains of mice is conferred by the chromosome 5 locus *flv*, while some susceptible mouse strains have a nonsense mutation in this gene.[23] Strains of MVE-susceptible mice harbor a high viral RNA load in their brains. Viral load was reduced in the cortex, olfactory bulb, thalamus, and hypothalamus of congenic resistant mice with an active *flv* gene. Low amounts of MVEV RNA from resistant mice carrying the *flv* gene were confined to the cerebral cortex, thalamus, and olfactory tuberculum. No viral RNA was detected in the hippocampus, pons, medulla oblongata, or cerebellum of resistant mice. The brains of resistance mice also had only mild inflammation, with lower numbers of inflammatory cells, and lower induction of the *IFN I/II* and *TNF-α* genes than in mice lacking functional *flv*.[23]

THE VIRUS

Contributions of MVEV E and NS1 Proteins to Disease

Flaviviruses' E protein not only takes part in viral tropism and pathogenesis, but also serves as a primary target for neutralizing antibodies. Its hinge region at the base of domain II permits the pH-dependent conformational change required for endosomal fusion and hemagglutination activity.[14,24] A MVEV neutralization escape variant with a substitution of a hydrophobic for the normally hydrophilic E protein residue 277 has low neuroinvasiveness and neurovirulence in mice inoculated intraperitoneally, but not following intracerebral inoculation. It also exhibits low hemagglutination activity. This variant replicates more slowly in cell culture early during infection compared to wild-type virus. While it enters human and mosquito cells in vitro at the same rate as wild-type virus, it has reduced pH-dependent fusion to endosomal membranes during receptor-mediated endocytosis, requiring pH 6.2, rather than pH 6.4, for activity.[25] Specific mutations in this E protein gene region attenuate the virus and block neuroinvasion.[26] The tip of domain II also plays a role in fusion, while the highly hydrophilic lateral face of domain III may or may not be vital to integrin binding to the virus' cell receptor and subsequent entry into target cells, dependent upon host cell type.[26,27]

Another MVEV variant differs from wild-type virus by a single substitution at residue l41 of the E protein, leading to a 100-fold decrease in neuroinvasiveness, but not neurovirulence, in 21-day-old mice inoculated intraperitoneally.[28] This variant also has decreased infectivity and viral yield in mosquito cells in vitro.

In general, the flaviviruses' NS1 protein translocates to the lumen of the endoplasmic reticulum and forms a stable homodimer. Dimerization changes NS1 from a hydrophilic to amphipathic protein associated with cell membranes. Dimerization or oligomerization is believed to be necessary for MVEV replication. By contrast, substitution of a proline at residue 250 in NS1 of Kunjin virus eliminated dimerization without loss of virus replication. The same substitution in an infectious clone of MVEV produced high levels of monomeric, but not dimeric NS1.[29] Replication of this mutant occurs slowly in cultured cells and is accompanied by loss of neuroinvasiveness in weanling mice inoculated intraperitoneally. Residue 250 in NS1 thus appears to be required for the dimerization of at least several members of the Japanese encephalitis virus complex.

MVEV Vectors and Transmission

MVEV is the most important cause of arbovirus encephalitis in Australia.[30] It is maintained by an enzootic cycle of infection between mosquitoes and waterfowl, particularly members of the avian order Ciconiiformes, such as herons and egrets, which are the major vertebrate hosts. This endemic cycle is found in the Kimberley region of Western Australia, the tropical Top End of the Northern Territory, and northern Queensland. The virus periodically expands out of these areas when flooding allows infected migrating waterfowl to introduce the virus into other bird and mosquito populations.[6] While *Cx. annulirostris* is the major vector of MVEV in Australia, several other mosquito genera, including *Anopheles* and *Ochlerotatus*, also transmit the virus.[6] *Cx. fatigans*, *Cx. australicus*, *Aedes notoscriptus*, *Ae. sagax*, and *Ae. vigilax* may also transmit MVEV. The latter has also been infected by feeding on a viremic chicken. Infected male *Ae. tremulus* mosquitoes have been trapped in the Kimberley region as well,[31,32] suggesting that transovarial transmission may occur in at least this mosquito species.

New Zealand lies in close proximity to Australia and is only known to harbor one endemic arbovirus, Whataroa virus, an alphavirus. Two Australian mosquito species that are able to transmit MVEV were introduced into New Zealand—*Ae. notoscriptus* and *Cx. quinquefasciatus*.[33] *Ae. notoscriptus* was introduced

during the 1920s and resides predominantly in urban and semiurban areas throughout the North Island and isolated areas of the South Island. While these mosquitoes may become infected with MVEV, they do not disseminate the virus in the cool temperatures present in New Zealand. *Cx. quinquefasciatus* mosquitoes were first found in New Zealand in 1848. They are present on the North and the South Islands, typically in and around urban settings, and overwinter as larvae from May to September. It appears to be the only mosquito species known to be a potential, competent vector for MVEV in New Zealand.[33]

MVEV in Humans and Other Mammals

Between 1989 and 1993, a cross-sectional and longitudinal study of a remote Aboriginal community of 250–300 people in northwestern Australia was tested annually for antibodies to MVEV.[34] Of the 249 people tested, 52.6% were seropositive, with a high proportion of the population seroconverting during the course of the study until almost everyone tested positive. The proportion of seropositive people increased with age, and males were slightly more likely to be seropositive than females.[34] Additionally, the clinical/subclinical ratio in this location and time frame was lower than was previously reported. Mosquito collections during a time of heavy rainfall in May 1993 revealed a very high minimum infection rate of 8.9/1000 mosquitoes, particularly *Cx. annulirostris*.[34]

In addition to humans, other mammals may be infected by MVEV.[35] When inoculated intracranially, MVEV causes fatal disease in suckling and weaned mice, infant rats, infant and adult sheep, horses, monkeys, young chickens, domestic ducks, and silver gulls. Several types of young animals that were infected by exposure to infected *Cx. annulirostris* mosquitoes were placed into four groups, dependent upon their viremic responses. Gray kangaroos ($n = 14$) and rabbits ($n = 24$) were placed in the high viremic group; pigs ($n = 24$), dogs ($n = 11$), and chickens ($n = 12$) were in the moderate group; and calves ($n = 12$), lambs ($n = 36$), and Agile wallabies ($n = 9$) were in the group with lowest viremia.[1,35,36]

Genetic Variance and MVEV Virulence

Analysis of 21 isolates of MVEV from Australia and Papua New Guinea from 1972 to 1984 revealed that most Australian isolates can be grouped into clusters linked by a similarity coefficient of greater than 75%, indicative of substantial homogeneity.[37] Previous studies of the genetic differentiation of 12 MVEV isolates found substantial genetic and phenotypic homogeneity among various MVEV isolates that differed greatly in geographic location and time. One MVEV variant found in various parts of Western Australia between 1972 and 2003 was nearly identical to a variant from northern Queensland, with only a 3.9% change in the E protein during that time period.[38,39] Greater divergence was found between some isolates from Papua New Guinea and Australia.[38] Interestingly, some MVEV isolates from the Western Province of Papua New Guinea in 1998 had greater similarity to Australian isolates than to other Papua New Guinea isolates from 1956 and 1966. This suggests a more recent flow of MVEV between these two parts of Oceania, perhaps due to the movement of wild waterbirds.[39] A separate, less virulent MVEV variant is restricted to the northeast Kimberley region of Western Australia.[39] It differs from other isolates in virulence and replication efficiency. By contrast, the molecular weight and peptide maps of the E and C proteins from MVEV, WNV, and Rocio virus differ greatly from each other, despite their being closely related serologically and belonging to the same flavivirus serocomplex.[40]

Despite the pronounced general homogeneity among MVEV isolates, several naturally occurring variants of MVEV do, nevertheless, exist with minor genetic differences that have led to major differences in virulence. McMinn et al.[25] compared two MVEV variants: a pathogenic field variant with a high level of neuroinvasiveness and a variant having a low level of neuroinvasiveness. The former differs from the latter by a single amino acid at residue 277 of the E glycoprotein. In weanling Swiss mice infected with these variants via the footpad route, the pathogenic form was present in draining lymph nodes by 24 h postinoculation, in serum between 36 and 72 h, and in the CNS by day 4, reaching maximum CNS titers (10^9 plaque-forming units/g) between days 6 and 9. All mice developed encephalitis and died prior to day 10. These mice had inflammatory cell infiltration into the cerebral cortex. CNS pathogenesis involved virus- and cytokine-mediated neuron toxicity and inflammatory edema. The attenuated MVEV variant, by contrast, was never detected in the draining lymph nodes of infected mice and was found in the serum between 60 and 72 h, and in the CNS by day 7, with a 300-fold lower titer than that of the pathogenic form. It could not be isolated from any host tissue after day 10. Most mice infected with this variant developed a subclinical infection with a mortality rate of less than 1%. Recovery was associated with the appearance of a high-titer serum anti-MVEV IgG response. Delayed entry into the CNS appeared to allow the production of neutralizing antibodies soon enough to prevent or mitigate neurological disease. Although both viral variants entered the CNS via the olfactory lobes, the pathogenic form spread throughout the CNS, while the attenuated form did not leave the olfactory lobes or adjacent structures.[24] Interestingly, viral growth rates, percentages of mortality, and average survival times were similar for these two variants when inoculated into mice intracranially.

A separate study attenuated the MVEV prototype strain in vitro by multiple passages through human cells and found several variants with alterations in residue 390 (normally Asp390) in the E protein, part of an Arg-Gly-Asp (RGD) sequence in a highly conserved, strongly hydrophilic region in flaviviruses.[41] Three mutants (Gly390, Ala390, and His390) had pronounced growth differences in comparison with wild-type virus when propagated in mammalian or mosquito cells. The alterations in cell tropism correlate with differences in entry kinetics and result in greater dependence on glycosaminoglycans during attachment to different mammalian cell types, as evidenced by their increased susceptibility to heparin during infection. These differences result in a 50- to 100-fold growth decrease in Vero and C6/36 cells and a 10-fold enhancement of growth in SW13 cells. Additionally, the Gly390 and His390 mutants are not virulent in mice, due to their loss of neuroinvasiveness and, perhaps, inefficient replication in extraneural tissues.[27]

Glycosaminoglycan-binding variants are removed 20 times more rapidly from the bloodstream of inoculated mice than from wild-type viruses. They are unable to spread into the brain following extraneural inoculation, likely due to the lack of sufficient magnitude or duration of viremia necessary for entry into the brain parenchyma. Since these variants have substitutions in Asp390, they have higher net positive charges. This residue may be part of a receptor-binding domain involved in virus attachment to sulfated proteoglycans.[42] In addition to demonstrating the relevance of this portion of the E protein to virulence, the above studies also suggest the possibility of adopting this type of attenuated MVEV variant for vaccination purposes. Along this line, it is important to note that viral variants selected by serial passage in different cell lines that were derived from different animal species lead to different genetic changes in the E protein.[28] During vaccine development, passage through some cell lines may result in variants that provide better protection against MVEV infection or pathology than do others, perhaps due to differences in the animal species of origin or in the cell types themselves.

MVEV Genotypes

MVEVs may be divided into four genotypes, G1–G4, with G1 and G2 being of more contemporary origin. G1 is the dominant genotype in mainland Australia and, recently, has been found in Papua New Guinea. G2 consists almost exclusively of mosquito isolates from the Kimberley region of Western Australia plus one reported human case.[39,43] G3 and G4 originated in Papua New Guinea and are each represented by a single strain. Both G3 and G4 virus genotypes are believed to be either not currently circulating or extinct.[44] Williams et al.[45] determined the full-length genomic sequences of the prototype strains of each genotype. The G2 strain was isolated from *Cx. annulirostris* mosquitoes from the Kimberley region in 1973. The only known G3 strain was isolated from the brain of a fatal human case in Port Moresby in 1956, while the only known G4 Papua New Guinea strain was isolated from a mixture of trapped culicine mosquitoes from the Sepik River region in 1966. The RNA of each strain was prepared from extracts of infected Vero kidney cell culture supernatants. These sequences are available on GenBank.[45] Among other findings, the G2 strain's genome was found to be the shortest by approximately 50 nucleosides and has a 63-nucleoside deletion in the highly variable region downstream of the open reading frame.[45] A recent study sequenced the complete genome of a MVEV G2 genotype from a patient in the Northern Territory.[43] This is the first such complete sequence of MVEV from CSF as well as the first demonstrated human infection by a G2 genotype virus. It should be pointed out that while the location, date of original isolation, and host species differ among the viral genotypes, in addition to possible alterations during passage through Vero cells prior to analysis, having complete genomes may allow possible links in RNA sequences to be associated with viral virulence.

Williams et al.[44] sequenced the entire prM and E genes from 66 MVEV strains, which had been isolated over 60 years (1951–2011) from various Australian regions. G1 was divided into two distinct sublineages (1A and 1B), with G1A containing Australian and Papua New Guinea strains. Australian G1A virus is found only in Kimberly in northwest Australia, while G1B has the most widespread distribution in Australia. Molecular clock analysis suggests that G2 is the oldest lineage, while G1 viruses diverged more recently. Both older and more recent G2 isolates have relatively low virulence following intraperitoneal inoculation into mice.[44] Both G1 and G2 contemporary lineages are present in the Kimberley region, suggesting that MVEV's enzootic focus is in northwestern Australia, following the construction of the Ord River Dam and the creation of Lake Argyle in the early 1970s. These environments attract large numbers of waterbirds and provide year-round conditions amenable to maintaining the MVEV transmission cycle.[32] Taken together, the above studies should aid in future research to identify factors influencing genetic evolution and variation within and between the MVEV genotypes over time and in different locations.

Superinfection Exclusion

A new group of insect-specific flaviviruses has been recently discovered. One novel species, Palm Creek virus, is present in Australia and was isolated from *Coquillettidia xanthogaster* mosquitoes. Prior infection of a mosquito cell line with Palm Creek virus suppressed subsequent replication of MVEV 10- to 43-fold, indicative of superinfection exclusion.[46] It should be noted that this species of mosquito is not a known vector of MVEV.

IMMUNE RESPONSE

While an intact immune response is necessary for viral clearance, it may also be pathological, leading to inflammation or antibody-dependent enhancement (ADE) of infection, as exemplified by different dengue serotypes. Replication of flaviviruses in the CNS leads to an intense meningeal, perivascular, and parenchymal inflammatory cell response. Injury and destruction of neurons are due, in part, to the adherence of phagocytic neutrophils and macrophages of the innate immune system to infected neurons. Following peripheral infection of weanling mice with MVEV, viruses enter the CNS, and within 5 days, the mice develop encephalitis. This is associated with a primarily neutrophilic inflammatory response in the infected perivascular regions and the brain parenchyma induced by increased levels of the proinflammatory cytokine tumor necrosis factor-α and the neutrophil-attracting chemokine N51/KC in the CNS. The neutrophils then activate their inducible nitric oxide synthase (iNOS), leading to the production of reactive nitrogen species nitric oxide within the CNS. Nitric oxide impairs neuronal functions and increases permeability of the BBB. Either depletion of neutrophils or inhibition of iNOS activity prolongs survival time in mice and decreases mortality, thus implicating neutrophils and reactive nitrogen species in neuronal cell death.[47] Inhibition of iNOS has similar effects in TBEV-infected mice.[48] Interestingly, less than 0.1% of MVEV-infected neurons become apoptotic.[47] This is in contrast to mice infected by DENV or JEV, in which apoptosis plays an important role in neuronal death. It also conflicts with the numerous apoptotic neurons found by Mathews[15] in several regions of the hippocampus of MVEV-infected mice.

Vaccines and Adaptive Immunity

Several vaccination strategies against MVEV were tested in mouse model systems and helped to delineate the aspects of adaptive immunity that are important for protection against MVEV infection and disease. A vaccine incorporating the structural proteins prM and E as well as the nonstructural proteins NS1 and NS2A was inoculated by the intracranial route into hybrid mice that are heterozygous for the flavivirus resistance allele flv^r. Vaccination resulted in reduced viral replication in the brain. These vaccinated mice were completely protected from challenge with 1000 infectious units of MVEV. The protection in this model system was mediated by neutralizing antibody to the E protein, without the necessity for a $CD8^+$ T killer cell response.[49] It should be noted, however, that studies using these hybrid mice may not reflect MVEV infection in normal or immunocompromised animals.

Other studies examined possible production of cross-protective immunity following immunization with JEV. One such study revealed that mice immunized with JEV actually died much sooner after challenge with MVEV than mock-immunized mice, suggesting possible development of ADE.[50] Passive immunization of mice with subneutralizing concentrations of heterologous JEV antiserum was subsequently found to result in increased viremia and mortality after subsequent challenge with MVEV in vivo, despite the lack of significant differences in the time taken during virus entry or in the magnitude of virus replication in the brain compared to control animals. In contrast, when higher, neutralizing levels of JEV antiserum were used, protective immunity was achieved.[23] Passive immunization of young mice with IgG from MVEV-immune human sera or sera from adult mice infected with sublethal amounts of MVEV also protected them from lethal intraperitoneal challenge.[50] These findings indicate that caution is needed in designing JEV and MVEV vaccination programs in regions, such as Australia and Papua New Guinea, in which MVEV and other JEV flavivirus family members cocirculate.[51]

Lobigs et al.[52] examined several other JEV-based vaccines for cross-protective activity against MVEV. One of these (ChimeriVax-JE) is a chimeric vaccine composed of the yellow fever virus 17D vaccine cDNA whose prM and E proteins are replaced by those from an attenuated JEV strain. A single dose of this live, chimeric vaccine completely protected animals upon subsequent challenge with MVEV in two mouse model systems (high-dose extraneural challenge of adult B6 mice and low-dose challenge of immunodeficient mice lacking type I IFN activity). It is also cross-protective against WNV. This vaccine elicits humoral and cellular immunity, both of which are protective following lethal challenge with MVEV. Importantly, this vaccine is safe to use in immunodeficient mice. A licensed, inactivated JEV vaccine tested in parallel (JE-Vax), however, led to ADE in mice upon challenge with MVEV when the vaccine was given on a low-dose schedule.[52]

Using a different strategy, vaccinating mice with either vaccinia vectors or naked DNA vectors encoding the MVEV prM and E proteins produces long-lived MVEV-neutralizing, protective humoral immunity.[49,53] DNA vectors delivered intradermally to mice using a gene gun produced long-lived, virus-neutralizing IgG1 antibody responses that protected all mice from death following challenge with high-titer MVEV. Gene gun inoculation also stimulates the production of the Th2 cytokine interleukin-4 (IL-4). While intramuscular DNA inoculation by needle also induced MVEV-specific antibodies able to resist challenge with live virus, they did not reduce virus infectivity in vitro. Needle inoculation produces IgG2a subclass antibodies as well as the Th1 cytokines IFN-γ and IL-2, the major factors in the anti-MVEV T cell response.[53] These MVEV DNA-mediated vaccine strategies also produce cross-protective immunity against high-dose challenge with JEV, with survival rates of 100% in normal versus 65% in nonimmunized mice.[54] Infection with live virus induces MVEV-specific antibodies that are predominately of the IgG2a and IgG2b subclasses with no or little IgG1 or other classes of antibodies.[53] It should be noted that the type and magnitude of humoral and Th cytokine production are dependent on the mouse strain employed.

Immunization with ultraviolet light-inactivated MVEV results in ADE and increases viral load, disease severity, and mortality upon challenge with sublethal levels of JEV.[54] It is quite possible that differences in the quality and magnitude of antibody responses would yield a range of cross-reactive homologous and heterologous results that would produce either protective or infection-enhancing activities against MVEV and other members of the JEV serocomplex. It should also be mentioned that a much earlier study found that when high-titer chicken antisera against MVEV were incubated with homologous virus, it neutralized MVEV and decreased the number of plaques on chicken embryo monolayers, but plaque numbers increased when low antibody concentrations were used. Similar findings are seen using rodent antiserum to passively protect rodent cells. IgG is the responsible antibody class and its Fc terminus is required for ADE to occur. Low numbers of Fc-bearing mononuclear phagocytes were present in the chicken monolayers, suggesting that low levels of homologous antibody may also lead to ADE during MVEV infection.[55]

Transfection of a murine fibroblast cell line with a recombinant MVEV E protein expression system leads to the secretion of subviral particles containing MVEV prM and E. The particles are active and induced low-pH-dependent membrane fusion and hemagglutination activity similar to that induced by normal virions. The MVEV E protein is present on the surface of the particles, undergoes the same posttranslational modifications, and has the same conformation as typical MVEV E proteins.[56] These particles protect BALB/c mice from lethal challenge with virulent MVEV. Protection correlates with the development of a neutralizing humoral immune response. Similar subviral particles have been developed that are protective against JEV, TBEV, and DENV-1 challenge.

T lymphocyte responses are also important in protection against MVEV. Several synthetic MVEV E protein peptides prime CD4[+] T helper lymphocytes for in vitro antiviral proliferative responses in three strains of mice with different MHC haplotypes. The T helper cell response was usually accompanied by an antibody response as well.[57] One of the E protein peptides contains multiple T cell epitopes and is recognized by various MVEV strains and Kunjin virus T helper cell clones, indicating at least some degree of cross-reactivity among flaviviruses in the JEV serocomplex. One peptide from the MVEV E protein also primes T helper cells in vivo in the same manner as the analogous peptide from DENV-2 primes anti-DENV-2 T helper cell responses.[58] The primed T cells both proliferate and produce interleukins and respond not only to viral peptides, but also to the whole native form of MVEV as well. The effective peptides must be collinearly linked to a B cell epitope from either MVEV or DENV-2 in order to enhance protective antibody responses and can be produced by simply mixing peptides containing free sulfhydryl groups. Interestingly, the peptide from DENV-2 more effectively primes T helper cells than the homologous peptide from MVEV.[58] Later work by the above laboratory found that primary inoculation of C57BL/6 mice with a relatively conserved peptide (amino acids 230–251) from the MVEV E protein stimulated reciprocal T helper cell and B cell reactivity against native MVEV. This peptide contains at least two B cell epitopes that induce antibodies, which neutralize MVEV at low titer

and are active against other JEV serocomplex viruses.[59] Two T cell elements are also present in the peptide's carboxyl terminus and activate protective antibodies in C3H, BALB/c, C57BIJ6, and B10 congenic mice. These inbred mice contain different major histocompatibility complex (MHC) class II molecules, and the responding T cells are able to recognize native virus in vivo. The T lymphocyte epitopes in this peptide have vaccine potential, which might be better realized if synthetic forms could be constructed which only induce Th2 responses and increase antibody titer, but not potentially harmful IFN-γ production.[59] Immunodominant CD8[+] T killer cell determinants for MHC class I-restricted elements, by contrast, are present in viral NS3 protein.[60]

PREVENTION

Sentinel chicken flocks are used to warn of the presence of MVEV and Kunjin virus in an area by testing for seroconversion against general or specific flavivirus types and by their increased susceptibility to heparin.[6] Mosquito pools are also tested in at-risk areas. In a 13-year (1989–2001) study of MVEV in an Aboriginal community in the tropical Kimberly region of Western Australia, virus was isolated from seven regional mosquito species. More than 90% of these mosquitoes were *Cx. annulirostris*, particularly in years with higher than average rainfall and flooding, leading to increased numbers of this mosquito species.[34] Over that time period, larger than normal numbers of human cases were only found in 1993. Interestingly, incidence of MVE only partially correlated with wet season rainfall and flooding, suggesting that other factors must also influence MVEV activity and need to be defined when attempting to predict human outbreaks. One possible factor is the lack of sufficient nonimmune bird hosts to allow amplification in a mosquito-bird cycle. Other mosquitoes, including *Aedes normanensis*, are also infected with MVEV in Australia.[61] It is possible that MVEV may be reactivated in arid regions after a heavy rainfall since vertical transmission may occur in the desiccation-resistant eggs of *Ochlerotatus* and *Aedes* mosquitoes.[34]

An "insect-specific" flavivirus lineage that contains at least 10 members is able to survive in mosquitoes without requiring vertebrate hosts. Palm Creek virus, isolated from *C. xanthogaster* mosquitoes in Australia in 2010, is a member of this lineage and is not known to cause disease in mosquitoes or vertebrates.[46] It has 63.7% nucleotide identity and 66.6% amino acid identity with Nakiwogo virus from *Mansonia* species mosquitoes in Uganda, its closest known relative. Infection of cultured mosquito cells with Palm Creek virus blocked the subsequent replication of either MVEV or WNV by superinfection exclusion as described above, despite large differences in their genetic material. Viruses similar to Palm Creek virus have been found in other *Coquillettidia* and *Culex* mosquito species in Australia as well.[46]

The salt-marsh Ilparpa Swamp is 10 km from the urban area of Alice Springs, Northern Territory. Wet season rainfall in the swamp, followed by effluent discharges from the adjacent sewage treatment plant, provides excellent conditions for the development of the immature stages of *Cx. annulirostris*. During the early 1970s, sewage discharge altered the swamp ecosystem, resulting in bulrush reeds and grasses becoming the dominant vegetation. The swamp area was also enlarged. Numbers of *Cx. annulirostris*, which had no natural predators in the region, increased, as did numbers of migratory birds. Several methods of decreasing numbers of infectious female mosquitoes were attempted, including development of evaporation ponds, sprinkler irrigation systems at an adjacent park, and using pipes to redirect the effluent. Other chemical and biological interventions included a regular adult mosquito insecticide fogging program and occasional aerial larval spraying with the synthetic bacterium *Bacillus thuringiensis* var. *israelensis* during high-risk disease periods.[62] While these interventions did decrease numbers of reported human MVE cases, they did not affect virus detection in the sentinel chickens. A drainage system was created in the Ilparpa Swamp in early 2002 in response to increased reports of MVE cases in 2000 and 2001. As the swamp area subsequently decreased, mosquito numbers fell dramatically and remained low.[63] More importantly, no seroconversions were detected in sentinel chickens to either MVEV or Kunjin virus and no human infections were reported in the Alice Springs urban region or surrounding rural areas.[63] It will be important for future studies to examine how the drainage system affects other swamp flora and fauna and whether the original plant and animal species are returning to levels seen prior to the effluent release. Making major changes to an ecosystem often is accompanied by potentially harmful unintended consequences.

Other means of mosquito reduction in swamps include ditching, runnelling, and impounding, whose use depends upon differing water retention issues, especially in salt-marsh or tidal habitats. Disadvantages of these methods are soil or water content changes, which impact fauna and flora, particularly ditching. While these habitat modification tactics are well documented for long-term mosquito control in salt-marshes, they have not been shown to be the most practical options for use in extensive freshwater environments.[63] Other types of habitat modification that decrease mosquito levels may be more "eco-friendly" than chemical applications, as well as being more practical and cost-effective as long-term solutions. One such modification is reducing water sources by draining or filling larval habitats. Such programs have been used to reduce the mosquito malarial vectors in Africa. Additionally, effluent releases currently occur more often in the winter months or intermittently, resulting in periods of wetness followed by drying. Improved sewage treatment is also important.[63]

TREATMENT

Treatment relies upon supportive therapy in intensive care units. The case-fatality rate during the 2011 outbreak was 18%, similar to the 20% case-fatality rate during the major outbreak of MVE in 1974. The similarity in mortality rates may be due to the continuing lack of specific, approved drug treatments for MVE.[8] Due to the low number of human cases, MVE-specific drug development has been minimal; however, this flavivirus may respond to drugs developed for use against other flaviviruses, such as JEV.

Some of the drug development work has focused upon the MVEV serine protease NS2B/NS3, critical for cleavage of the viral polyprotein into its individual, functional proteins. The crystal structures of the MVEV protease-helicase complex have been determined,[64] while Joy et al.[65] characterized the biochemical properties and substrate preferences of the MVEV protease.[65] This trypsin-like enzyme is specific for substrates with two consecutive basic residues and cleaves the C-terminal portion of the polyprotein's P1 arginine. This specificity is unusual for mammalian proteases, making it an attractive drug target. Armed with this knowledge, several MVEV protease inhibitors have been developed. Using structure–activity relationship studies, Ang et al.[66] designed a structurally constrained agmatine peptidomimetic inhibitor that has a three-fold increase in potency against the MVEV NS2B/NS3 protease ($IC_{50} = 4.9 \pm 0.4 \mu M$).

Dipeptides containing a C-terminal agmatine (decarboxylated arginine) inhibit the WNV protease with an inhibitory concentration$_{50}$ (IC_{50}) in the μM range.[67] Since an 85.3% cleavage sequence and cofactor homology exists between the WNV and MVEV NS2B/NS3 protease complex, Ang et al.[68] compared the P2 and P3 residue preferences of the two proteases using a series of C-terminal agmatine dipeptides. Both enzymes are highly specific to lysine at both the P2 and

P3 positions, suggesting that a single peptidomimetic viral protease inhibitor may be active against both viruses. This would be very useful since the presence of both MVEV and Kunjin virus overlaps in some regions of Australia.

Based upon the previously determined ability of D-arginine-based peptides to potently inhibit the WNV protease, Joy et al.[65] assessed the anti-MVEV activity of a known D-arginine peptide and found that it inhibits the MVEV protease with an IC_{50} of 72 nM. The viral inhibitor aprotinin, however, is much less effective against the MVEV protease than it is against proteases of other flaviviruses with an IC_{50} of 8 μM. Hopefully, protease inhibitors developed against some other members of the JEV serocomplex will prove more useful against MVEV.

SUMMARY OVERVIEW

Diseases: asymptomatic to life-threatening, potentially permanent encephalitis, including cognitive impairment, seizures, hypotonia, and quadriplegia

Causative agent—Murray Valley encephalitis virus

Vectors: Culex annulirostris, Cx. fatigans, Cx. australicus, Aedes notoscriptus, Ae. sagax, Ae. vigilax, and some members of the Anopheles and Ochlerotatus genera

Common reservoirs: waterfowl, particularly herons and egrets

Mode of transmission: mosquito bite

Geographical distribution: Australia and Papua New Guinea

Year of emergence: 1916

REFERENCES

1. Mackenzie, Broom AK. Australian X disease, Murray Valley encephalitis and the French connection. *Vet Microbiol.* 1995;46:79–90.
2. Doherty RL, Carley JG, Kay BH, Filippich C, Marks EN. Murray Valley encephalitis virus infection in mosquitoes and domestic fowls in Queensland, 1974. *Aust J Exp Biol Med Sci.* 1976;54(3):237–243.
3. Selvey LA, Johansen CA, Broom AK, et al. Rainfall and sentinel chicken seroconversions predict human cases of Murray Valley encephalitis in the north of Western Australia. *BMC Infect Dis.* 2014;14:672.
4. Broom AK, Lindsay MD, Johansen CA, Wright AE, Mackenzie JS. Two possible mechanisms for survival and initiation of Murray Valley encephalitis virus activity in the Kimberley region of Western Australia. *Am J Trop Med Hyg.* 1995;53:95–99.
5. Cordova SP, Smith DW, Broom AK, Lindsay DL, Dowse GK, Beers MY. Murray Valley encephalitis in Western Australia in 2000, with evidence of southerly spread. *Commun J Dis Intell.* 2000;24(12):368–372.
6. Brown A, Bolisetty S, Whelan P, Smith D, Wheaton G. Reappearance of human cases due to Murray Valley encephalitis virus and Kunjin virus in Central Australia after an absence of 26 years. *Commun Dis Intell.* 2002;26:39–44.
7. Mackenzie JS, Lindsay MDA, Smith DW, Imrie A. The ecology and epidemiology of Ross River and Murray Valley encephalitis viruses in Western Australia: examples of One Health in action. *Trans R Soc Trop Med Hyg.* 2017;111:248–254.
8. Selvey LA, Dailey L, Lindsay M, et al. The changing epidemiology of Murray Valley encephalitis in Australia: the 2011 outbreak and a review of the literature. *PLoS Negl Trop Dis.* 2014;8:e2656.
9. Stich A, Günther S, Drosten C, et al. Clinical and laboratory findings on the first imported case of Murray Valley encephalitis in Europe. *Clin Infect Dis.* 2003;37:e19–e21.
10. Niven DJ, Afra K, Iftinca M, et al. Fatal infection with Murray valley encephalitis virus imported from Australia to Canada. *Emerg Infect Dis.* 2003;223(2):280–283.
11. Burrow NC, Whelan PI, Kilburn CJ, Fisher DA, Currie BJ, Smith DW. Australian encephalitis in the Northern Territory: clinical and epidemiological features 1987-1996. *Aust N Z J Med.* 1998;28:590–596.
12. Robertson G. Murray Valley encephalitis: pathological aspects. *Med J Aust.* 1972;1:107–110.
13. Brown A, Krause V. Central Australian MVE update, 2001. *Commun Dis Intell.* 2001;25:49–50.
14. McMinn PC, Lee E, Hartley S, Roehrig JT, Dalgarno L, Weir RC. Murray Valley encephalitis virus envelope protein antigenic variants with altered hemagglutination properties and reduced neuroinvasiveness in mice. *Virology.* 1995;211:10–20.
15. Mathews V, Robertson T, Kendrick T, Abdo M, Papadimitriou J, McMinn P. Morphological features of Murray Valley encephalitis virus infection in the central nervous system of Swiss mice. *Int J Exp Pathol.* 2000;81:31–40.
16. Speers DJ, Flexma J, Blyth CC, et al. Clinical and radiological predictors of outcome for Murray Valley encephalitis. *Am J Trop Med Hyg.* 2013;88(3):481–489.
17. Einsiedel L, Kat E, Ravindran J, Slavotinek J, Gordon DL. MRI findings in Murray Valley encephalitis. *Am J Neuroradiol.* 2003;24:1379–1382.
18. Wong SH, Smith DW, Fallon MJ, Kermod AG. Murray Valley encephalitis mimicking herpes simplex encephalitis. *J Clin Neurosci.* 2005;12(7):822–824.
19. Lindsey NP, Hayes EB, Staples JE, Fischer M. West Nile virus disease in children, United States, 1999–2007. *Pediatrics.* 2009;123:e1084–e1089.
20. Selvey A, Speers DJ, Smith DW. Long-term outcomes of Murray Valley encephalitis cases in Western Australia: what have we learnt? *Intern Med J.* 2016;46(2):193–201.
21. Anastasiadou A, Kakoulidis I, Butel D, Kehagia E, Papa A. Follow-up study of Greek patients with West Nile virus neuroinvasive disease. *Int J Infect Dis.* 2013;17:494–497.
22. Murray KO, Garcia MN, Rahbar MH, et al. Survival analysis, long-term outcomes, and percentage of recovery up to 8 years post-infection among the Houston West Nile virus cohort. *PLoS One.* 2014;9:e102953.

23. Silvia OJ, Pantelic L, Mackenzie JS, Shellam GR, Papadimitriou J, Urosevic N. Virus spread, tissue inflammation and antiviral response in brains of flavivirus susceptible and resistant mice acutely infected with Murray Valley encephalitis virus. *Arch Virol*. 2004;149:447–464.

24. McMinn PC, Dalgarno L, Weir RC. A comparison of the spread of Murray Valley encephalitis viruses of high or low neuroinvasiveness in the tissues of Swiss mice after peripheral inoculation. *Virology*. 1996;220:414–423.

25. McMin PC, Weir RC, Dalgarno L. A mouse-attenuated envelope protein variant of Murray Valley encephalitis virus with altered fusion activity. *J Gen Virol*. 1996;75:2085–2088.

26. Hurrelbrink RJ, McMinn PC. Attenuation of Murray Valley encephalitis virus by site-directed mutagenesis of the hinge and putative receptor-binding regions of the envelope protein. *J Virol*. 2001;75(16):7692–7702.

27. Lee E, Lobigs M. Substitutions at the putative receptor-binding site of an encephalitic flavivirus alter virulence and host cell tropism and reveal a role for glycosaminoglycans in entry. *J Virol*. 2000;7:8867–8875.

28. McMinn PC, Marshall LD, Dalgarno L. Neurovirulence and neuroinvasiveness of Murray Valley encephalitis virus mutants selected by passage in a monkey kidney cell line. *J Gen Virol*. 1995;76:865–872.

29. Clark DC, Lobigs M, Lee E, et al. *In situ* reactions of monoclonal antibodies with a viable mutant of Murray Valley encephalitis virus reveal an absence of dimeric NS1 protein. *J Gen Virol*. 2007;88:1175–1183.

30. Russell RC, Dwyer DE. Arboviruses associated with human disease in Australia. *Microbes Infect*. 2000;2:693–704.

31. Kay BH, Fanning ID, Mottram P. The vector competence of *Culex annulirostris, Aedes sagax* and *Aedes alboannulatus* for Murray Valley encephalitis virus at different temperatures. *Med Vet Entomol*. 1989;3(2):107–112.

32. Mackenzie JS, Broom AK. Ord River irrigation area: the effect of dam construction and irrigation on the incidence of Murray Valley encephalitis virus. In: Kay BH, ed. *Water Resources: Health, Environment and Development*. E & FN; 1998:108–122.

33. Kramer LD, Chin P, Cane RP, Kauffman EB, Mackereth G. Vector competence of New Zealand mosquitoes for selected arboviruses. *Am J Trop Med Hyg*. 2011;85(1):182–189.

34. Broom AK, Lindsay MDA, Plant AJ, Wright AE, Condon RJ, Mackenzie JS. Epizootic activity of Murray Valley encephalitis virus in an Aboriginal community in the Southeast Kimberley Region of Western Australia: results of cross-sectional and longitudinal serologic studies. *Am J Trop Med Hyg*. 2002;67(3):319–323.

35. Kay BH, Young PL, Hall RA, Fanning ID. Experimental infection with Murray Valley encephalitis virus. Pigs, cattle, sheep, dogs, rabbits, macropods and chickens. *Aust J Exp Biol Med Sci*. 1985;63(pt. 1):109–126.

36. Holmes JM, Gilkerson JM, el Hage CL, Slocombe RF, Muurlink MA. Murray Valley encephalomyelitis in a horse. *Aust Vet J*. 2012;90(7):252–254.

37. Coelen RJ, Mackenzie JS. Genetic variation of Murray Valley encephalitis virus. *J Gen Biol*. 1988;69:1903–1912.

38. Lobigs M, Marshall ID, Weir RC, Dalgarno L. Genetic differentiation of Murray Valley encephalitis virus in Australia and Papua New Guinea. *Aust J Exp Biol Med Sci*. 1986;64:571–586.

39. Johansen CA, Susai V, Hall RA, et al. Genetic and phenotypic differences between isolates of Murray Valley encephalitis virus in Western Australia, 1972-2003. *Virus Genes*. 2007;35:147–154.

40. Heinz FZ, Kunz C. Homogeneity of the structural glycoprotein from European isolates of tick-borne encephalitis virus: comparison with other flaviviruses. *J Gen Virol*. 1981;57:263–274.

41. Lobigs R, Nestorowicz UA, Marshall ID, Weir RC, Dalgarno L. Host cell selection of Murray Valley encephalitis virus variants altered at an RGD sequence in the envelope protein and in mouse virulence. *Virology*. 1990;176:587–595.

42. Lee E, Lobigs M. Mechanism of virulence attenuation of glycosaminoglycan-binding variants of Japanese encephalitis virus and Murray Valley encephalitis virus. *J Virol*. 2002;76(1):4901–4911.

43. Russell JS, Caly L, Kostecki R, et al. The first isolation and whole genome sequencing of Murray Valley encephalitis virus from cerebrospinal fluid of a patient with encephalitis. *Viruses*. 2018;10:319.

44. Williams DT, Diviney SM, Niazi A-u-R, et al. The molecular epidemiology and evolution of Murray Valley encephalitis virus: recent emergence of distinct sub-lineages of the dominant genotype 1. *PLoS Negl Trop Dis*. 2015;9(11), e0004240.

45. Williams DT, Diviney SM, Corscadden KJ, Chua BH, Mackenzie JS. Complete genome sequences of the prototype isolates of genotypes 2, 3, and 4 of Murray Valley encephalitis virus. *Genome Announc*. 2014;2(3):e0051814.

46. Hobson-Peters J, Yam AWY, Lu JWF, et al. A new insect-specific flavivirus from northern Australia suppresses replication of West Nile virus and Murray Valley encephalitis virus in co-infected mosquito cells. *PLoS One*. 2013;8(2):e56534.

47. Andrews DM, Matthews VB, Sammels LM, Carrello AC, McMinn PC. The severity of Murray Valley encephalitis in mice is linked to neutrophil infiltration and inducible nitric oxide synthase activity in the central nervous system. *J Virol*. 1999;73(10):8781–8790.

48. Kreil TR, Eibl MM. Nitric oxide and viral infection: no antiviral activity against a flavivirus *in vitro*, and evidence for contribution to pathogenesis in experimental infection *in vivo*. *Virology*. 1996;219:304–306.

49. Hall RA, Brand TNH, Lobigs M, Sangster MY, Howard MJ, Mackenzie JS. Protective immune responses to the E and NS1 proteins of Murray Valley encephalitis virus in hybrids of flavivirus-resistant mice. *J Gen Virol*. 1996;77:1287–1294.

50. Broom AK, Wallace MJ, Mackenzie JS, Smith DW, Hall RA. Immunisation with gamma globulin to Murray Valley encephalitis virus and with an inactivated Japanese encephalitis virus vaccine as prophylaxis against Australian encephalitis: evaluation in a mouse model. *J Med Virol*. 2000;61(2):259–265.

51. Wallace MJ, Smith DW, Broom AK, et al. Antibody-dependent enhancement of Murray Valley encephalitis virus virulence in mice. *J Gen Virol.* 2003;84:1723–1728.

52. Lobigs M, Larena M, Alsharifi M, Lee E, Pavy M. Live chimeric and inactivated Japanese encephalitis virus vaccines differ in their cross-protective values against Murray Valley encephalitis virus. *J Virol.* 2009;83(6):2436–2445.

53. Colombage G, Hall R, Pavy M, Lobigs M. DNA-based and alphavirus-vectored immunisation with prM and E proteins elicits long-lived and protective immunity against the flavivirus, Murray Valley encephalitis virus. *Virology.* 1998;250:151–163.

54. Lobigs M, Pavy M, Hal R. Cross-protective and infection-enhancing immunity in mice vaccinated against flaviviruses belonging to the Japanese encephalitis virus serocomplex. *Vaccine.* 2003;21:1572–1579.

55. Kliks SC, Halstead SB. Role of antibodies and host cells in plaque enhancement of Murray Valley encephalitis virus. *J Virol.* 1983;46(2):394–404.

56. Kroeger MA, McMinn PC. Murray Valley encephalitis virus recombinant subviral particles protect mice from lethal challenge with virulent wild-type virus. *Arch Virol.* 2002;147:1155–1172.

57. Mathews JH, Allan JE, Roehrig JT, Brubaker JR, Uren MF, Hunt AR. T-helper cell and associated antibody response to synthetic peptides of the E glycoprotein of Murray Valley encephalitis virus. *J Virol.* 1991;65(10):5141–5148.

58. Roehrig JT, Johnson AJ, Hunt AR, Beaty BJ, Mathews JN. Enhancement of the antibody response to flavivirus B-cell epitopes by using homologous or heterologous T-cell epitopes. *J Virol.* 1992;66(6):3385–3390.

59. Mathews JH, Roehrig JT, Brubaker JR, Hunt AR, Allan JE. A synthetic peptide to the E glycoprotein of Murray Valley encephalitis virus defines multiple virus-reactive T- and B-cell epitope. *J Virol.* 1992;66(11):6555–6562.

60. Lobigs M, Arthur CE, Müllbacher A, Blanden RV. The flavivirus nonstructural protein NS3 is a dominant source of cytotoxic T cell peptide determinants. *Virology.* 1994;202(1):195–201.

61. Broom AK, Wright AE, MacKenzie JS, Lindsay MD, Robinson D. Isolation of Murray Valley encephalitis and Ross River viruses from *Aedes normanensis* (Diptera: Culicidae) in Western Australia. *J Med Entomol.* 1989;26(2):100–103.

62. Kurucz N, Whelan PI, Porigneaux P. Mosquito control in Ilparpa Swamp—a big step forward. Mosquito bites in the Asia Pacific Region. *Bull Mosquito Control Assoc Aust.* 2002;14:1–2.

63. Jacups S, Kurucz N, Whitters R, Whelan P. Habitat modification for mosquito control in the Ilparpa Swamp, Northern Territory, Australia. *Aust J Vector Ecol.* 2011;36(2):292–299.

64. Assenberg R, Ren J, Verma A, et al. Crystal structure of the Murray Valley encephalitis virus NS5 methyltransferase domain in complex with cap analogues. *J Gen Virol.* 2007;88:2228–2236.

65. Joy J, Mee NF, Kuan WL, Perlyn KZ, Wen TS, Hill J. Biochemical characterisation of Murray Valley encephalitis virus protease. *FEBS Lett.* 2010;584:3149–3152.

66. Ang MJY, Yong JHG, Poulsen A, et al. Substrate-based peptidomimetic inhibitors of the Murray Valley encephalitis virus NS2B/NS3 serine protease: a P1-P4 SAR study. *Eur J Med Chem.* 2013;68:72–80.

67. Lim HA, Joy J, Hill J, Chia CSB. Novel agmatine and agmatine-like peptidomimetic inhibitors of the West Nile virus NS2B/NS3 serine protease. *Eur J Med Chem.* 2011;46:3130–3134.

68. Ang MJY, Li Z, Lim HA, et al. A P2 and P3 substrate specificity comparison between the Murray Valley encephalitis and West Nile virus NS2B/NS3 protease using C-terminal agmatine dipeptides. *Peptides.* 2014;52:49–52.

CHAPTER 8

Other Neglected Mosquito-Borne Flaviviruses: Ilhéus, Bussuquara, Rocio, Kokobera, Stratford, and Wesselsbron Viruses

NEGLECTED FLAVIVIRUSES OF LATIN AMERICA

Ilhéus and Bussuquara Viruses

Ilhéus virus (ILHV) is found in humans and animals and is distributed over large areas of South and Central America, including Brazil, Peru, French Guyana, Columbia, Ecuador, Bolivia, Guatemala, Panama, and Trinidad.[1–8] A large study of the seroprevalence of ILHV in Trinidad, however, failed to detect ILHV-specific antibodies in horses ($n = 506$), cattle ($n = 163$), sheep ($n = 198$), goats ($n = 82$), pigs ($n = 184$), or wild birds although low levels of two other flaviviruses, Saint Louis encephalitis virus (SLEV) and WNV, were found.[9]

A closely related Brazilian flavivirus, Bussuquara virus, belongs to a separate clade of flaviviruses. This virus caused one case of an acute febrile disease in a person in Brazil in 1956. The fever was accompanied by anorexia, joint pain, chills, profuse sweating, and headache of 4-day duration.[10] *Culex* mosquitoes serve as the vector for Bussuquara virus, and the virus has also been isolated from sentinel and wild *Proechimys* species rodents in the Amazon region.[11] Given the paucity of known human disease, Bussuquara virus is more of a potential, than actual, threat to humans currently.

History of ILHV

In 1944, ILHV was isolated from *Aedes* and *Psorophora* species mosquitoes in Bahia, on the eastern coast of Brazil. Its identification was later confirmed by viral isolation from female *Aedes scapularis* in the wetlands of the Pantanal in center-west Brazil.[12,13] It is also found in *Culex, Sabethes, Haemagogus,* and *Trichoprosopon* mosquitoes as well as some bird species in Latin America.[7,13–18] Neutralizing antibodies against ILHV may be found in sentinel monkeys, birds, and horses.[13,19,20] In a recent serosurvey, 10.3%–10.7% of the tested horses from two different subregions of the Pantanal wetlands ($n = 760$) were seropositive for ILHV, 7.8% for St. Louis encephalitis virus (SLEV), and 3.2% for West Nile virus (WNV).[20,21] No tested sheep ($n = 283$) were infected with ILHV.

ILHV-Association Disease

ILHV only sporadically infects humans and has not caused any epidemics. Consequences of infection range from asymptomatic to a severe febrile, encephalitis-like syndrome.[1,3,5,6,11,22,23] Mild cases involve gastrointestinal or respiratory symptoms of approximately 1-week duration. The central nervous system (CNS) and the cardiovascular system may be involved in severe cases, but no long-term sequelae or deaths have been reported in humans.[4]

Typically, patients with ILHV develop mild febrile illness with malaise; headache; muscle, bone, and joint pain; and photophobia. Infection by ILHV may be mistaken for infection by other flaviviruses that are associated with severe disease, including dengue virus (DENV), SLEV, and yellow fever virus (YFV), with which it cross-reacts in serological assays.[11] Other symptoms of ILHV infection of humans include vesicular rash, sore throat, retroocular pain, conjunctival injection, facial swelling, earache, nausea and vomiting, jaundice, and abdominal pain.[3] In the case of a 15-year-old farmer from northern Bolivia, no cardiac, neurologic, or renal pathology was present and he fully recovered soon afterward.[4] The region where the disease was contracted is near the border of Brazil and is surrounded by rivers and chestnut fields. Fishing and agriculture are the primary sources of income in the area.

Ilhéus and Bussuquara Viruses

Based upon a 600-nucleotide sequence of the NS5 gene, ILHV has been classified as a member of the Japanese

Zika and Other Neglected and Emerging Flaviviruses. https://doi.org/10.1016/B978-0-323-82501-6.00010-4

encephalitis virus (JEV) complex of mosquito-borne flaviviruses, which include Bussuquara, Rocio, Cacipacore, and Iguape viruses. Several of these have only been detected in South America.[24] ILHV is most closely related to Rocio virus (ROCV).[3,25,26] While Ilhéus, Rocio, and Bussuquara viruses are the causative agents of acute febrile illness in humans, the other above listed viruses are not currently known to cause human disease.[24]

Bussuquara virus-infected murine peritoneal macrophages develop a flattened shape with a high number of large spikes of cytoplasm prolongations within 3 days of infection.[27] This is also found in YFV-, ROCV-, and SLEV-infected cells. Enlarged, hypertrophic rough and smooth endoplasmic reticula are abundant as well as many free, cytoplasmic ribosomes. Spherical objects are present in the cytoplasm, usually found inside vesicles. These structures may represent viral particles.

ILHV is primarily maintained in a sylvatic, enzootic cycle between birds and mosquitoes, especially *Psorophora ferox* mosquitoes, but has also been reported in *Psorophora lutzii*, *Psorophora varipes*, *Sabethes chloropterus*, *Haemagogus spegazzinii*, and *Trichoprosopon* mosquitoes.[7,15,17,28] Two strains of ILHV have been isolated from the double-collared seedeater and the shiny cowbird in Brazil as well. Several other bird species are seropositive for ILHV, including the ruddy ground dove, the diamond dove, and the saffron finch.[29]

Several tested species of nonhuman primates in Northeast Brazil produce neutralizing antibodies against ILHV, including marmosets (*Callithrix jacchus* and *Callithrix penicillata*), coati (*Nasua nasua*), and black-striped (*Sapajus libidinosus*) and blond (*Sapajus flavius*) capuchin monkeys. In addition to potential public health concerns, the latter findings have implication for animal conservation, since *S. flavius* is a critically endangered species and the area of collection was near the epicenter of the concurrent Zika virus (ZIKV) outbreak in mid-2015–January 2016.[29-31] A 2017 report detected low incidence of ILHV- and virus-specific neutralizing antibodies in black howler monkeys (*Alouatta caraya*) in Argentina, 1 of 108 tested monkeys. Bussuquara virus-specific antibodies were detected in 1 of 189 Argentine military recruits.[32,33] ILHV- and Bussuquara-specific hemagglutination-inhibiting antibodies have also been in 7.4% and 0.3% of water buffaloes (*Bubalus bubalis*), respectively, in the Brazilian Amazon ($n = 654$).[34]

Vaccination—ILHV

Intraperitoneal infection of 6-week-old C57BL/6 mice with ILHV induces protective cross-reactive neutralizing antibodies against challenge with a lethal dose of ROCV with a 100% survival rate. Prior infection of the mice with SLEV also produces cross-protective immunity, although it is less effective than that induced by ILHV. Other Brazilian flaviviruses, including all four serotypes of DENV, YFV, and ZIKV, do not protect against ROCV.[35] ROCV is more closely related to ILHV and SLEV than other flaviviruses, having high amino acid sequence similarities.[26,36] Since ROCV can cause severe encephalitis in humans, immunization with attenuated ILHV has potential for vaccination against ROCV.[35]

Rocio Virus
History of Rocio Virus

From 1975 to 1980, ROCV caused severe outbreaks of encephalitis in at least 23 municipalities in the Ribeira Valley along the southeastern coast of Brazil. Retrospective serological studies indicate that ROCV encephalitis had previously been present in seven febrile patients during 1973 and 1974 as well.[37] Presently, a total of over 1000 ROCV encephalitis cases have been reported and are known to have resulted in approximately 100 deaths. Over 200 additional people developed serious sequelae.[11] A large epidemic occurred in 1975–76 in São Paulo, the current Brazilian capital, affecting 465 people with 61 deaths (fatality rate of 13%). ROCV was isolated from 10 of the patients, but only from those who died within 5 days of disease onset.[38] The greatest numbers of cases were in those aged 15–30 years. Young males were also disproportionally affected.[39] No further cases of ROCV infection have been reported since 1980, despite the presence of seropositive humans and animals in different regions of Brazil, including eight people in Bahia who had either IgG or IgM antibodies and from two children in the Ribeira Valley.[35,37,40,41] The presence of IgM is indicative of recent infection. Since Bahia is 1200 km from São Paulo, ROCV has a large range and has been proposed to be spread by migratory birds.[4,42] Further outbreaks may occur in humans due to environmental modifications, such as conversion of forest into agricultural areas, which bring humans into greater contact with the mosquito vector and reservoir hosts.[42]

Rocio Virus-Associated Disease

After a 7- to 14-day incubation period, infection with ROCV may result in severe encephalitis of 1- to 2-week duration. The symptoms include fever, headache, anorexia, nausea and vomiting, myalgia, and malaise. This is followed by encephalitis, characterized by confusion, altered reflexes, motor impairment, meningeal irritation, convulsions, and cerebellar syndrome.

Abdominal distension and urinary retention may also occur. Serious sequelae include meningeal irritation (57.3%), alteration of consciousness (51%), and motor abnormalities (49.7%), such as abnormal gait and equilibrium. Visual, olfactory, and auditory dysfunction; difficulty in swallowing; incontinence; and memory problems have also been reported.[37]

Rocio Virus

ROCV is a member of the JEV serocomplex that is restricted to Brazil.[36] It is present in the cisternae of the endoplasmic reticulum and Golgi apparatus of suckling mice neurons, but does not appear to bud from these cells.[43]

Some reports have characterized ROCV as a subtype of ILHV, based upon serological findings.[44] Some evidence suggests otherwise, however. The first complete nucleoside sequence was performed on a ROCV strain (SPH 34675) isolated in 1975 from the cerebellum and upper spinal cord of an agricultural worker from São Paulo.[36] An annotated version of the sequence was published recently.[45] Other strains have also been sequenced. Partial characterization of the nucleotide sequences of the NS5 alone or together with the E gene indicates a close relationship to pathogenic and nonpathogenic JEV complex members, including SLEV, ILHV, and Bussuquara virus. It is also closely related to Cacipacore and Iguape viruses, which are not currently known to cause human disease.[24] ROCV and ILHV form a distinct subclade of the JEV serocomplex.[42] Since ROCV and ILHV have a nucleoside sequence identity of 72.5% of the full-length NS5 gene, they are two distinct species. Additionally, ROCV is linked to epidemics of encephalitis, while ILHV infection generally causes sporadic febrile illness with only minor neurological disease.[16,46]

ROCV occurs primarily as a sylvatic zoonosis that occasionally infects humans and domestic animals exposed to its ornithophilic (bird-loving) mosquito vectors. The virus was isolated from a pool of 19 *P. ferox* mosquitoes ($n = 47$ pools), but not in 2183 pools of some other mosquito species.[47] *A. scapularis* mosquitoes, nevertheless, are also believed to be involved in ROCV transmission.[47-49] ROCV is also able to infect *Culex* species mosquitoes and cultured *Aedes albopictus* cells in the laboratory as well, but it is unknown whether they infect mosquitoes naturally and, if so, whether they serve as vectors for zoonotic transmission.[50,51]

Among vertebrates, ROCV has been isolated from a wild rufous-collared sparrow (*Zonotrichia capensis*), which may serve as one of its reservoir hosts.[38] Experimental infection of house sparrows (*Passer domesticus*) results in a low to moderate level of viremia of 2- to 3-day duration in two-thirds of nestling and adult sparrows. While prior SLEV infection prevents detectable levels of viremia in sparrows that are later challenged with ROCV, ROCV infection does not protect against subsequent SLEV infection.[52] Since house sparrows are relatively inefficient viremic hosts, it is unlikely that they would play a significant role in ROCV transmission if the virus were introduced into the United States.

Several species of mammals also host ROCV that is acquired either naturally or experimentally. In a serosurvey of horses from various regions of Brazil ($n = 753$), 82% of the serum samples were positive for ROCV and SLEV, suggesting antigenic cross-reactivity or prior infection with both viruses. Anti-ROCV IgG was found in 6.1% of tested horses. No CNS symptoms were present; however, so many horses appear to have had asymptomatic infection.[53] A separate study conducted in the Pantanal in west-central Brazil found only 0.1% of the horses were seropositive for ROCV, while 10.3% were seropositive for ILHV ($n = 760$). None of the 283 tested sheep were seropositive for either virus.[21]

ROCV was isolated from sentinel mice during the outbreak in São Paulo.[38] Six-week-old C57BL/6 mice experimentally infected intraperitoneally may serve as a good animal model for the study of ROCV-induced disease.[35] Mice infected with 2.76×10^4 to 2.76×10^8 plaque-forming units of ROCV have significant weight loss and a high fatality rate (90%–100%). BALB/c mice are also used as animal models of ROCV-induced disease, as described below.

ROCV infection of golden hamsters (*Mesocricetus auratus*) causes intense tissue damage to the liver, lung, kidney, brain, heart, pancreas, and spleen, with the brain, heart, and pancreas sustaining the greatest damage. Within 72 h following intracranial infection, necrosis is found throughout the heart. Extensive necrosis is also seen in both endocrine and exocrine areas of the pancreas. Viral particles in the pancreas are primarily found in the zymogen granules within acinar cells, in beta cells of the islets of Langerhans, and in vacuoles of unmyelinated nerves supplying this organ.[54] ROCV can also persist and be recovered for at least 3 months from the brain, blood, and liver of hamsters infected intraperitoneally.[55]

Immune Response to Rocio Virus

Since cross-protective immunity exists among flaviviruses, immunity to other Brazilian flaviviruses may at least partially explain the disappearance of ROCV disease after 1980. Indeed, cross-protection against ROCV infection is seen in C57BL/6 mice previously exposed to ILHV or SLEV. Prior ILHV infection or prior infection with a sublethal dose of ROCV led to 100% survival of ROCV-challenged mice.[35] No such cross-protection occurs in mice exposed to other flaviviruses found in Brazil (the four DENVs, YFV, or Bussuquara, Cacipacore, and Iguape viruses). Interestingly, prior exposure to YFV actually resulted in higher mortality and loss of body weight, perhaps due to a form of antibody-dependent enhancement, as is seen when infection with one serotype of DENV is followed by infection with a different DENV serotype.

When young adult BALB/c mice are infected with ROCV by the intraperitoneal route, all animals die within 9 days. Using immunohistochemistry and molecular biology, ROCV is found in neurons, astrocytes, microglia, endothelium, and macrophages/monocytes at day 4 of infection in the spinal cord, entering the brain by day 8.[56] Inflammatory damage in the CNS is accompanied by an influx of neutrophils and mononuclear leukocytes, including CD8[+] T lymphocytes. Levels of CNS interferon (IFN)-α mRNA and protein increase in less than 24 h after the virus enters the spinal cord and remain at high levels until death. IFN-γ and interleukin (IL)-1β mRNA are found in nervous tissue days 2–4 after infection. At days 4–6, mRNA for the T helper 2 (Th2) cytokine IL-4, as well for the T regulatory cytokines IL-10 and transforming growth factor-β (TGF-β), is present in neural tissues. These regulatory cytokines may be produced in an unsuccessful attempt to control the inflammatory response.

Murine peritoneal macrophages are infected by high concentrations of ROCV in vitro. Infected macrophages exhibit hypertrophy, enlargement of membranous structures, increased numbers of lysosomes, and extensive phagosome production. Infection of macrophages decreases the synthesis of protective cytokines, such as lipopolysaccharide-stimulated TGF-β and, at high levels, reduces IL-1β production. In contrast, the closely related, but less pathogenic, Bussuquara virus enhances the production of IL-1β by stimulated macrophages. These alterations are not seen in unstimulated cells. The production of protective IFN-α, but not proinflammatory TNF-α, increases in ROCV-infected cells within 48 h.[57]

A chimeric, nonpathogenic Kunjin form of WNV virus containing the ROCV prM-E genes inhibits IFN-α, IFN-β, and Janus kinase-signal transducer and activator of transcription (JAK–STAT) signaling and enhances viral replication and virulence in young C57BL/6 mice.[58] Such inhibition of type I IFN

pathways is caused by proteins of other flaviviruses as well, including DENV, JEV, TBEV, and WNV.[58]

Infection of peritoneal macrophages also stimulates the synthesis of reactive nitrogen species, including the antiviral compound nitric oxide (NO) after 24 h; however, experimentally reducing NO synthesis by the inducible nitric oxide synthase (iNOS) gene fails to decrease viral death, suggesting that NO does not play a major role in killing ROCV.[57] While NO is generally neuroprotective, excessive levels lead to neuronal death. A recent study found that increased expression of iNOS gene and the corresponding overproduction of NO levels contribute to brain injury in BALB/c mice.[59] Even though CNS tissue damage is greater in iNOS[−/−] mice, they are more resistant to ROCV-related encephalitis and death. NO induction is mediated by the Th1 cytokine IFN-γ, which is down-modulated by IL-33 and its receptor, ST2.[59] IL-33 belongs to the IL-1 cytokine family that is highly expressed in the CNS. It can be produced by astrocytes and microglia and other monocyte-derived cells. ROCV infection increases the expression of the IL-33 and ST2 genes. ST2 is present on the surface of Th2, but not Th1, cells, where it serves as an important Th2 effector molecule that helps to maintain a proper Th1/Th2 balance. ST2 regulates antiviral CD8[+] T killer cell activity as well. Infected ST2[−/−] mice have greater tissue damage, massive leukocyte infiltration, and higher viral load in the CNS, accompanied by increased TNF-α and IFN-γ levels.[59]

Leukocyte infiltration during ROCV infection involves the CC-chemokine receptor 5 (CCR-5) and its ligand, macrophage inflammatory protein 1 alpha (MIP-1α), which contribute to ROCV-induced CNS pathology by stimulating migration of infected cells into the brain. CCR5/MIP-1α is particularly important in recruiting cells to sites containing several virus groups, including WNV.[60] A deficiency in this chemokine/chemokine receptor pathway in infected mice decreases CNS inflammation, lowers viral load, and increases survival time.[61] The CCR5 receptor is expressed on CD8[+] T killer cells and Th1 lymphocytes, granulocytes, macrophages (including microglia), and dendritic cells. CNS infiltration during ROCV infection begins with an influx of IL-33-producing macrophages, followed by infiltration of T and B lymphocytes and NK cells. The T cells and NK cells produce high levels of inflammatory IFN-γ and TNF-α, which stimulate neuronal degeneration and death by upregulating iNOS gene expression and generating larger amounts of NO, as described above.[56]

Degeneration of neurons, but not infected astrocytes, occurs in the hippocampus, dentate gyrus, and CA3 region and is postulated to result from direct infection of these cells. Increasing numbers of caspase 3-producing apoptotic cells are present throughout the CNS late during infection and include neurons and lymphomononuclear and endothelial cells. These neurological changes are followed by acute flaccid hind limb paralysis, muscle weakness, tremors, and loss of balance. Mouse model systems provide a convenient way in which to study the pathogenesis and physiopathology seen during ROCV-induced human meningoencephalomyelitis.[56]

NEGLECTED FLAVIVIRUSES OF AUSTRALIA AND THE PACIFIC ISLANDS
Kokobera and Stratford Viruses
History of Kokobera and Stratford viruses
Kokobera virus (KOKV) was isolated in 1960 from *Culex annulirostris* mosquitoes in northern Queensland, Australia.[62] Stratford virus (STRV) was isolated in 1961 from Cairns, Bainyik virus in 1966 from Papua New Guinea, a single isolate of New Mapoon virus in 1998 in northern Queensland (the most divergent member of the group), and Torres virus in 2000 from Saibai Island in the Torres Strait, Queensland.[62–66] At least some of the anti-KOKV monoclonal antibodies cross-react with STRV.[67]

STRV is endemic in parts of Queensland and Papua New Guinea. It was first isolated from *Aedes vigilax* Skuse mosquitoes in Far North Queensland[62] and is endemic in Australia. The major periods of STRV cases reported in humans occurred in 2006 ($n=14$), 2010 ($n=11$), and 2013 ($n=11$).[68] Several studies have found STRV in several mosquito species in coastal regions, including *Ae. vigilax* Skuse in Queensland, and STRV-infected *Ae. vigilax*, *Ae. procax*, *Ae. notoscriptus*, *Ae. aculeatus*, *Ae. alternans*, and *Anopheles annulipes* in New South Wales.[68,69] Interestingly, no STRV isolates were found in *Cx. annulirostris* in New South Wales even though *Cx. annulirostris* was still common in coastal regions of New South Wales during that time period and the environmental conditions were favorable. Moreover, STRV was isolated from other mosquito species in these locations.

Ae. vigilax, responsible for 46.5% of the STRV detected, is the most important vector pest mosquito in Australia and is found in tidally influenced estuarine wetlands, with the exception of the most southern coastal regions of Australia.[70] In some parts of the continent, it is extremely abundant. *Ae. procax* (34.9% of STRV isolates) is present in areas having freshwater to brackish water.[71] It is locally abundant in some of these regions. *Ae. notoscriptus* (11.6% of STRV isolates) is often present in natural and artificial water-holding containers throughout urban Australia.[72] STRV RNA is also found in mosquito expectorate collected from sites in South Australia.[73] The observed increase in localized STRV activity may be due to factors affecting the reservoir host and environmental conditions influencing mosquito abundance.[68]

In 2002–03, eight STRV isolates were derived from *Aedes camptorhynchus* and *Aedes ratcliffei* in Western Australia,[74] while in 2014, three STRV isolates were found in South Australia from *Ae. notoscriptus*.[73]

Kokobera and Stratford viruses and disease
The KOKV group of mosquito-borne flaviviruses belongs to the JEV complex. KOKV and STRV are distantly related to other members of the JEV complex, averaging only 50% nucleoside homology to the other subgroups, including Usutu virus (USUV), Alkhurma hemorrhagic fever virus (ALFV), and Koutango virus.[75] The KOKV complex contains three members. The first of these is the Kokobera virus, first isolated in Oceania in 1960. Its primary vector is *Cx. annulirostris*. Its major wildlife reservoir hosts are marsupials, including kangaroos, wallabies, and other macropods, all of which are seropositive for KOKV. More recent studies indicate that KOKV is now limited primarily located in regions containing Australian marsupials.[66] Horses may be domestic reservoirs as well.[76] A single KOKV isolate was also found in *Ochlerotatus vigilax* mosquitoes.[77]

KOKV and STRV typically cause a mild, febrile disease in humans. The other members of the group, New Mapoon, Bainyik (previously known as strain MK7979), and Torres (previously known as strain TS5273) viruses, are also present in Oceania but have not been reported to cause any human illness,[64,69] although Bainyik virus causes encephalitis in mice and thus should be monitored for possible zoonotic disease in humans as well.[65] Three patients with acute polyarticular illnesses from southeastern Australia were found to be seropositive for KOKV during the summers in the 1980s and are the first people reporting disease associated with infection by this virus.[76,78,79] There is only one reported case of KOKV-induced encephalitis and myelitis. Two members of the YFV group of flaviviruses, Edge Hill virus from Australia, transmitted by *Aedes* species mosquitoes, and Sepik virus from New Guinea, transmitted by *Ficalbia* species mosquitoes and *Culex sitiens*, were isolated in the 1960s and are associated with febrile disease in humans as well.[79]

KOKV is enzootic to Australia and Papua New Guinea and has been present in Australia from at least the year 1606 and the European discovery of the continent. It was additionally found in Aboriginal people prior to

European colonization.[66] Of the KOKV isolates, one is present in Queensland and New South Wales, another from Northern Territory and Western Australia, and the last in Papua New Guinea. The Western Australia group is composed of northern and southwest isolates and is the group that was present in Aboriginal people prior to European colonization.[66,75,80] It exists in several different genetic subtypes in different regions and may be divided into two clades that diverged in the 1950s.[66,81]

KOKV is present in very low numbers in the islands in Northern Australia.[82] One isolate of KOKV was isolated from over 80,000 tested mosquitoes from a small island off the coast of northern Australia during January and February 2000, in addition to one isolate of JEV and four Kunjin virus isolates.[82] All infected mosquitoes were members of the Weidemann subgroup of *Cx. sitiens*. Given the size of the island and the limited number of immunologically naïve hosts, these mosquitoes may have introduced from an enzootic area, such as Papua New Guinea or the Australian mainland.[83] The emergence of KOKV into new regions of Australia may be related to tidal swamping of lands, which lead to a corresponding increase in potential mosquito breeding sites.[81]

NEGLECTED FLAVIVIRUS OF AFRICA
Wesselsbron Virus
Introduction and history of Wesselsbron virus
Wesselsbron virus (WSL virus) is a mosquito-borne virus in Africa that occasionally causes zoonotic infection. The virus typically is linked to abortions and teratogenic effects in sheep, West African dwarf goats, and other ruminants.[84]

WSL virus was first found in a newborn lamb in South Africa in 1956.[85] Infection kills newborn lambs and kids, while causing clinically inapparent infection in adult sheep and goats.[85,86] The disease also struck lambs in that country in 1996. Two human WSL virus disease cases were later discovered during an investigation of the 2010–11 Rift Valley fever epidemic and were the first confirmed human cases of WSL virus disease reported in South Africa since 1996.[87]

Wesselsbron disease
Fever and myalgia are the most common symptoms in humans.[84] The disease is more severe in goats and sheep, leading to listlessness, infertility, abortion, or death of newborns. In cattle, WSL virus causes mild febrile illness and may, occasionally, lead to more serious disease. Additionally, WSL appears able to cross the placental barrier in cattle and cause disease of the

fetal calves, although WSL-related abortions appear to be uncommon in cattle.[88]

Goats and sheep are much more susceptible to WSL virus-associated severe disease than humans or cattle, especially the Nigerian viral strains. Baba[89,90] found that experimentally infected young goats become viremic after 1–3 days and remain so for another 3–4 days, with a coinciding biphasic febrile response. Other symptoms include rough hair coat, weakness, swaying of the hindquarters, mucoid diarrhea, and edema of the head.[90] Fatal infection occurs in half of the infected young goats. WSL virus may be reisolated in mice inoculated with all of the tested tissues from dead goats, including the liver, spleen, lungs, brain, kidneys, adrenal glands, lymph nodes, and heart. While complement-fixing and HI antibodies are present in all animals, neutralizing antibody is only found in surviving goats.[90]

The course of WSL disease differs in adult and young sheep and goats. Experimentally infected adult sheep and goats become viremic 2 days postinfection and develop moderate to severe fever several hours afterward.[91] Necropsy reveals small necrotic foci in the liver that are associated with localized Kupffer cell activity. Acidophilic bodies and foci of necrotic hepatocytes are also present. Pyknosis and karyorrhexis are present in the nucleus of lymphocytes undergoing apoptosis in the spleen and lymph nodes.[91] By contrast, infected lambs develop viremia 1 day after infection, soon followed by biphasic fever. Virus may be reisolated from mice inoculated with every tested tissue from infected lambs, as was seen with the goats, despite the lack of pathology in the lambs in areas other than the liver and lymphatic tissue.[92]

Wesselsbron virus
WSL virus is transmitted through the bite of mosquitoes, particularly those of the *Aedes* genus. During a study of floodwater mosquitoes in South Africa ($n = 4732$), WSL was detected in five *Aedes* species. This study also found Middelburg virus and five unidentified viruses in these mosquitoes. In a study of almost 3500 *Aedes mcintoshi/luridus* and *Aedes juppi/caballus* mosquitoes, 10 tested positive for WSL virus and 2 for Middleburg virus. Six unidentified viruses were also found in these mosquitoes.[93] Of the local sheep, 59% had WSL-specific HI antibody and another 48% had anti-Middelburg virus antibody, demonstrating that the *Aedes* species vectors are capable of transmitting virus to susceptible mammals.[93] During the course of this study, a researcher underwent seroconversion and developed WSL fever, emphasizing the possibility of zoonotic transmission. Virus has also been isolated in

Aedes vexans in Senegal and Mauritania.[94] Interestingly, WSL was isolated from *Aedes circumluteolus* mosquitoes in 1989 in Madagascar, an isolated island off of the East Coast of Africa.[95] *Ae. circumluteolus* are also capable of transmitting WSL virus to mice in a laboratory setting,[96] while the transmission rate from *Aedes caballus*, *Aedes aegypti*, *Culex theileri*, and *Culex quinquefasciatus* to rodents is very low.[97,98] Other countries in which mosquitoes are either seropositive or infected include Botswana, Zimbabwe, Uganda, Mozambique, and the Democratic Republic of the Congo.[84,94]

In addition to sheep, goats, and cattle, WSL virus infects a wide range of animals. It has been isolated from black rats, horses, donkeys, zebras, camels,[99] a cape short-eared gerbil, and an ostrich.[84,100] Seropositive lemurs, a form of nonhuman primate, are also present in Madagascar, suggesting the potential for zoonotic transmission there as well.[95] In addition to South Africa, WSL virus is present in animals throughout Africa, including Ethiopia,[101] the woodland savannahs of Gabon,[102] the Central African Republic,[103] Zimbabwe,[88] Nigeria,[104] Guinea, and Cote d'Ivoire.[90]

Human infection and disease, while rare, have occurred in several areas of Africa, including South Africa, Senegal, and Cameroon.[105] People in other areas of Africa are also seropositive. While there are no records of human WSL disease in Nigeria, 67% of the population in the Oyo State were seropositive,[106] indicating that the people were exposed to viral antigens. No virus could be isolated from the sera of this group of people, indicating that infection may not have occurred or that the virus is either absent or present in low levels in sera. In Cameroon, sera from 102 febrile people were tested for antibodies against flaviviruses and 1.3% of the sera were positive for WSL virus. Antibodies against other flaviviruses, such as ZIKV, YFV, DENV-1, and DENV-2, were also present in people in this country,[105] complicating diagnosis due to antigenic cross-reactivity. In a small study of 30 people from Mozambique, neutralizing antibodies against WSL virus were present in 15.9% of those tested.[107]

Many strains of WSL virus have been reported. In Senegal and Mauritania alone, 51 strains of WSL virus have been isolated from *Ae. vexans* mosquitoes.[94] How many of these strains are capable of infecting and causing disease in humans is unknown. The black rat may serve as a WSL virus reservoir host, since they are an urban species and human cases in Senegal have 99%–100% nucleoside similarity to the strain from these rats.[84]

Flaviviruses frequently demonstrate serological cross-reactivity, as mentioned above. No significant HI or complement-fixing antigenic variation was detected among WSL, YFV, and Potiskum virus by testing for

either of those types of antibodies. Differences were, however, found between the above viruses and the human pathogen ZIKV and Uganda S and Banzi viruses (not known to cause disease in humans). A better understanding of cross-reactivity between pathogenic and nonpathogenic human flavivirus species will aid in diagnosis in regions that are endemic for more than one flavivirus species.[108] Microneutralization tests in kidney cell cultures appear to be species-specific[88] and may be useful in differentiating regional flaviviruses of animals and humans.

SUMMARY OVERVIEW OF ILHÉUS VIRUS

Diseases: asymptomatic to severe febrile, encephalitis-like syndrome

Vectors: *Psorophora ferox* and possibly *Aedes* species of mosquitoes

Common reservoirs: birds and possibly horses and non-human primates

Mode of transmission: mosquito bite

Geographical distribution: South and Central America

Year of emergence: 1944

SUMMARY OVERVIEW OF BUSSUQUARA VIRUS (ONE HUMAN CASE)

Diseases: acute febrile disease accompanied by anorexia, joint pain, chills, profuse sweating, and headache

Vectors: *Culex* mosquitoes

Common reservoirs: *Proechimys* species rodents

Mode of transmission: mosquito bite

Geographical distribution: Brazil (one asymptomatic infection in a human in Argentina)

Year of emergence: 1956

SUMMARY OVERVIEW OF ROCIO VIRUS

Diseases: acute febrile illness; severe encephalitis; sequelae include CNS sensory, and motor abnormalities and incontinence

Vectors: *Psorophora ferox* and *Aedes scapularis* mosquitoes

Common reservoirs: birds, particularly sparrows

Mode of transmission: mosquito bite

Geographical distribution: Brazil

Year of emergence: 1973

SUMMARY OVERVIEW OF KOKOBERA VIRUS

Diseases: usually mild febrile disease; rarely, acute poly-articular illness, encephalitis, myelitis

Vectors: *Culex annulirostris*
Common reservoirs: marsupials and possibly horses
Mode of transmission: mosquito bite
Geographical distribution: Australia and Papua New Guinea
Year of emergence: 1960

SUMMARY OVERVIEW OF STRATFORD VIRUS

Diseases: usually mild, febrile disease
Vectors: *Aedes* species mosquitoes
Common reservoirs: unknown
Mode of transmission: mosquito bite
Geographical distribution: Papua New Guinea and Australia
Year of emergence: 1961

SUMMARY OVERVIEW OF WESSELSBRON VIRUS

Diseases: rarely lead to a mild, febrile disease with myalgia in humans: abortions and teratogenic effects occur in sheep and goats
Vectors: *Aedes* species mosquitoes
Common reservoirs: black rat
Mode of transmission: mosquito bite
Geographical distribution: throughout Africa
Year of emergence: 1956 (in lambs)

REFERENCES

1. Nassar ES, Coimbra TL, Rocco IM, et al. Human disease caused by an arbovirus closely related to Ilhéus virus: report of five cases. *Intervirology.* 1997;40:247–252.
2. Panon G, Fauran P, Digoutte JP. Isolation of Ilhéus virus in French Guyana. *Bull Soc Pathol Exot Filiales.* 1979;72(4):315–318.
3. Johnson BW, Cruz C, Felices V, et al. Ilhéus virus isolate from a human, Ecuador. *Emerg Infect Dis.* 2007;13:956–958.
4. Venegas EA, Aguilar PV, Cruz C, et al. Ilhéus virus infection in human, Bolivia. *Emerg Infect Dis.* 2012;18(3):516–518.
5. Srihongse S, Johnson CM. Isolation of Ilhéus virus from man in Panama. *Am J Trop Med Hyg.* 1967;16:516–518.
6. Spence L, Anderson CR, Downs WG. Isolation of Ilhéus virus from human beings in Trinidad, West Indies. *Trans R Soc Trop Med Hyg.* 1962;56:504–509.
7. de Rodaniche E, Galindo P. Isolation of Ilhéus virus from *Sabethes chloropterus* captured in Guatemala in 1956. *Am J Trop Med Hyg.* 1957;6(4):686–687.
8. Aitken TH, Anderson CR, Downs WG. The isolation of Ilhéus virus from wild-caught forest mosquitoes in Trinidad. *Am J Trop Med Hyg.* 1956;5(4):621–625.
9. Thompson NN, Auguste AJ, Coombs D, et al. Serological evidence of flaviviruses and alphaviruses in livestock and wildlife in Trinidad. *Vector Borne Zoonotic Dis.* 2012;12(11):969–978.
10. Pinheiro FP. *CRC Handbook Series in Zoonosis, Viral Zoonosis.* CRC Press; 1981.
11. Figueiredo LT. The Brazilian flaviviruses. *Microbes Infect.* 2000;2:1643–1649.
12. Laemmert HW, Hughes T. The virus of Ilhéus encephalitis: isolation, serological specificity and transmission. *J Immunol.* 1947;55:61–67.
13. Pauvolid-Corrêa A, Kenney JL, Couto-Lima D, et al. Ilhéus virus isolation in the Pantanal, West-Central Brazil. *PLoS Negl Trop Dis.* 2013;7(7), e2318.
14. Shope RE. *The Flaviviruses: Detection, Diagnosis and Vaccination Development.* Academic Press; 2003.
15. de Rodaniche E, Galindo P. Isolation of the virus of Ilhéus encephalitis from mosquitoes captured in Panama. *Am J Trop Med Hyg.* 1961;10(3):393–394.
16. Vasconcelos PFC, Travassos da Rosa AP, Pinheiro FP, et al. *An Overview of Arbovirology in Brazil and Neighbouring Countries.* Instituto Evandro Chagas; 1998.
17. Turell MJ, O'Guinn ML, Jones JW, et al. Isolation of viruses from mosquitoes (Diptera: Culicidae) collected in the Amazon Basin region of Peru. *J Med Entomol.* 2005;42(5):891–898.
18. Karabatsos N. *International Catalogue of Arboviruses Including Certain Other Viruses of Vertebrates.* 3rd ed. American Society of Tropical Medicine & Hygiene; 1985.
19. Iversson LB, Silva RAMS, Travassos da Rosa APA, Barros VLRS. Circulation of Eastern equine encephalitis, Western equine encephalitis, Ilhéus, Maguari and Tacaiuma viruses in equines of the Brazilian Pantanal, South America. *Rev Inst Med Trop Sao Paulo.* 1993;35(4):355–359.
20. Pauvolid-Corrêa A, Morales MA, Levis S, et al. Neutralising antibodies for West Nile virus in horses from Brazilian Pantanal. *Mem Inst Oswaldo Cruz.* 2011;106(4):467–474.
21. Pauvolid-Corrêa A, Campos Z, Juliano R, Velez J, Nogueira RMR, Komar N. Serological evidence of widespread circulation of West Nile virus and other flaviviruses in equines of the Pantanal, Brazil. *PLoS Negl Trop Dis.* 2014;8(2), e2706.
22. Prías-Landónez E, Bernal-Cubides C, Morales-Alarcon A. Isolation of Ilhéus virus from a man in Colombia. *Am J Trop Med Hyg.* 1968;17:112–114.
23. Causey OR, Causey CE, Maroja OM, Macedo DG. The isolation of arthropod-borne viruses, including members of two hitherto undescribed serological groups, in the Amazon Region of Brazil. *Am J Trop Med Hyg.* 1961;10:227–249.
24. Baleotti FG, Moreli ML, Figueiredo LTM. Brazilian flavivirus phylogeny based on NS5. *Mem Inst Oswaldo Cruz.* 2003;98(3):379–382.
25. Cruz AC, da Rosa AP, Ferreira II, Albuquerque MM, Galler R. Ilhéus virus (Flaviviridae, Flavivirus) is closely related to Japanese encephalitis virus complex. *Intervirology.* 1997;40(4):220–225.

26. Kuno G, Chang G, Tsuchiya K, Karabatsos N, Cropp C. Phylogeny of the genus Flavivirus. *J Virol.* 1998;72(1):73–83.

27. Barros VE, Thomazini JA, Figueiredo LT. Cytopathological changes induced by selected Brazilian flaviviruses in mouse macrophages. *J Microsc.* 2004;216(pt. 1):5–14.

28. Pinheiro F, Travassos da Rosa A. *CRC Handbook of Zoonoses.* CRC Press; 1994.

29. Pereira LE, Suzuki A, Coimbra TLM, de Souza RP, Chamelet ELB. Ilhéus arbovirus in wild birds (*Sporophila caerulescens* and *Molothrus bonariensis*). *Rev Saude Publica.* 2001;35(2):119–123.

30. Laroque PO, Valença-Montenegro MM, Ferreira DR, et al. Epidemiologic survey for arbovirus in Galician capuchin monkeys (*Cebus flavius*) free living in Paraíba and captive Capuchin monkey (*Cebus libidinosus*) from Northeast Brazil. *Pesqui Vet Bras.* 2014;34:462–468.

31. de Oliveira-Filho EF, Oliveira RAS, Ferreira DRA, et al. Seroprevalence of selected flaviviruses in free-living and captive capuchin monkeys in the state of Pernambuco, Brazil. *Transbound Emerg Dis.* 2017;65:1094–1097.

32. Morales MA, Fabbri CM, Zunino GE, et al. Detection of the mosquito-borne flaviviruses, West Nile, dengue, Saint Louis encephalitis, Ilhéus, Bussuquara, and yellow fever in free-ranging black howlers (*Alouatta caraya*) of Northeastern Argentina. *PLoS Negl Trop Dis.* 2017;11, e0005351.

33. Glowacki G, Spinsanti L, Basualdo MA, Díaz G, Contigiani M. Prevalence of flavivirus antibodies in young voluntary recruits to military service in the province of Formosa, Argentina. *Rev Argent Microbiol.* 1998;30(4):170–175.

34. Casseb AR, Cruz AV, Jesus IS, et al. Seroprevalence of flaviviruses antibodies in water buffaloes (*Bubalus bubalis*) in Brazilian Amazon. *J Venom Anim Toxins Incl Trop Dis.* 2014;20:9.

35. Amarilla AA, Fumagalli MJ, Figueiredo ML, et al. Ilhéus and Saint Louis encephalitis viruses elicit cross-protection against a lethal Rocio virus challenge in mice. *PLoS One.* 2018;13(6), e0199071.

36. Medeiros DBA, Nunes MRT, Vasconcelos PFC, Chang G-JJ, Kuno G. Complete genome characterization of Rocio virus (Flavivirus: Flaviviridae), a Brazilian flavivirus isolated from a fatal case of encephalitis during an epidemic in São Paulo State. *J Gen Virol.* 2007;88:2237–2246.

37. Iversson LB. *The Arboviruses: Epidemiology and Ecology.* CRC Press; 1988.

38. de Souza Lopes O, Coimbra TLM, Sacchetta LA, Calisher CH. Emergence of a new arbovirus disease in Brazil. I. Isolation and characterization of the etiologic agent, Rocio virus. *Am J Epidemiol.* 1978;107:444–449.

39. de Souza Lopes O, de Abreu Sacchetta L, Coimbra TL, Pinto GH, Glasser CM. Emergence of a new arbovirus disease in Brazil. II. Epidemiologic studies on 1975 epidemic. *Am J Epidemiol.* 1978;108(5):394–401.

40. Iversson LB, Travassos da Rosa AP, Rosa MD. Recent occurrence of human infection by Rocio arbovirus in the Valley of Ribeira region. *Rev Inst Med Trop Sao Paulo.* 1989;31:28–31.

41. Straatmann A, Santos-Torres S, Vasconcelos PF, da Rosa AP, Rodrigues SG, Tavares-Neto J. Serological evidence of the circulation of the Rocio arbovirus (Flaviviridae) in Bahia. *Rev Soc Bras Med Trop.* 1997;30(6):511–515.

42. Coimbra TLM, Santos RN, Petrella S, Nagasse-Sugahara TK, Castrignano SB, Santos CLS. Molecular characterization of two Rocio flavivirus strains isolated during the encephalitis epidemic in São Paulo State, Brazil and the development of one-step RT-PCR assay for diagnosis. *Rev Inst Med Trop Sao Paulo.* 2008;50(2):89–94.

43. Tanaka H, Weigl DR, de Souza Lopes O. The replication of Rocio virus in brain tissue of suckling mice: study by electron microscopy. *Arch Virol.* 1983;78(3–4):309–314.

44. ICTV. *Virus Taxonomy: Eighth Report of the International Committee on the Taxonomy of Viruses.* Elsevier; 2005.

45. Setoh YX, Amarilla AA, Peng NY, et al. Full genome sequence of Rocio virus reveal substantial variations from the prototype Rocio virus SPH 34675 sequence. *Arch Virol.* 2018;163:255–258.

46. Vasconcelos PFC, Travassos da Rosa APA, Dégallier N, Travassos da Rosa JFS, Pinheiro FP. Clinical and eco-epidemiological situation of human arboviruses in Brazilian Amazonia. *Cienc Cult.* 1992;44:117–124.

47. de Souza Lopes O, de Abreu Sacchetta L, Francy DB, Jakob WL, Calisher CH. Emergence of a new arbovirus disease in Brazil. III. Isolation of Rocio virus from *Psorophora ferox* (Humboldt, 1819). *Am J Epidemiol.* 1981;113(2):122–125.

48. Mitchell CJ, Forattini OP. Experimental transmission of Rocio encephalitis virus by *Aedes scapularis* (Diptera: Culicidae) from the epidemic zone in Brazil. *J Med Entomol.* 1984;1(1):34–37.

49. Mitchell CJ, Forattini OP, Miller BR. Vector competence experiments with Rocio virus and three mosquito species from the epidemic zone in Brazil. *Rev Saude Publica.* 1986;20:171–177.

50. Mitchell CJ, Monath TP, Cropp CB. Experimental transmission of Rocio virus by mosquitoes. *Am J Trop Med Hyg.* 1981;30:465–472.

51. White LL. Susceptibility of *Aedes albopictus* C6/36 cells to viral infection. *J Clin Microbiol.* 1987;25(7):1221–1224.

52. Monath TP, Kemp GE, Cropp CB, Bowen GS. Experimental infection of house sparrows (*Passer domesticus*) with Rocio virus. *Am J Trop Med Hyg.* 1978;27(6):1251–1254.

53. Silva JM, Romeiro MF, de Souza WM, et al. A Saint Louis encephalitis and Rocio virus serosurvey in Brazilian horses. *Rev Soc Bras Med Trop.* 2014;47(4):414–417.

54. Harrison AK, Murphy FA, Gardner JJ, Bauer SP. Myocardial and pancreatic necrosis induced by Rocio virus, a new flavivirus. *Exp Mol Pathol.* 2014;32:102–113.

55. Henriques DF, Quaresma JAS, Fuzii HT, et al. Persistence of experimental Rocio virus infection in the golden hamster (*Mesocricetus auratus*). *Mem Inst Oswaldo Cruz.* 2012;107(5):630–636.

56. Barros VED, Saggioro FP, Neder L, et al. An experimental model of meningoencephalomyelitis by Rocio

flavivirus in BALB/c mice: inflammatory response, cytokine production, and histopathology. *Am J Trop Med Hyg.* 2011;85(2):363–373.

57. Barros VED, Ferreira BR, Livonesi M, Figueiredo LTM. Cytokine and nitric oxide production by mouse macrophages infected with Brazilian flaviviruses. *Rev Inst Med Trop Sao Paulo.* 2009;51(3):141–147.

58. Amarilla AA, Setoh YX, Periasamy P, et al. Chimeric viruses between Rocio and West Nile: the role for Rocio prM-E proteins in virulence and inhibition of interferon-α/β signaling. *Sci Rep.* 2017;7:44642.

59. Franca RF, Costa RS, Silva JR, et al. IL-33 signaling is essential to attenuate viral-induced encephalitis development by downregulating iNOS expression in the central nervous system. *J Neuroinflammation.* 2016;13(1):159.

60. Glass WG, Lim JK, Cholera R, Pletnev AG, Gao JL, Murphy PM. Chemokine receptor CCR5 promotes leukocyte trafficking to the brain and survival in West Nile virus infection. *J Exp Med.* 2005;202:1087–1098.

61. Chavez JH, Franca RF, Oliveira CJ, et al. Influence of the CCR-5/MIP-1 α axis in the pathogenesis of Rocio virus encephalitis in a mouse model. *Am J Trop Med Hyg.* 2013;89:1013–1018.

62. Doherty RL, Carley JG, Mackerras MJ, Marks EN. Studies of arthropod-borne virus infections in Queensland. III. Isolation and characterisation of virus strains from wild-caught mosquitoes in North Queensland. *Aust J Exp Biol Med Sci.* 1963;41:17–39.

63. Poidinger M, Hall RA, Mackenzie JS. Molecular characterization of the Japanese encephalitis serocomplex of the *Flavivirus* genus. *Virology.* 1996;218:417–421.

64. Nisbet DJ, Lee KJ, van den Hurk AF, et al. Identification of new flaviviruses in the Kokobera virus complex. *J Gen Virol.* 2005;86:121–124.

65. May FJ, Clark DC, Pham VK, et al. Genetic divergence among members of the Kokobera group of flaviviruses supports their separation into distinct species. *J Gen Virol.* 2013;94:1462–1467.

66. Blasi A, Presti AL, Cella E, Angeletti S, Ciccozzi M. The phylogenetic and evolutionary history of Kokobera virus. *Asian Pac J Trop Med.* 2016;9(10):968–972.

67. Hall RA, Burgess GW, Kay BH, Clancy P. Monoclonal antibodies to Kunjin and Kokobera viruses. *Immunol Cell Biol.* 1991;69(1):47–49.

68. Toi CS, Webb CE, Haniotis J, Clancy J, Doggett SL. Seasonal activity, vector relationships and genetic analysis of mosquito-borne Stratford virus. *PLoS One.* 2017;12(3), e0173105.

69. Mackenzie JS, Williams DT. The zoonotic flaviviruses of Southern, South-Eastern and Eastern Asia, and Australasia: the potential for emergent viruses. *Zoonoses Public Health.* 2009;56:338–356.

70. Russell RC, Kay BH. Medical entomology: changes in the spectrum of mosquito-borne disease in Australia and other vector threats and risks, 1972-2004. *Aust J Entomol.* 2004;43:271–282.

71. Ryan PA, Kay BH. Emergence trapping of mosquitoes (Diptera: Culicidae) in brackish forest habitats in Maroochy Shire, South-East Queensland, Australia, and a management option for *Verrallina funereal* (Theobald) and *Aedes procax* (Skuse). *Aust J Entomol.* 2000;39:212–218.

72. Kay BH, Watson TM, Ryan PA. Definition of productive *Aedes notoscriptus* (Diptera: Culicidae) habitats in Western Brisbane, and a strategy for their control. *Aust J Entomol.* 2008;47:142–148.

73. Flies EJ, Toi C, Weinstein P, Doggett SL, Williams CR. Converting mosquito surveillance to arbovirus surveillance with honey-baited nucleic acid preservation cards. *Vector Borne Zoonotic Dis.* 2015;5(7):397–403.

74. Johansen C, Maley F, Broom AK. Isolation of Stratford virus from mosquitoes collected in the southwest of Western Australia. *Arbovirus Res Aust.* 2005;9:164–166.

75. Mackenzie JS, Lindsay MD, Coelen RJ, Broom K, Hall RA, Smith DW. Arboviruses causing human disease in the Australasian zoogeographic region. *Arch Virol.* 1994;136(3–4):447–467.

76. Doherty R, Gorman BM, Whitehead RH, Carley JG. Studies of epidemic polyarthritis: the significance of three Group A arboviruses isolated from mosquitoes in Queensland. *Australas Ann Med.* 1964;3:322–327.

77. Johansen CA, Nisbet DJ, Zborowski P, van den Hurk AF, Ritchie SA, Mackenzie JS. Flavivirus isolations from mosquitoes collected from Western Cape York Peninsula, Australia, 1999-2000. *J Am Mosq Control Assoc.* 2003;19(4):392–396.

78. Hawkes RA, Boughton CR, Naim HM, Wild J, Chapman B. Arbovirus infections of humans in New South Wales. Seroepidemiology of the flavivirus group of togaviruses. *Med J Aust.* 1985;143(12–13):555–561.

79. Boughton CR, Hawkes RA, Naim HM. Illness caused by a Kokobera-like virus in South-Eastern Australia. *Med J Aust.* 1986;145(2):90–92.

80. Russell RC. Arboviruses and their vectors in Australia: an update on the ecology and epidemiology of some mosquito-borne arboviruses. *Rev Med Vet Entomol.* 1995;83:141–158.

81. Poidinger M, Hall RA, Lindsay MD, Broom AK, Mackenzi JS. The molecular epidemiology of Kokobera virus. *Virus Res.* 2000;68:7–13.

82. Johansen CA, Nisbet DJ, Foley PN, et al. Flavivirus isolations from mosquitoes collected from Saibai Island in the Torres Strait, Australia, during an incursion of Japanese encephalitis virus. *Med Vet Entomol.* 2004;18:281–287.

83. Johansen CA, Farrow RA, Morrisen A, et al. Wind-borne mosquitoes: could they be a mechanism of incursion of Japanese encephalitis virus into Australia? *Arbovirus Res Aust.* 2001;8:180–186.

84. Diagne MM, Faye M, Faye O, et al. Emergence of Wesselsbron virus among black rat and humans in Eastern Senegal in 2013. *One Health.* 2017;3:23–28.

85. Weiss KE, Haig DA, Alexander RA. Wesselsbron virus—a virus not previously described associated with

abortion in domestic animals. *Onderstepoort J Vet Res.* 1956;27:183–195.

86. Weiss KE. Wesselsbron virus disease. *Bull Epizoot Dis Afr.* 1957;5:431–458.

87. Weyer J, Thomas J, Leman PA, Grobbelaar AA, Kemp A, Paweska JT. Human cases of Wesselsbron disease, South Africa 2010-2011. *Vector Borne Zoonotic Dis.* 2013;13(5):330–336.

88. Blackburn NK, Swanepoel R. An investigation of flavivirus infections of cattle in Zimbabwe Rhodesia with particular reference to Wesselsbron virus. *J Hyg (Camb).* 1980;85:1–33.

89. Baba SS, Fagbami AH, Omilabu SA. Wesselsbron virus infection in West African dwarf goats (*Fouta djallon*): virological and immunological studies. *Acta Virol.* 1989;33(1):81–86.

90. Baba SS. Virological and immunological studies of Wesselsbron virus in experimentally infected red Sokoto (Maradi) goats. *Vet Microbiol.* 1993;34:311–320.

91. Coetzer JA, Theodoridis A. Clinical and pathological studies in adult sheep and goats experimentally infected with Wesselsbron disease virus. *Onderstepoort J Vet Res.* 1982;49:19–22.

92. Theodoridis A, Coetzer JA. Wesselsbron disease: virological and serological studies in experimentally infected sheep and goats. *Onderstepoort J Vet Res.* 1980;47:221–229.

93. Jupp PG, Kemp A. Studies on an outbreak of Wesselsbron virus in the Free State Province, South Africa. *J Am Mosq Control Assoc.* 1998;14(1):40–45.

94. Diallo M, Nabeth P, Ba K, et al. Mosquito vectors of the 1998–1999 outbreak of Rift Valley fever and other arboviruses (Bagaza, Sanar, Wesselsbron and West Nile) in Mauritania and Senegal. *Med Vet Entomol.* 2005;19(2):119–126.

95. Morvan J, Fontenille D, Digoutte JP, Coulanges P. The Wesselsbron virus, a new arbovirus for Madagascar. *Arch Inst Pasteur Madagascar.* 1990;57:183–192.

96. Muspratt J, Smithburn KC, Paterson HE, Kokernot RH. Studies on arthropod-borne viruses of Tongaland. X. The laboratory transmission of Wesselsbron virus by the bite of *Aedes (Banksinella) circumluteolus* Theo. *S Afr J Med Sci.* 1957;22:121–126.

97. Kokernot RH, Paterson HE, De Meillon B. Studies on the transmission of Wesselsbron virus by *Aedes* (*Ochlerotatus*) *caballus* (Theo.). *S Afr Med J.* 1958;32:546–548.

98. Simasathien P, Olson LC. Factors influencing the vector potential of *Aedes aegypti* and *Culex quinquefasciatus* for Wesselsbron virus. *J Med Entomol.* 1973;10(6):587–590.

99. Kemp GE, Causey OR, Moore DL, O'Connor EH. Viral isolates from livestock in Northern Nigeria: 1966-1970. *Am J Vet Res.* 1973;34:707–710.

100. Allwright DM, Geyer A, Burger WP, Williams R, Gerdes GH, Barnard BJ. Isolation of Wesselsbron virus from ostriches. *Vet Rec.* 1995;136:99.

101. Ardoin P, Rodhain F, Hannoun C. Epidemiologic study of arboviruses in the Arba-Minch district of Ethiopia. *Trop Geogr Med.* 1976;28:309–315.

102. Jan C, Languillat G, Renaudet J, Robin Y. A serological survey of arboviruses in Gabon. *Bull Soc Pathol Exot Filiales.* 1978;1:140–146.

103. Guilherme JM, Gonella-Legall C, Legall F, Nakoume E, Vincent J. Seroprevalence of five arboviruses in Zebu cattle in the Central African Republic. *Trans R Soc Trop Med Hyg.* 1996;90:31–33.

104. Baba SS, Fagbami AH, Ojeh CK, Olaleye OD, Omilabu SA. Wesselsbron virus antibody in domestic animals in Nigeria: retrospective and prospective studies. *New Microbiol.* 1995;18(2):151–162.

105. Fokam EB, Levai LD, Guzman H, et al. Silent circulation of arboviruses in Cameroon. *East Afr Med J.* 2010;87(6):262–268.

106. Fagbami A. Human arthropod-borne virus infections in Nigeria. Serological and virological investigations and Shaki, Oyo State. *J Hyg Epidemiol Microbiol Immunol.* 1978;22:184–189.

107. Gudo ES, Falk K, Cliff J. Historical perspective of arboviruses in Mozambique and its implication for current and future epidemics. *Adv Exp Med Biol.* 2018;1062:11–18.

108. Baba SS, Fagbami AH, Olaleye OD. Antigenic relatedness of selected flaviviruses: study with homologous and heterologous immune mouse ascitic fluids. *Rev Inst Med Trop Sao Paulo.* 1998;40(6):343–349.

CHAPTER 9

Tickborne Encephalitis Virus

INTRODUCTION TO TICKBORNE ENCEPHALITIS VIRUS AND ITS HISTORY

Tickborne encephalitis virus (TBEV) is one of the most important tickborne arboviruses in Central and Eastern European countries, Russia, and parts of Asia, infecting at least 13,000 people annually despite the fact that it is not a reportable disease in China. There has been a 300% increase in human infections during the 10 years preceding 2018.[1–4] At least three groups of this virus exist: TBEV-European (TBEV-Eur), TBEV-Siberian (TBEV-Sib), and TBEV-Far Eastern (TBEV-FE). The viruses' range is increasing and now includes parts of France, Sweden, Finland, Norway, Italy, and the Netherlands.[5–8] This increase may be due to the growing numbers and spread of its tick vectors, which may reflect climatic changes as well as changes in the land usage.[9,10] TBEV has been placed into category C of the CDCs list of potential bioterrorism agents due to its availability, ease of production and dissemination, and potential for high morbidity and mortality.[11]

Social and political factors contribute to disease incidence. For example, reported tickborne encephalitis (TBE) incidence increased from 2- to 30-fold in many Central and Eastern European countries as they gained their independence from Soviet rule. This led to the subsequent breakdown of medical and public health institutions in addition to decreased income and availability of food. In Latvia, high-risk behavior included harvesting food from tick-infested forests and decreased vaccination. In eight Eastern European countries, national socioeconomic conditions, such as poverty and household expenditure on food, strongly correlate with the extent of TBE incidence.

In many endemic regions, TBEV distribution is highly focal. The spatiotemporal heterogeneities in TBE epidemiology in these countries appear to better explain the differences in national disease incidence patterns than those detected by climate change alone, since it is uniform across the affected areas. The apparent increases in TBEV incidence may also reflect more accurate reporting of current disease incidence in humans than was the case when these countries were part of the former Soviet Union.[12]

A study of TBEV-FE in China between 2003 and 2016 found that the disease is reemerging and that its range is expanding. Approximately 99% of the cases in humans are reported in the forested areas of the northeastern part of China and 93% of them occur from May to July.[13] The spatial distribution of human TBE in this area of China is associated with land use and the amounts of broad-leaved forest and mixed broadleaf-conifer forests, distribution of *Ixodes persulcatus* ticks, altitudes between 400 and 600 m, and climate. In contrast, disease incidence in northwestern China is highest in areas with altitudes between 1400 and 1700 m, while it is found between altitudes of 2000–3000 m in the southwestern endemic areas of the country. The differences in altitude correspond to *Ix. persulcatus* distribution. In a natural focus of TBEV-FE in southwestern China, 8.3% of the regional adult *Ixodes ovatus* ticks are infected. Temperature, relative humidity, rainfall, and sunshine hours also potentially affect the tick life cycles and viral replication in the tick.[13] Relative humidity of 75%–90% is also important in increasing the activity of *Ixodes ricinus* nymphs and the subsequent TBEV-Eur incidence in humans in southern Poland.[14]

In addition to recent increases in the range of TBEV-FE, changes in pathogenicity have been occurring in the populations of TBEV. A TBEV-FE strain that causes high morbidity and mortality in the large Japanese field mouse was isolated in Japan in 2008. A far less virulent strain with 36 nucleoside differences and 12 amino acid changes in the gene encoding the NS5 protein had been previously isolated from wild rodents in 1995. The more pathogenic strain 2008 strain underwent greater viral multiplication and inflammatory responses in the brains of mice than the earlier strain.[15]

The reemergence of human infection in China may have at least partially resulted from the "Greening" Program, instituted in the mid-1900s that returned agricultural lands to forests and grasslands.[16] While forestry workers are at high risk of infection, an increasing proportion of disease is occurring among farmers and domestic workers who perform pot herb-picking activities in the spring and summer. The latter two groups are less experienced in avoiding tick bites and also have

Zika and Other Neglected and Emerging Flaviviruses. https://doi.org/10.1016/B978-0-323-82501-6.00012-8

a much lower rate of TBEV vaccination than do forestry workers.[13] It should be noted, however, that TBE is not a notifiable disease in China, which may result in underreporting, especially in the more remote regions where tick-human contact is greater than found in urban areas.

TBEV NEUROLOGICAL DISEASE AND VIRAL STRUCTURE

In experimentally infected bank voles, all three TBEV subtypes cause viremia. They are also highly neurotropic, infecting only neurons and not neuroglia, first in the cortex and hippocampus, and later appearing in Purkinje cells of the cerebellum, similar to viral distribution in experimentally infected mice.[17,18] Mice infected with low doses of TBEV by the subcutaneous route may also develop systemic inflammatory thymic and splenic atrophy as well as stress responses, including increased serum levels of corticosterone (a stress hormone that downregulates some parts of the immune response) and tumor necrosis factor-α (TNF-α) (a powerful inflammatory cytokine).[18] Humans develop nonspecific, microscopic lesions throughout the gray matter of the brainstem, cerebrum, cerebellar cortex, pons, cerebellum, thalamus, and anterior horns of the spinal cord.[18-22] Degenerative changes in the cerebral cortex are confined to the pyramidal cells of the motor area where lymphocytes accumulate and glial cells proliferate near the surface of the cerebrum.[21,23] Viral RNA, but not viral antigen, remains in the brain for up to 168 days after infection, but may or may not be infective throughout this time period. TBEV-Eur causes a biphasic disease in most regions outside of China, initially presenting with flu-like symptoms. In 20%–30% of cases, patients enter into the second phase of infection.[24] This phase is characterized by central nervous system (CNS) involvement, including ataxia, paralysis of the limbs, meningitis, encephalitis, meningoencephalitis, or polioencephalomyelitis, primarily in the spinal cord, brainstem, and cerebellum, associated with infiltration of inflammatory cells into the CNS.[10,21,25-30] Epilepsia partialis continua is a rare variant of simple focal motor status epilepticus and is reported in people infected by either TBEV-FE or TBEV-Eur.[31] Neurons may be damaged by a combination of viral infection, infiltrating CD8+ T cells, proinflammatory cytokines, and activated microglial cells.[18] Neighboring cells may also be damaged, presumably due to bystander effects.[32] The virus is present in serum in the first, febrile phase, but only rarely in the second, neurological phase.[33]

During infection with TBEV-FE, 31%–64% of patients develop focal encephalitic symptoms, 26% develop meningeal disease, 14%–16% become febrile, and only 3%–8% develop biphasic disease.[22] The fatality rate is as high as 35%, and complete recovery only occurs in 25% of the patients; however, less than 0.5% of those infected develop chronic disease. Focal encephalitic symptoms are found in 5% of patients infected by TBEV-Sib: 47% develop meningeal disease, 40% become febrile, and 21% develop biphasic disease. The fatality rate is 2%, and complete recovery from this virus type occurs in 80% of the patients. During TBEV-Eur infection, 72%–87% of patients develop biphasic disease.[22] In adults, the fatality rate is generally less than 2%, but a focus of highly virulent TBEV-Eur has been reported in southern Germany that had a fatality rate of 33%.

Variations in the E and nucleocapsid proteins affect virulence. The strain responsible for the high fatality rate in Germany is a TBEV-Eur variant. It has two unique amino acid substitutions in the E protein that are not found in typical TBEV-Eur strains.[34] Additionally, as many as 50% of TBEV-Eur patients develop residual sequelae, even in people infected by normal, low-mortality strains. The risk of developing severe disease, higher mortality rates, and long-lasting sequelae increases with age. Permanent sequelae are seen in as many as 46% of the patients and include cognitive and neuropsychiatric complaints, balance disorders, headache, dysphasia, hearing defects, and spinal paralysis.[22,23] Infection with TBEV-Eur is generally more common in adults than children. Children typically develop milder disease, although severe illness and permanent sequelae occasionally occur. Prognosis is favorable in children.[35,36]

TBEV-FE variants differ in their pathogenic potential, with many seropositive, yet healthy people found in China. Nevertheless, TBEV-FE produces a more prolonged viremia in comparison with the other TBEV variants.[17] In addition to nervous system disease, severe cases of TBE in China report paralysis, disturbance of consciousness, difficulties in swallowing and verbal communication, myocardial damage, and liver dysfunction.[37] The wide range of differences in pathogenicity appears to be at least partially due to single amino acid substitutions in the E protein that are associated with low levels of neuroinvasion, limited peripheral replication, and lessened pathogenicity in mice.[38,39] Differences in the host's major histocompatibility complex (MHC) molecules or regional human activities, including occupational variation within a given area, may also contribute to disease severity and neuroinvasiveness. At least three specific amino acid substitutions in TBEV-Eur's E protein are known to result in decreased disease in vivo. One of these substitutions (Glu122 → Gly), found in both TBEV-FE and TBEV-Eur, is associated with binding to host heparan sulfate during viral entry into its target cells.[38]

Isolating and sequencing of strains of TBEV-FE from patients with varying degrees of severity (encephalitic, febrile, and subclinical) indicate that the nucleocapsid protein also influences pathogenicity. The nucleocapsid is involved in viral budding during transit of virus between the endomembranous components (endosomes, the endoplasmic reticulum, and Golgi apparatus) of the host cell. Several amino acid substitutions in the viral nonstructural NS3 or NS5 proteins decrease TBEV-FE virulence.[40] Additionally, four amino acids in the C-terminus of NS5's polymerase are important in neuronal degeneration as well as neuronal dysfunction, including decreased neurite differentiation and outgrowth. These NS5 alterations do not directly affect viral replication or the host inflammatory response. They may do so, however, by altering interactions between NS5 and host PDZ domain-containing proteins, effecting synaptic plasticity and axonal degeneration in the nervous system.[41]

TBEV's NS5 contains 2 PDZ binding motifs.[42,43] PDZ domains are often present in host multidomain scaffolding proteins in the CNS. These scaffolds are important for the regulation of synaptic plasticity and synaptic vesicle dynamics. The NS5 methyltransferase and RNA polymerase domains inhibit neuronal differentiation by binding to the host PDZ domain protein Scribble and outcompete the binding of the host Rho GTPase Ras-related C3 botulinum toxin substrate 1 (Rac1) and the guanine nucleotide exchange factor, PAK-interacting guanine nucleotide exchange factor (βPIX).[44] Rac1 is critical in regulating cytoskeletal actin rearrangements in cells, including axon guidance and neurite outgrowth. Its activity is controlled by βPIX. NS5 is able to bind to several other host proteins as well, including those regulating synaptic membrane exocytosis-2, zonula occludens-2, GIAP glutamate receptor-interacting protein 2, GIAP C-terminus-interacting protein, the calcium/calmodulin-dependent serine protein kinase, and interleukin-16 (IL-16).[43]

The 3'-untranslated region (UTR) of TBEV-FE is also involved in pathogenesis. Partial deletions and the addition of poly A's in the variable 5'-terminal of the 3'-UTR increase virulence in mouse brains, while decreasing viral multiplication in the periphery, without effecting the induction of interferon (IFN) or IFN-stimulated genes (ISGs).[45] Such alterations in the 3'-UTR's variable region are also present in TBEV strains passaged in mammalian cell cultures in vitro as well as in TBEV-Eur strains isolated from humans.[46-48] Moreover, deletions in this region are associated with disease severity in the highly virulent TBEV-FE strain Sofjin-HO and the low virulent strain Oshima 5-10 in mice.[49] This region of Sofjin-HO contains fewer stem-loop structures than Oshima 5-10.[45] Host cell proteins, including La, p100, fructose-bisphosphatase 1 (FBP1), and Mov34, bind to the viral 3'-UTRs as well.[45]

Infiltrating inflammatory cells cross the blood–brain barrier (BBB) as they enter the CNS. TBEV entry into the brain precedes BBB disruption. BBB permeability increases during later stages of infection in the presence of high virus loads in the brain.[50] Among patients with neuroinvasive infection, 25%–40% of the survivors develop long-lasting neurological sequelae, which include severe headaches and decreased quality of life.[10,23,51] Although only about 5% of primary human microvascular endothelial cell cultures are infected in vitro, the infection is persistent and yields high TBEV titers (over 10^6 plaque-forming units/mL), without causing cytopathic effect. The low infection rate in the brain microvascular endothelial cells may partially explain why only some TBEV-infected individuals develop CNS infection.[52] Astrocytes, glial cells which help to maintain the BBB, may be infected by TBEV as well.

Unlike some mosquito-borne flaviviruses, including WNV, no changes are found in the expression of key tight junction proteins, such as occludin and zonula occludens-1, cell adhesion molecules, or alterations in the intercellular junctions between these brain endothelial cells. Moreover, in in vitro models, TBEV crosses the BBB using a transcellular pathway that does not compromise the cellular monolayer integrity, is independent of TBEV strain virulence, and also is found during infection with several other flaviviruses, including WNV and JEV.[52] CD8+ T killer cells, however, alter BBB tight junction proteins and increase CNS vascular permeability, but not in infected perforin-deficient mice.[53] Increased BBB permeability, however, still occurs in the absence of CD8+ T killer cells, suggesting the involvement of additional factors, including proinflammatory cytokines, chemokines, and matrix-degrading metalloproteinase-9 (MMP-9).

Increased BBB permeability in mice additionally corresponds to high levels of mRNA for TNF-α, IL-6, IFN-γ, ICAM-1 (intercellular adhesion molecule), RANTES (regulated upon activation, normal T cell expressed, and secreted), MCP-1 (macrophage chemotactic protein-1), MIP-1α (migration inhibitory protein),

MIP-1β, and IP-10 (interferon gamma-induced protein 10).[50] In humans, serum levels of the proinflammatory cytokines TNF-α and IL-6 peak during the first week of hospitalization. Reducing levels of these cytokines and chemokines is associated with quicker improvement and faster recovery in vivo. Moreover, TBE patients' CSF contains increased levels of MCP-1 and RANTES.[54,55] In humans, high levels of MMP-9 are also present in the serum[56] and CSF.[57]

In vitro, TBEV infection of several types of cultured human neural cell lines (neuroblastoma, medulloblastoma, and glioblastoma) leads to very high viral titers. Proliferation of rough ER membranes, especially in the perinuclear region, and extensive rearrangement of the cytoskeleton occur in both medulloblastoma and glioblastoma, but not neuroblastoma, cell lines.[32] A dense network of microtubulin is found in areas in which viral E protein accumulates, suggesting that the host cytoskeleton may be involved in the TBEV maturation process. While a large number of apoptotic signs are present in neuroblastoma cells, including condensation, margination, and fragmentation of chromatin; vacuolation of the cytoplasm; dilatation of the ER cisternae; and shrinkage of cells, the neuroblastoma cells primarily die by necrosis rather than by apoptosis.[32]

Host cell genes affect disease severity as well. At least 140 genes are involved in the human cellular response to TBEV. The effects of any of these single genes upon disease severity in humans are difficult to determine since virulence may be multifactorial, with more than one host gene contributing to the overall extent of pathology.[58] In Russia and Lithuania, a variety of innate immune system-related genes contain deletions or single-nucleotide polymorphisms that are associated with predisposition to TBEV infection or to the development of severe neurological disease. These virulence-associated nucleoside alterations are present in the following host cell genes: oligoadenylate synthase 2 (OAS2) and 3 (OAS3), the dendritic cell-specific intercellular adhesion molecule (ICAM)-3 grabbing nonintegrin (DC-SIGN), interleukin 28B/interferon lambda 3 (IL28B/IFNL3), IL-10, chemokine receptor 5 (CCR5), MMP9, and AT-rich DNA-interacting domain-containing protein.[58–65] A polymorphism in the Toll-like receptor 3 (TLR3) gene correlates with more severe disease as well.[62,65] MMPs degrade extracellular matrix proteins that are important in cellular development and morphogenesis, in addition to activating the production of cytokines and chemokines involved in tissue remodeling. High levels of these molecules are present during inflammation and in the serum and CSF of TBE patients.[57,63,66] Increased activity of these proteinases

may aid in the disruption of the BBB by degrading the barrier's protein connections, allowing leukocytes to enter the CNS and cause local inflammatory reactions.

Ixodes species ticks are vectors for a number of neurological diseases of viral and bacterial origin, including TBE and neuroborreliosis caused by the Lyme disease spirochete. Levels of serum HMGB-1 (high-mobility group box 1) early during diseases aid in differentiation between these tickborne microbes and help to indicate appropriate treatment for people with neurological disease following tick bites.[67]

THE VIRUS
Viral Subtypes

According to the International Committee on Taxonomy of Viruses, TBEV is divided into three subtypes (TBEV-Eur, TBEV-FE, and TBEV-Sib), which differ in amino acid 206 of the E protein. European strains contain Val at this position, Siberian strains contain Leu, and Far-Eastern strains contain Ser.[68] TBEV-Eur is primarily transmitted by *Ixodes ricinus* hard ticks. These ticks are found throughout Europe and transmit almost all of the TBEV-Eur in Europe. TBEV-Eur RNA is detectable by PCR in samples of both human clinical sera and urine, but not in the CSF. This type of TBEV may also be found when performing typical immunological tests for other conditions, suggesting a higher incidence of TBEV in humans than that which is being reported.[69] Several other TBEV subtypes have also been proposed based on nucleoside and amino acid differences. One such potential new subtype, containing the 886-84-like virus strains, is proposed to be named TBEV-Baikalian (TBEV-Bkl) and is related to TBEV-Sib, with both TBEVs having a Leu at position 206 of the E protein.[70] An additional proposed rodent subtype, subtype Himalayan TBEV, was detected in 200 marmots in Qinghai–Tibet Plateau in China.[71] This subtype needs to be monitored for possible zoonotic transmission to humans, especially those handling muskrats, muskrat hides, or their bodily fluids.

TBEV-Eur appears to cause a milder disease than other TBEV subtypes.[72] In the Republic of Korea, numbers of human encephalitis cases of unknown origin are being increasingly detected. While no confirmed human cases of TBE have been reported in that country, nevertheless, TBEV-Eur is present in its tick populations, including the primary vectors, *Haemaphysalis longicornis* (Fig. 9.1) and *Haemaphysalis flava*, *Ixodes nipponensis*, *Amblyomma testudinarium*, and *Haemaphysalis phasiana* may also, rarely, act as vectors as well.[37] TBEV-Eur incidence in humans is linked to host-seeking

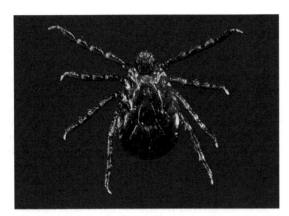

FIG. 9.1 Adult female *Haemaphysalis longicornis* tick, the primary vector of TBEV-Eur.(Credit: CDC/DBVD—Content provider; James Gathany—Photo credit).

activity of nymphal *Ix. ricinus.* Interestingly, while the ratio of TBE cases to questing nymphs is highest during summer-autumn seasons, the numbers of questing nymphs are highest during the spring–summer period. Discrepancies between TBE incidence in humans and abundance of host-questing nymphs may be due to temperature-related differences of virus replication in their tick vectors.[73] Extrinsic climatic conditions also affect the infection of the *Ix. persulcatus* vector of TBEV-FE.[74,75]

TBEV-Sib and TBEV-FE are present in *Ix. ricinus.*[37] Strains of TBEV-Sib and TBEV-FE have also been isolated from *Aedes vexans nipponii* mosquitoes in Russia, but their relevance as viral reservoirs or possible agents of zoonotic disease is unknown. Based on genetic comparison of five TBEV-Eur strains from humans with severe disease, the emergence of TBEV-Eur in Central Europe appears to have been due to a pool of viral strains whose nucleotide identity ranges from 97.5% to 99.6%, despite the fact that these strains were all isolated in 1953 in Central Bohemia, Czechoslovakia, after only a few passages in cell culture. The TBEVs isolated from this region vary greatly in length, from 445 to 751 nucleosides, and differ among themselves by three to nine unique amino acid substitutions.[46] All of these sequenced strains have large deletions in their 3′ noncoding regions, an area associated with strain multiplication and virulence in mouse brains in TBEV-FE.[46,76]

TBEV-Sib has a large range and is the dominant viral type in many parts of Russia and neighboring countries. It is, moreover, slowly replacing the two other subtypes in Northern Europe.[7,77] It is less neuroinvasive than TBEV-FE, especially in children, and has a mortality rate of 2%–3%. TBEV-Sib is, however, more likely to cause recurrent infection or chronic disease than TBEV-Eur.[77–79] TBEV-Sib has at least three lineages that infect humans: the Asian, South-Siberian, and Baltic lineages, plus a suggested East-Siberian lineage.[70] Based upon sequences of their TBEV E genes, the first three of these subtypes are present in the Crimean peninsula in southeastern Europe.[80] TBEV-Sib is typically transmitted by *Ix. persulcatus,* whose range extends from Eastern Europe to China and Japan.[68,79]

TBEV-FE is found predominantly in Far-Eastern Russia, China, and Japan. It is present in at least three species of ticks: *Ix. persulcatus* (its predominant vector), *D. reticulatus,* and *Haemaphysalis punctate* in Moldova.[81] In addition to *Ix. persulcatus* (infection rate = 7.9%), a recent study revealed additional arthropod vectors for TBEV-FE in the Far East of Russia, *Haemaphysalis concinna* (infection rate = 5.6%), *Haemaphysalis japonica douglasi* (infection rate = 2.0%), and *Dermacentor silvarum* (infection rate = 1.3%), in addition to a pool of *Aedes vexans* mosquitoes.[80] In the northern part of Hokkaido, the northernmost Japanese island, *Ix. persulcatus* is the primary vector for TBEV-FE, while *Ix. ovatus* serves this role in the southern part of the island.[37] The range of TBEV-FE may thus be larger than reported, especially if the virus is present in as-yet-unknown tick species.

Among the tick vector species, *Ix. ricinus* may pose the greatest risk to animal and human health since they remain attached to the vertebrate hosts for up to 10 days and transmit the largest variety of pathogens, including other viruses, bacteria, and protozoa. They also take blood meals as larvae and nymphs, as well as adult females. *Ix. ricinus* feeds on almost all wild or domestic animals living in woods and pastures, while humans serve as incidental hosts upon entering tick habitats.[82] In a study conducted in 2012 in France, half of all these ticks (*n* = 267) carried one or more pathogens. Half of the infected ticks hosted at least two pathogens and, in some instances, were infected by as many as five pathogenic microbes, in addition to symbiotic organisms.[83] Human infection by multiple tickborne pathogens might result in a synergistic increase in disease severity since some of the pathogens are immunosuppressive. While TBEV RNA was not detected in this study, future studies in ticks should be conducted in regions where TBE is endemic and in surrounding areas so as to take measures to prevent zoonotic spread over a larger region of Eurasia.

Intriguingly, TBEV-FE is found in a mosaic pattern in various European regions of the former Soviet Union, the Urals, and Siberia.[68] It has been suggested that the odd distribution of pockets of TBEV-FE strains in

Europe and Siberia, thousands of kilometers away from its endemic range, may be due to a massive westward redistribution of game animals, including roe deer, wild boars, and game fowl, in the former Soviet Union, especially since the western distribution of this subtype ends in European part of the former Soviet Union and it has not expanded into the neighboring European countries.[84]

It has been suggested that migratory birds carrying infected ticks may spread various subtypes of TBEV over long distances. In support of this hypothesis, infected *Ix. ricinus* larvae are found on some migrating birds, including tree pipits and European robins.[84,85] However, adult *Ix. ricinus* very seldom parasitize birds, except for large ground-dwelling birds, such as pheasants, so that birds appear to be incompetent hosts for transmitting TBEV to ticks.[85] Additionally, bird migration patterns are typically along longitudinal, not latitudinal, directions. Moreover, in a Swedish study that tested 13,260 migrating birds, only 4 bore TBEV-infected *Ix. ricinus* nymphs.[85] It is thus unlikely that birds from the Russian Far East or East Siberia would migrate to the Urals, the Ukraine, or Estonia or be the primary driver behind the development of the widely separated TBEV clines in these areas.[86] This may not be the case in other areas where the virus is endemic. Based on phylogeny, TBEV-FE may have been exported to Japanese islands by migratory birds from Far-Eastern Russia.[87] Similarly, the reemergence and spread of TBEV in northeastern Germany may be due to migrating birds or to a multiyear persistence of low levels of virus.[88] After the establishment of new disease foci, TBEV persistence may rely on the presence of transmission-competent small mammals, especially mice, bank voles, and some hedgehogs.[89]

Vectors and Vertebrate Hosts

The above information suggests that migratory birds may or may not be responsible for widespread distribution of at least some of the TBEV subtypes. Other nonmigratory wild birds, however, may be involved in the regional spread of TBEV. In a study conducted in Tomsk, Western Siberia between 2006 and 2011, TBEV RNA and antigen were detected in 9.7% and 22.8%, respectively, of samples obtained from wild birds. TBEV was also detected in 14.1% of *Ix. persulcatus*, 5.2% of *Ix. pavlovskyi*, and 4.2% of *Ix. plumbeus* ticks taken from wild birds. TBEV-FE was the major subtype found in these ticks, while the remaining viruses were of the TBEV-Sib subtype.[90] In general, TBEV-Sib predominates in suburban foci.[91,92] TBEV-FE in this region of Russia, however, is prevalent in urban foci, where *Ix. pavlovskyi*

is the major tick species and feeds primarily on birds throughout its life cycle. *Ix. pavlovskyi* and wild birds, particularly fieldfares, may have a role of maintaining TBEV circulation in the cities of the region, including Novosibirsk and its suburbs.[90,93-95] Fieldfares migrate from Siberia to Europe, including Italy, France, and Belgium, for wintering. These birds also migrate from Western Siberia to Crimea[96] and may have introduced TBEV-FE to the Black Sea basin. Nevertheless, the major TBEV vectors and hosts in Siberia are *Ix. persulcatus* and small rodents, respectively. While several other ixodid ticks in this region also serve as TBEV hosts, of these, only *D. reticulatus* feeds on humans.[91]

Ix. ricinus survival requires a high relative humidity ($\geq 85\%$) at ground level; thus, the amount of precipitation may affect tick density and geographical distribution. Temperature also affects the development rate and questing activity of ticks. Several parameters help to determine TBE incidence in humans, including the density of infected nymphs and the extent of human exposure to these nymphs.[90] Since questing nymphs climb high on vegetation, they are influenced by multiple environmental factors, especially to desiccation, which occurs when the relative humidity drops below 80%. Warmer, drier weather is associated with rapid decreases in nymph numbers, so few ticks are found in the coastal regions of Slovenia.[92] Tick larvae, however, remain on or just below ground level. In drier conditions, nymphs also spend more time questing on or close to the ground and are more likely to infest shrews or other small rodents.[3]

The density of the nymphs is also influenced by the population densities of tick maintenance hosts, especially roe and red deer, in the preceding year. These deer are not competent transmission hosts, since their degree of viremia is too low to permit viral transmission, but they still play an important role in the tick life cycle by supporting populations of these disease vector ticks.[97] The numbers of roe deer increased in the 1990s, resulting from reduced predation due to low numbers of red fox and lynx, mild winters, and reduced competition for food, resulting from the increased hunting of Eurasian elk.[98] Red foxes are important predators of young roe deer and small mammals, many of which serve as important reservoirs for other tickborne human pathogens, including *Borrelia* and *Rickettsia* bacterial species.[3] An interesting relationship exists between deer, small mammal, and red fox numbers since nymphal ticks feeding on deer (incompetent hosts) lower the numbers of nymphs feeding on small mammals (competent vectors). Red foxes prey upon both animal types.[3]

In a highly endemic area of Sweden, numbers of roe deer, red deer, mountain hares, and European hares showed positive covariance with TBE incidence; wild boar, lynx, and red foxes had no covariance; and the Eurasian elk and fallow deer had negative covariance.[89] The recent presence of high-density populations of roe deer may drive the younger deer to migrate to other areas in search of food, thus creating new TBEV foci and increasing the viruses' range. Reduction in deer abundance may not, however, decrease TBE incidence in humans since, in search of new blood donors, the ticks may increase their feeding on humans and actually increase the incidence of human TBE.[87]

The abundance of roe deer is not always linked to TBE incidence in humans. In Sweden, two harsh winters greatly reduced roe deer numbers, leading ticks to feed on an abundant number of bank voles at that time.[3] In Norway and Slovenia, high TBE incidence correlates with densities of red deer and farm animals. The density of red deer has been increasing since the 1970s in some European countries.[98] By contrast, in the Swedish Baltic Island, mountain hares are the sole maintenance hosts for the ticks, while in South Wales, tick densities are related to grazing livestock in grassland regions in the absence of deer.[89]

While deer, hares, boars, and ground-feeding birds host nymphs or adult ticks, the numbers and availability of small mammals, especially shrews, bank voles, and other rodents, in the previous season are of greater importance since these animals are the primary hosts for tick larvae.[99–101] TBEV-Sib is also vertically transmitted in northern red-backed voles.[101] Yellow-necked mice also permit nonviremic transmission between *Ix. ricinus* ticks better than bank voles and are important hosts in European deciduous forests.[102] Rodent density is affected by the production of the fruits of oak, beech, and chestnut trees. Interestingly, climate conditions in the center of *Ix. ricinus'* range appear to be of lesser importance for TBE incidence in humans than changes in land use, host animal populations, human living conditions, and societal factors. The effects of changing climate are more clearly evident along the growing northern edge of *Ix. ricinus'* range.[89,103]

Adult ticks feed on other large animals as well. Dogs, horses, and monkeys may develop symptomatic infection. Cattle, goats, and sheep, as well as wild boars and roe deer, may be seropositive without developing neurological disease. The above domestic animals are used as sentinel animals to aid in the discovery of new TBEV risk areas.[104–106] Screening of over 7000 sheep and goats in Germany revealed substantial differences in seroprevalence among flocks (0%–43%), confirming the patchy pattern of viral foci. Screening of the domestic animals, especially sheep, may be more effective and less time-consuming and expensive than screening ticks.[104]

TBEV Life Cycle and Interaction With Its Hosts

The TBEV life cycle requires ticks, which may serve as both viral vectors and reservoirs and small rodent tick hosts.[100] Humans, who are primarily infected by the bite of an infected tick, are only incidental hosts. Human behavior influences TBE incidence: good weather increases the chance of people encountering ticks, as evidenced by long warm autumns which increase human outdoor recreational activities and lead to spikes in TBE incidence.[107] This was seen in Sweden in 2011, when the unusually warm, humid weather prolonged the vegetation period. Regions with a yearly vegetation period of at least 180 days have greater tick abundance than regions with shorter growing seasons.[108] This allowed for both tick questing behavior and large numbers of people spending time outdoors to coincide nearly year-round. Under these conditions, 284 human cases of TBE were reported in Sweden during 2011. Spring climate conditions also affected TBE incidence. Warm weather during that spring, followed by generous levels of precipitation in June and July, led to abundant mushroom growth. Mushroom-picking and berry-picking are among the risk factors for acquiring TBE.[3]

Following the bite of an infected tick nymph, TBEV begins to replicate in the local skin immune cells, such as macrophages, neutrophils, and Langerhans cells. Stimulation of Langerhans cells by hosts TLR3, TLR7, and TLR9 is impaired by components in tick saliva.[109,110] Tick saliva also decreases natural killer (NK) cell activity in vitro.[111] TBEV reproduction and viability as well as their expression of viral E protein are enhanced by *Ix. ricinus* saliva.[112] In TBEV-infected Langerhans cells, tick saliva increases activation of the Akt pathway with its antiapoptotic and prosurvival effects on host target cells. The immune molecules signal transducer and activator of transcription 1 (STAT1) and nuclear factor κ of B cells (NF-κB) are also raised, resulting in increased TBEV replication and transmission.[113] In mouse fibroblasts and splenic dendritic cells (DCs), *Ix. ricinus* saliva blocks IFN activity against TBEV.[112] In the splenic DCs, TBEV also decreases cell surface expression of the IFN-α and IFN-β receptor, thus escaping the host's powerful antiviral IFN pathway.[114] STAT1 phosphorylation, secretion of TNF-α and IL-6, and apoptosis of TBEV-infected cells are inhibited by tick saliva.[109] Tick saliva also impairs DC migration and antigen presentation to CD4+

T helper cells and reduces T cell differentiation toward the antiinflammatory Th2 responses.[115]

TBEV-infected Langerhans cells enter the draining lymph nodes and pass first into lymphatic vessels and then into the circulatory system via the thoracic duct. Virus is found in blood leukocytes within days after the tick bite. During the viremic phase, peripheral immune system tissues are infected, particularly the spleen and bone marrow, and also enter into the liver.[10,22,116,117]

The immunoglobulin-like domain III of the viral E protein binds to the highly negatively charged polysaccharide heparan sulfate, found on a large variety of vertebrate and tick cells. Viral mutations that induce a more positive charge in this E protein domain increase neuroinvasiveness. Following the binding of the E protein to heparan sulfate, the virus enters host cells via clathrin-dependent endocytosis. This form of cell entry also occurs in other flaviviruses that use a different host protein as their host cell receptor.[118] TBEV is also brought into cells via endocytosis in the presence of nonneutralizing antibodies via antibody-dependent enhancement (ADE), in which antibodies enhance rather than inhibiting viral infection of host cells, as has been well characterized during dengue virus (DENV) infection.[119] During DENV infection, ADE is mediated by virus–antibody complexes binding to host cell Fc receptors. In the case of TBEV, however, entry is independent of Fc receptors and is believed to occur by antibody-mediated exposure of the E protein's fusion loop.[120] Within the acidic endosome, E proteins form a trimer via interactions of its fusion loops.[121] Changes in pH inhibit these necessary E protein structural rearrangements since the rearrangements rely on the low pH that is typically found in the endosomal environment.[122]

Domain II of the E protein contains a highly conserved loop that is involved in the fusion of viral and host membranes during TBEV entry into target cells. This domain also possesses the sole glycosylation site in the mature virus. In addition to entry into cells, domain II is involved in neurovirulence and viral exit from mammalian cells.[121] Other studies have suggested that several host proteins play a role in neuroinvasiveness as well. These host proteins include a 35 kDa protein, a 110 kDa glycoprotein, and a 67 kDa protein, possibly the nonintegrin laminin receptor.[123–126]

Mutations in the TBEV E protein affect viral fusion and entry into the host target cell, while mutations in the 3' core of the noncoding region decrease viral replication and neuroinvasiveness.[126] Mutation of the capsid protein partially disrupts viral assembly, reduces production of infectious virus particles, and

decreases spread of TBEV from its peripheral entry site.[126] Additionally, neuropathogenesis is decreased if the virus has mutations that alter the glycosylation sites of the viral prM, E, or NS1 proteins or the prM's furin-cleavage site.[127]

TBEV and the CNS

In humans with fatal TBEV-induced disease, neurons are the primary targets in the brain. In this site, TBEV replicates at a 10,000-fold higher rate in neuronal, than in epithelial, cells.[32] Astrocytes, the most abundant glial cell type, are also infected by TBEV, resulting in reactive astrogliosis.[20] Soon after their infection, cultured primary cortical astrocytes produce and secrete IFN-α, which protects the surrounding cells from viral infection.[128] The infected astrocytes also increase their expression of the activation marker glial fibrillary acidic protein as well as MMP-1. Rat astrocytes themselves are not killed by cytopathic effect due to their expression of the IFN receptor IFNAR, but do experience changes in the rat's astrocyte actin cytoskeleton microfilaments. However, unlike the case in human astrocytes, no changes are found in their microtubules. Infection also does not alter the astrocytes' shape.[10,66,129] Loss or blockage of the IFNAR leads to high levels of viral replication and virus-induced cytopathic effects in these cells.[128] Astrocytes also serve as a reservoir of dormant TBEV during chronic CNS infection.[129]

TBEV infects cultured human neuroblastoma, medulloblastoma, and glioblastoma cell lines in vitro. In these cells, virus activity is associated with host cell rough ER proliferation, an extensive rearrangement of the cells' cytoskeletal structures, and the rounding of the cells which is characteristic of apoptosis.[129] Electron tomography reveals connections between microtubules and vacuoles in which viral proteins, produced in the neurons' cell bodies during early stages of infection, accumulate in neuronal dendrites. In the dendrites, the viral proteins inhibit neurite outgrowth and disrupt host mRNA transport along dendrites.[44,130,131] These events occur to a greater extent during TBEV infection of CNS cells than they do during the infection of CNS cells by other flaviviruses.[132,133] TBEV replication stimulates the formation of characteristic ultrastructural membrane alterations in neurites, the laminal membrane structures.[132] Assemblages of membranous whorls and autophagic vacuoles are present in infected human neurons. TBEV replication sites are present in these autophagosomes, where they associate with lipid droplets. The lipid may serve as an energy source for viral replication. In human neuroblastoma cells, stimulating autophagy increases TBEV production and its inhibition decreases numbers of infectious viruses.[132]

Infection of astrocytes also induces growth and rearrangements of the rough ER similar to those described above. Unique tubule-like structures 17.9 ± 0.15 nm in diameter are formed that directly connect to viral particles and provide sites for the concentration of the TBEV replication machinery into replication vesicles. They enhance viral RNA replication and protein synthesis in addition to sequestering dsRNA from the host innate immune sensors.[66,134,135] Some swollen mitochondria have also been detected in the brains of those with TBE.[66] Alterations include a spherical invagination that is connected to the cytoplasm by a pore. The replication vesicles produce vesicle packets, followed by the formation of convoluted membranes and paracrystalline arrays that are part of a single ER-derived membrane network upon which virion assembly occurs. The virions acquire their envelope during budding into the ER lumen and are subsequently transported to the Golgi apparatus where the E and prM proteins are modified and the latter is cleaved by furin. From the Golgi apparatus, virions are transported to and released from the cell's surface.[136,137]

TBEV Transmission

TBEV transmission to humans is unusually rapid, occurring within minutes after a tick bite, and causes disease in about one-third of infected people. Viral spread between ticks occurs vertically (female-to-offspring), horizontally (between ticks feeding at the same site of an infected host as described below), and transstadially (carried from one tick stage to the next). While one study reported that 0.5%–2% of unfed tick nymphs were TBEV-infected, the rate was 7%–20% in fed ticks removed from humans.[3,138] These differences in tick infection rates were not, however, found in a later study.[88]

The major route of TBEV transmission between ticks occurs by cofeeding of infected and noninfected ticks, which feed in clumps on the same host.[102,135] During this blood meal, 30%–50% of the ingested material and any microbes contained within it are released back into the host and may be taken up by an uninfected neighboring tick. This process of passing virus from infected to uninfected ticks may continue for 2 or more weeks.[137] Cofeeding begins at temperatures over 9 °C for nymphs and larvae, suggesting that increased numbers of days with temperatures greater than 9 °C increase the instance of cofeeding and the subsequent transmission of virus to previously uninfected ticks. Studies indicate, however, that even though the mean annual temperature increased suddenly at the end of the 1980s and has remained warm such then, there was no significant correlation between the incidence of human TBE in Sweden and France and mean annual temperatures or numbers of days with temperature of greater than 9 °C.[98]

People may also be infected by blood transfusion or solid organ transplantation, such as kidney or liver transplants.[139] The latter route of infection is typically fatal due to the administration of immunosuppressants to the organ recipients. Hundreds of people have also become infected by consuming unpasteurized goat milk or cheese.[140–143] TBEV has been found in milk from experimentally infected cows and also in sheep that have subclinical infection.[144,145] The association between milk and disease has been known since the1950s and was named "biphasic milk fever."

THE IMMUNE RESPONSE TO TBEV
Adaptive Immune Responses

Even though leukocytes are not typically present in the CNS (with the exception of microglia), both CD4+ T helper 1 (Th1) and CD8+ T killer lymphocytes are present in the CSF during TBEV infection and may play a role in neuronal damage. Far fewer numbers of B lymphocytes are present in the CSF, but their activity may be protective.[21,146–148] The increased levels of IL-5 found during infection may play a role in the migration of lymphocytes into CSF.

While interactions between TBEV infection and antibody responses are complex, nevertheless, some trends are discernable. Serum levels of anti-TBEV IgG and IgM antibodies correlate with good clinical outcome, and serum IgM levels correlate with attenuated BBB disruption. Both IgM and IgG are in CSF as well as in the serum of infected people.[110] While produced well after IgM, antiviral IgG provides long-term or perhaps lifelong immunity to TBEV.[149] Comparison of mice with varying degrees of resistance to TBEV indicates that resistant mice have a strong neutralizing antibody response, which is lacking in TBEV-sensitive mice. Interestingly, in both resistant and sensitive mice strains, virus replication rate does not appear to be the major factor influencing mean survival time.[150] The administration of intravenous TBEV-specific neutralizing antibodies to infected mice, however, does increase their survival after viral challenge.[151] In humans with TBE, failure to produce neutralizing antibodies is associated with a very severe disease course. The presence or absence of anti-TBEV neutralizing antibodies is also important to consider when testing TBEV vaccine efficacy.

In humans, levels of serum and CSF IgM are lower in older patients. Accordingly, increased age is associated with a greater risk of severe neurological disease and poor prognosis during TBEV infection.[152] The presence of anti-TBEV IgM in the CSF of humans, however, correlates with greater CSF inflammation upon hospital admission, but also with more complete disease resolution.[148] Additionally, concentrations of the Th2 cytokine IL-5 are increased in the CSF, but not serum, during TBEV infection. Levels of this Th2 cytokine did not correlate with clinical presentation or anti-TBEV IgM and IgG titers, even though IL-5 induces differentiation of B cells to Ig-secreting plasma cells.[149]

Anti-TBEV antibodies in the serum and CSF of infected persons are directed against the E protein and against some nonstructural and hydrophobic intracellular viral proteins, including NS1, NS2A, NS3, NS4B, and NS5. These antibodies may persist for over 2 months in patients with acute disease. Serum IgM antibodies appear early during infection and appear to be protective.[55,153–155] IgG antibody levels peak during the convalescent phase. Low levels of CSF IgM and low levels of anti-TBEV neutralizing antibody during week 2 of disease are linked to moderate to severe encephalitis and adverse disease course.[156] The IgM response appears to be more relevant to favorable clinical outcome than does the IgG response.[148] In people with chronic disease, IgM may persist for a year or more in the absence of appreciable levels of IgG.[157] A separate study, however, reports that protective levels of IgG may be lifelong.[154,157] Antibodies produced in response to infection by one TBEV subtype or to some current vaccination formulations are able to cross-neutralize most of the other TBEV serotypes as well as KFDV and AHFV, but not Powassan virus (POWV).[153] This is of great importance since licensed vaccines against KFDV and its AHFV variant are either not readily available or have very limited distribution.

Production of the correct type of CD4+ T helper cell-derived cytokines is necessary to produce neutralizing antibody; however, only a small number of studies report on numbers and functions of T lymphocytes during TBEV infection. While the CD4+ T helper cells play a minor role at best during acute disease, CD8+ T killer cells are reported to be strongly activated within 1 week after TBEV-related hospitalization. At the peak of the immune response during the second phase of TBEV infection, these T killer cells express both Ki67 and CD38 molecules that are indicative of an effector cell.[158] Many of the CD8+ T killer cells express high levels of perforin and granzyme B and low levels of antiapoptotic Bcl-2, suggesting their readiness to kill infected cells. The T killer cells then gradually differentiate into T memory cells.[158] Patients with severe disease have low levels of T cell activity during acute infection, including suppressed mitogen-activated proliferation, suggesting an important role for T cells in controlling infection.[158,159]

Two chemokines that are involved in T cell recruitment to the nervous system, CXCL10 and CXCL11, are present in the CSF of TBE patients.[160] They may be at least partially responsible for the increased levels of T cells crossing the BBB and entering into the CSF during TBEV infection.[161] While T cells have important roles in clearing infection, they are similar to a double-edged sword since they also may contribute to immunopathology, especially the CD8+ T killer cells.[110] In addition to their presence in the CSF, increased levels of these cells are present in the CNS of TBE patients.[162] Granzyme B+ T killer cell infiltrates are associated with the death of infected human neuronal tissue.[21] Mice with deficiencies in T killer cells (such as severe combined immunodeficiency or CD8neg mice) survive longer during TBEV infection than immunocompetent mice receiving adoptively transferred T killer cells.[147] These findings are in accord with the decrease in severe neurological disease during infection with WNV or Murray Valley encephalitis virus in mice lacking T killer cells, perforin, or Fas ligand.[163] Inhibition of inducible nitric oxide synthase functioning along with the resulting decrease in nitric oxide levels also prolongs survival. Nitric oxide interferes with normal neuronal functions and may also be a factor in the increased permeability of the BBB during flavivirus infections.[162] By contrast, adoptive transfer of CD4+ T helper lymphocytes into TBEV-infected severe combined immunodeficiency mice is protective.[147] Postmortem tissues of humans with TBE also have large numbers of microglia in the brain parenchyma. These brain tissue macrophages may also contribute to neuron death or they may remove debris from dead or damaged cells.[21,157]

The Innate Immune Response to TBEV

NK cells present in the CSF of patients with TBE are activated prior to hospitalization.[158,161] These cells are predominantly highly differentiated CD57+ cells and CD56dim NK cells that are activated prior to their transformation into CD56bright NK cells.[153] Activated NK cells produce increased levels of cytokines, including IL-12, IL-15, IL-18, IFN-γ, and TNF-α. Interestingly, unlike their typical response to viruses, these activated NK cells express less perforin, granzyme B, and Bcl-2, indicating decreased NK cell activity against infected targets during acute disease. Within 3 weeks, however, NK cell responses return to normal levels.[158] Among people who are hospitalized with severe TBE, the proportion of NK cells is higher in the blood than in the CSF,[159] whereas in people having only mild, febrile infection, NK cell frequency decreases by 1 week postinfection and then returns to normal levels during the convalescent period.[164]

TBEVs enter and exit the cytoplasm of macrophages by localized destruction of the plasmalemma. Progeny viruses appear on the surface of the nucleocapsid.[165] Within 3 h of entering and reproducing in macrophages, the cells' respiratory burst is triggered, as evidenced by increased activity of the NADPH-oxidase complex, lactate dehydrogenase, succinate dehydrogenase, and cytochrome oxidase. Metabolites of the reactive nitrogen species nitric oxide accumulate between 5 and 48 h after infection, as the newly formed viruses exit the host cell and, between 1 and 4 days, superoxide dismutase and lysosomal enzymes, such as nonspecific esterase and acid phosphatase, become active.[165]

In the 1950s and 1960s, type I IFNs (IFN-α and IFN-β) were discovered to be secreted factors that interfere with viral replication. They were subsequently found to decrease replication of TBEV.[166] The IFN promoter stimulator 1 (IPS-1) pathway prolongs survival of TBEV-infected mice and its absence reduces the systemic IFN-α response, corresponding to higher viral replication in peripheral tissues as well as locally within the brain.[10,167] TBEV-induced IFN expression depends on the phosphorylation and nuclear localization of the transcription factor IFN regulatory factor 3 (IRF-3). TBEV delays IFN production by slowing gene induction by the IFN-β promoter. The differing levels of induction of type I IFNs by various TBEV-Eur strains are related to the degree of RNA replication. Levels of IFN transcripts remain below the threshold level for secretion for at least 24 h, by which time large amounts of TBEV have been produced, leading to the infection of neighboring cells.[136] Binding of secreted IFNs to their respective receptors activates the Janus kinase/STAT (JAK/STAT) pathway, which initiates the transcription of over 300 ISGs. Host cell recognition of TBEV dsRNA is delayed by sequestration of this RNA within the altered ER tubules, reducing its detection by cytoplasmic pathogen receptors and giving the viruses a head start of approximately 24 h before the beginning of an effective IFN response.[167]

All TBEV-infected mice that lack a functional gene for IPS-1 die early during the course of infection. The IPS-1 pathway relies upon the retinoic acid-inducible gene 1 (RIG-1).[168] RIG-1 localizes with stress granules produced in TBEV-infected cells in response to

the detection of dsRNA as part of the integrated stress response. Stress activates kinases that phosphorylate and inactivate eukaryotic translation initiation factor 2 (eIF2), which acts with the aggregated prion-like T cell-restricted intracellular antigen 1 (TIA-1) to form cytoplasmic stress granules that inhibit viral replication. Other granular components typically include the TIA-1-related (TIAR) protein, the Ras-GAP SH3 domain-binding protein (G3BP), and the translation elongation initiation factors eIF3 and eIF4B. Cytoplasmic TIA-1 and TIAR travel to viral replication vesicles where they bind to TBEV, specifically depleting TIA-1 from stress granules, while G3BP1 remains in the granules. The importance of TIA-1 in inhibiting TBEV production may be seen when levels of TIA-1 are decreased by increasing the levels of TIA-1-specific small interfering RNA (siRNA). This process alters viral replication and early translation and is also found during infection with other flaviviruses, including the mosquito-borne WNV and DENV.[169]

Infection by TBEV, as well as mosquito-borne WNV, DENV, and JEV, triggers an antiviral unfolded protein response (UPR) by increasing the levels of heat shock protein 72 and activating the transcription factor 6 pathway. This increases the expression of the spliced X box-binding protein 1 mRNA and protein. The inositol-requiring enzyme 1 pathway also plays a role in initiating the UPR during TBEV infection.[170] TBEV may, however, manipulate this response to facilitate its own replication since inhibition of the UPR reduces TBEV production.[137,170]

Several ISGs are upregulated following TBEV infection. These include the OASs and tripartite motif-79α (TRIM79α). OASs are activated by the presence of dsRNA and, in turn, activate RNase L, which degrades viral RNA. Several polymorphisms in the OAS genes correlate with severe TBE disease.[59] Mice do not naturally have the OAS1b isoform, but a congenic mouse strain containing a functional *OAS1b* gene is resistant to neurological damage by some, but not all, TBEV-FE strains.[171] Rodent-specific TRIM79α is an E3 ubiquitin ligase that inhibits TBEV function by inducing degradation of viral NS5 by lysosomes.[172]

TBEV also upregulates the expression of and is inhibited by the virus inhibitory protein ER-associated interferon inducible (viperin), another ISG that interferes with WNV and DENV reproduction as well.[10] Viperin targets TBEV's positive-sense RNA synthesis early during the course of infection in a manner that is dependent upon its [4Fe–4S] metalloclusters, held by its radical S-adenosyl-L-methionine domain.[173] One of the critical cytosolic iron–sulfur protein assembly molecules, CIAO1, is necessary for viperin stability and Fe–S cluster formation. Viperin also interacts with TBEV's prM, E, NS2A, NS2B, and NS3, leading to a viperin-NS3- and proteasome-dependent degradation of viral proteins.[174] Additionally, viperin interferes with TBEV assembly by inhibiting the activity of the cellular protein Golgi brefeldin A-resistant guanine nucleotide exchange factor 1, which is involved in the cellular secretory pathway. Viperin also blocks TBEV assembly, inducing the formation of noninfectious viral particles that are composed of only the capsid and envelope proteins. Taken together, these activities result in the secretion of noninfectious capsid particles.[175]

Viperin is expressed at high levels in olfactory bulb astrocytes in their basal state. Its expression is decreased in both the olfactory bulb and cerebrum of mice deficient in IPS-1.[24,128,168] Viperin decreases TBEV replication in astrocytes. In culture, viperin strongly inhibits TBEV replication in primary cerebral neurons, as is also the case for the mosquito-borne WNV and ZIKV, but does not inhibit viral replication in cerebellar granular cell neurons. Viperin also decreases replication of the similar, but typically nonpathogenic, Langat virus in the olfactory bulb and cerebrum, but not in the cerebellum or brainstem.[10] Cortical neurons rely completely on viperin for IFN-mediated inhibition of TBEV, while other ISGs may contribute to the antiviral effect in astrocytes.[24]

When TBEV-Sib infects a human medulloblastoma cell line derived from cerebellar neurons, it induces the expression of many ISGs and proinflammatory cytokines.[176] Infection of these cells also activates expression of type III IFN (IFN-λ), but not type I or II IFN genes. Only pretreatment with type I IFN, however, inhibits TBEV replication and downregulates a large group of proinflammatory cytokines in this medulloblastoma cell line.

TBEV utilizes several mechanisms in order to evade the IFN antiviral response.[10] One mechanism is to keep its dsRNA replication intermediates in vesicular structures inside the host ER membranes. This delays viral RNA recognition by cytosolic RIG-1-like receptors and subsequent IRF3 phosphorylation and type I IFN induction.[167,177,178] Along with other flaviviruses, TBEV's NS5 antagonizes interferon-alpha receptor (IFNAR) signaling by interacting with the cellular Scribble molecule. This aids in the localization of NS5 to the plasma membrane, which is required for NS5 to inhibit type I and type II IFN-mediated JAK–STAT signaling.[42,179] Experimental knockdown of Scribble interferes with NS5 transit to the plasma membrane, thereby blocking viral inhibition of JAK–STAT signaling.[42] Another evasive mechanism that is employed by the NS5s of both

TBEV and WNV is to decrease cell surface expression of an IFNAR1 subunit by binding to prolidase, a host peptidase that is required for IFNAR1 maturation and cell surface expression, as well as for IFN-β activity.[114]

TBEV and Cytokines and Chemokines

Serum levels of TNF-α, IL-1α, and IL-6 increase early during the course of TBE. Large increases in levels of MCP-1, found in brains of infected people, may help to disrupt the BBB. Strains of mice that are highly susceptible to TBEV pathology have greater amounts of MCP-1, as well as IFN-γ, interferon gamma-induced protein 10 (IP-10), migration inhibitory protein (MIP)-1α, and IL-5 in their brains than resistant mouse strains, while the most resistant mouse strains had the lowest levels of the following chemokines: RANTES, MIP-1α, and MIP-1 as well as IL-6 mRNA.[150] Infected astrocytes also express higher levels of the following inflammatory cytokines or chemokines: TNF-α, IL-1, IL-4, IL-6, IL-8, IL-12p40, IL-12p70, IP-10, and MIP.[133,180] The proinflammatory chemokines CXCL0, CXCL11, and RANTES are also present in CSF and serum from TBE patients.[54,161,180,181]

The inflammatory chemokine RANTES is upregulated in the brain, but not in peripheral tissues or sera, of the very young and adult mice infected with TBEV by the intracranial route.[181] It is among the most rapidly and rigorously induced molecules in the CNS of these mice. The viral NS5 protein increases RANTES production in primary astrocytes. NS5 activates the IRF-3 signaling pathway, leading to nuclear translocation of IRF-3 and its binding to the RANTES promoter.[148] The mosquito-borne flaviviruses JEV, WNV, ZIKV, and DENV also use NS5 to induce RANTES. Blocking IRF-3 activation drastically decreases RANTES expression.[181] RANTES may help induce macrophage- and T cell-mediated inflammatory responses in rodents in which, unlike humans, neutrophils are present in the CNS of infected mice. Increased levels of RANTES correlate with neuropathology in these mice, while antagonizing RANTES prolongs mouse survival and decreases cellular infiltration of the brain. Moreover, RANTES mRNA and protein levels increase in human brain-derived cell lines and primary progenitor-derived astrocytes, but only between 24 and 48 h after infection,[180] perhaps due to the delay in IFN induction during TBEV infection.[167,178] CCR5 serves as one of the receptors for RANTES. In humans, homozygosity for the CCR5Δ32 allele is linked with predisposition to clinical TBE in Lithuanians, but not Russians.[61,64,182]

Proinflammatory chemokines, some of which are produced in infected astrocytes, recruit T killer cells to the CNS, where they contribute to immunopathology during TBE, including the activation of apoptosis in neurons.[50,66,147] The chemokine IP-10 attracts activated T cells to the CNS and, at high levels, is a potent neurotoxin. IP-10 levels are also elevated in both the CSF and the serum of those with TBE.[160,180] The inflammatory response of astrocytes during TBEV infection may thus play a major role in neuronal degradation, as is also the case during infection with WNV or JEV.

Levels of both inflammatory cytokines and chemokines, as well as antiinflammatory cytokines and soluble cytokine receptors which are produced during the course of TBE, may be altered by antibiotics, such as the tetracyclines, which cross the BBB and moderate local inflammation in the CNS.[55] Soluble cytokine receptors act as competitive inhibitors to decrease the binding of the cytokines to their respective receptors on the surface of infected cells. This reduces the activation of the corresponding cytokine and decreases inflammation. Their levels, as well as levels of immunomodulatory IL-10, increase soon after hospitalization. Administration of tetracycline hydrochloride also appears to expedite the decrease in levels of IL-6 and IL-1β and lower the levels of these inflammatory cytokines. Additionally, after administration of tetracycline, levels of the antiinflammatory soluble IL-6 receptor (sIL-6R), the soluble TNF receptor 1 (sTNFR1), and the IL-1 receptor antagonist (IL-1 RA) rise more rapidly and to a greater degree than that seen in untreated patients.[55] Serum levels of IL-1RA and sTNFRI are 100-fold higher than the levels of IL-1β and TNF-α, while levels of sIL-6R are 1000-fold higher than IL-6.[55] The ratio of IL-1 to IL-1RA has a greater impact on disease outcome than does the concentration of IL-1 alone. This is also true of the ratio of IL-6 and TNF-α. While tetracycline-treated patients have higher levels of IL-6 than untreated patients, they also have a more favorable IL-6:sIL-6R ratio. Interestingly, in patients having elevated serum IL-6 levels, there was no correlation with gender or disease severity.[155] Elevated IL-6 levels did, however, correlate with age, with all of those under 26 years of age having normal levels of this cytokine, regardless of clinical presentation. Furthermore, in those patients having detectable levels of IgG, there is an inverse correlation with TBEV-specific IgG titer. Serum levels of IL-6 alone, therefore, are not a reliable indicator of disease outcome.[155]

Atrasheuskaya et al.[55] also reported that TBEV-infected children have higher levels of IL-6 than adults. IL-6 may either act in a proinflammatory manner when alone or may instead inhibit production of TNF-α; it is a part of an IL-6/sIL-6R complex. Infected children have more favorable IL-1α:IL-1RA and TNF-α:sTNFRI ratios

than adults. Notably, unlike adults, children in the study did not develop meningitis or meningoencephalitis.

When production of neopterin and β-2 microglobulin is measured in aseptic meningoencephalitis patients with ($n = 72$) or without ($n = 61$) TBEV infection, CSF neopterin and β-2 microglobulin levels are significantly higher in TBE than in non-TBE cases.[183] These levels return to normal levels after a year. The levels and duration of neopterin and β-2 microglobulin do not correlate to the clinical course. This long-lasting strong inflammatory reaction may have chronic clinical consequences, however.

Effects of TBEV on Expression of Immune System Genes

Using an ex vivo model system, human whole blood samples were infected with one of two TBEV-FE strains, which differ in virulence. In the highly pathogenic viral strain, expression of several immune system genes, including those involved in leukocyte adherence and activation, is downregulated. These molecules include CD11b, ICAM-1, and CD69 on monocytes and CD69, CD25, and CD95 on NK cells, and CD69 on CD8$^+$ T killer cells. Infection with the nonpathogenic TBEV strain instead increased innate defense mechanisms that rapidly eliminate the virus. In vivo, monocytes and neutrophils of asymptomatic patients have higher phagocytic and receptor activity than cells from symptomatic patients.[184]

Several forms of siRNA molecules alter the production of specific proteins by degrading their mRNA or by blocking translation. Both TBEV-infected *Ix. scapularis*- and *Ix. ricinus*-derived cell lines mount RNAi responses against TBEV. This miRNA response generally upregulates the production of proteins that are involved in immunity and metabolism. The downregulated molecules are generally involved in protein folding and cellular stress responses, including production of heat shock proteins, even though the precise transcripts and proteins are differentially expressed in cells from these two different tick species.[10,185] Viral subgenomic flavivirus RNA (sfRNA) is produced during TBEV infection by the incomplete degradation of genomic viral RNA by the cellular 5′-3′ exoribonuclease XRN1.[185,186] The resulting sfRNAs block the antiviral RNAi response in tick cells.[185]

Genetic Differences in Host Resistance to TBEV

Host genetic factors also influence resistance to TBEV. Some of the host gene products that are known to be involved in controlling the extent of pathology include the MHC class I molecules HLA-A and HLA-B, DC-SIGN, the innate immune system's pathogen recognition molecule TLR3, CCR5, and OAS.[150] The genomes of mice with varying resistance to TBE indicate differences in several of the genes that are found within a survival-controlling locus on mouse chromosome 7.[187] *CD33* and *SIGLEC E* are two of these genes that are present on microglia. They are immunoreceptor tyrosine-based inhibition motif (ITIM)-containing inhibitory receptors that negatively regulate various immune responses. The *CD33* gene carries a nonsense mutation in the most TBEV-susceptible mouse strain, while *SIGLEC E* has a single amino acid change in this mouse strain. Two other genes that differ in mice with varying TBEV susceptibility produce the serine proteases KLK1B22 and KLK1B16, which activate the complement system and stimulate the release of bradykinin, which alters vascular permeability. Other immune molecules that are produced by genes in the resistance/susceptibility chromosome 7 loci include FUT2, MKRN3, OTOG, GRWD1, and ABCC6.[187] Some of these gene products have also been implicated in resistance to other flaviviruses. Future studies are needed to better determine how alterations in these genes affect mouse responses to these viruses.

PREVENTION

Many European countries, including parts of Russia, Austria, Germany, Finland, Hungary, Latvia, Slovenia, Switzerland, and Italy, have governmental vaccination programs that vary in coverage and efficacy. In Austria, vaccine coverage is 88% and disease incidence is less than 1 per 100,000 people. The Czech Republic has vaccine coverage of 16% and incidence of 7.8 per 100,000, while Slovenia has 12% coverage and an incidence of 13.1 per 100,000.[188] As expected, encephalitis incidence is lower among the vaccines.

Many available TBEV vaccines are based on formalin-inactivated tissue culture-derived TBEV-FE and TBEV-Eur strains that are heterologous to most of the current TBEV isolates and were isolated 40–80 years ago.[189] These may or may not be active against TBEV-Sib or other, current, TBEV-FE or TBEV-Eur strains unless the vaccine incorporates a conserved region of these viruses. In the Far East of Russia in the 2000s, disease incidence following vaccination was 8.2% with a fatality rate of 0%. By contrast, between 2007 and 2011, in Russia, 23.79% patients with TBEV-Sib-associated encephalitis had previously been vaccinated with a TBEV-FE strain.[189] Human vaccination

with a heterologous TBEV strain thus may be less effective in reducing severe to fatal disease than homologous vaccine strains. The extent of cross-subtype protection is important since all three TBEV subtypes cocirculate in the Baltic States and some regions of European Russia.[188] Mice immunized subcutaneously with TBEV-FE or TBEV-Eur are partly protected against a heterologous TBEV-Sib reference strain. Protection correlates with levels of hemagglutination-inhibiting (HI) and neutralizing antibodies.[189]

More recent studies[190] examined TBEV-FE-based vaccine protection in mice against a large number of distinct viral strains isolated during different years and in different regions of Russia. Protective levels of neutralizing antibodies were achieved against all examined TBEV strains studied. Results for other flaviviruses present in the region were mixed: the vaccine-induced protective levels of neutralizing antibodies against Omsk hemorrhagic fever virus (OHFV), but not against POWV. Different levels and degrees of protection were seen among the tested viruses.[190] An 8-year study similarly showed that immunization of humans with a vaccine against TBEV-Eur resulted in the production of neutralizing antibodies against TBEV and OHFV in 100% and 86% of those immunized, respectively.[191] The presence of neutralizing antibodies, however, may not always reflect the extent of protection, especially against heterologous challenge viruses.[192] Protective efficacy relies more on individual properties of the vaccine and challenge virus strains than on the TBEV subtype. These properties include the speed and amount of viral replication early during infection and the rate at which the virus enters the cells (the length of time spent extracellularly, exposed to antibodies) as well as the viral strains modulation of various host immune factors.[190] Vaccine efficiency also depends on producing antibodies against particular viral epitopes, the amino acid composition of the virion surface, and intrinsic properties of the challenge viral strain's E protein structure, including amino acids localized on the viral surface and in the stem and anchor region, which interacts with the ectodomain, as well as certain point mutations.[190]

Administration of three doses of TBEV-Eur-based vaccines results in very high seroconversion or seropositivity rates against heterologous TBEV-FE and TBEV-Sib strains. Neutralizing activity against OHFV is also produced by these anti-TBEV vaccines, albeit at a lower level than is seen using TBEV subtypes. This vaccination strategy usually does not result in differences in the levels of neutralizing antibodies against homologous and heterologous challenge subtypes.[193,194] Additionally, while these vaccines slightly enhance ZIKV levels in human erythroleukemia cells in vitro, no significant differences are found in morbidity or mortality of ZIKV disease in TBEV-Eur-vaccinated immunodeficient mice.[195] A more recently developed subunit vaccine based on fusion of the several regions of the TBEV E protein with the OmpF porin of the *Yersinia pseudotuberculosis* bacterium only produced 60% protection against TBEV infection.[196]

Nonhuman primate models appear to yield results that are closer to those found in humans than when using mouse models. African green monkeys were used to determine whether particular vaccines could induce protective immunity against OHFV. Monkeys vaccinated subcutaneously with an inactivated TBEV vaccine produced high neutralizing antibody titers against both TBEV and OHFV. No TBEV was present in the spleen, lymph nodes, or CNS of the TBEV-immunized animals after challenge. However, while this vaccine protected monkeys against hemolytic disease following challenge with OHFV, it failed to prevent the reproduction of OHFV in the CNS and visceral organs. Crab-eating macaques also provide a permissive model for testing the protective efficacy of TBEV vaccines.[197]

Th1 cells secreting IFN-γ, TNF-α, and IL-2 (triple-positive cells) produce more IFN-γ than Th1 cells secreting only IFN-γ. Multicytokine-producing cells are more effective at controlling viral infections than are those producing only a single cytokine. Th1 cells that produce only IL-2 are better able to proliferate and produce long-term memory cells than single IFN-γ producers.[198] Tick saliva slants CD4$^+$ T helper cells toward a Th2-type response.[115] Formalin-inactivated TBEV vaccines also produce short-term immunological memory in mice, with a predominant Th2 immune response, whereas in natural infection, the Th1-derived cytokines IL-2, IFN-γ, and TNF-α predominate and the T cells may persist for decades.[189] Immunization of humans with a vaccine containing the TBEV capsid, prM/M, and E proteins also alters Th1 cytokine patterns from those normally produced in response to TBEV infection.[198] Following the full course of TBEV vaccination, the proportion of triple-positive cells and their ability to produce IFN-γ are lower, but the proportion of TNF-α$^+$ IL-2$^+$ IFN-γ^{neg} cells is higher than that present after natural infection.[198] Levels of serum TBEV-specific antibody titers correlate with the extent of IL-2 and TNF-α responses following vaccination, but no such correlation was found between the T helper cytokine subsets and TBEV-specific antibody levels in TBEV patients.[198] A separate study found that TBEV-specific CD4$^+$ T helper cell responses to the capsid and E proteins are significantly higher in those receiving some vaccine formulations than in patients following natural infection. Other formulations, however, induce only slight differences in both CD4$^+$ T helper and CD8$^+$ T killer cell responses.[199]

In the interests of safety and cost-effectiveness, a series of subunit vaccines were prepared using three variants of the recombinant domain III of the TBEV E protein from TBEV-Eur, TBEV-Sib, and TBEV-FE, which were immobilized on a dextran carrier using CpG oligonucleotides as an adjuvant.[200] The subunit vaccines induce production of low levels of neutralizing antibody against the three TBEV subtypes and are less protective against TBEV infection in mice than the currently available Tick-E-Vac vaccine.

In an attempt to develop a live, attenuated TBEV vaccine that is not neurovirulent, TBEV/DENV4 hybrid constructs were produced to contain a region that serves as a target of a miRNA that is highly expressed in brain tissues. This viral vaccine construct is not able to replicate in the brains of immunized animals but is still able to infect non-CNS tissues and induce a robust immune response. This approach to vaccine development may allow construction of a targeted live attenuated anti-TBEV vaccine that is not neurotropic or neurovirulent.[201]

Despite the effectiveness of some of the TBEV vaccines, a small number of vaccinees still become infected by TBEV, perhaps due to amino acid substitutions in some TBEV strains which inhibit the binding of the TBEV E protein with the vaccine-induced antibodies.[202] Indeed, approximately 20% of the genomic datasets for the Neudoerfl, K23, 205, and Sofjin TBEV strains contain two to three alterations that result in altered charge, polar characteristics, ability to form hydrogen bonds, or change of amino acid volume. These alterations may greatly impact the affinity between E protein antigens and antibodies.[203] Additional studies are needed in order to detect the optimal variants of the antigenic determinants that are needed to produce a universally effective, polyvalent vaccine against all of the TBEV subtypes.

TREATMENT

No specific anti-TBEV medication is currently approved for use in humans. Ribavirin, 6-azauridine, and mericitabine, while active against some flaviviruses, do not inhibit TBEV in vitro at low concentrations and 6-azauridine is cytotoxic to human neuroblastoma cells. Several nucleoside analogs, however, are highly effective in cell culture without producing detectable cellular toxicity.[203] One of these, 7-deaza-2′-C-methyladenosine, reduces neuroinfection and viral titers in brains of TBEV-infected mice and increases the rate of survival.[204,205] Unfortunately, treatment with nucleoside analogs frequently is typically accompanied by the production of drug-resistant viral escape mutants, primarily due to the high mutation rates associated with the viral RNA-dependent RNA polymerase. The high mutation rates of flaviviruses together with high viral replication rates complicate the production of long-term effective drugs. Two drug-resistant TBEV strains that have only one conservative amino acid substitution in the viral RNA polymerase convey resistance to a broad spectrum of 2'-methylated nucleoside inhibitors, but not to 4'-C-azidocytidine, suggesting that combination therapy might decrease the emergence of drug-resistant viruses.[204] Combination therapy is successfully used to treat HIV-infected people, and HIV mutates at a higher rate than flaviviruses.

BCX4430, an imino-C-nucleoside, inhibits TBEV at μM concentrations in vitro. Much higher concentrations are needed to inhibit tickborne KFDV than louping ill disease flaviviruses.[206] This compound also strongly inhibits mosquito-borne WNV.

Polyphenols have a wide range of anticancer and antiviral activities. The polyphenol complex derived from seagrass of the Zosteraceae family decreases the titer of a highly pathogenic TBEV-FE strain by 2.8–4 logs in tissue culture while producing minimal cytopathic effect.[205] Its major components are rosmarinic acid, luteolin, and luteolin disulfate. Other polyphenols, including those derived from turmeric, red wines, or green tea, also are active against some viruses and perhaps should be considered for use in combination therapy against flaviviruses, including TBEV subtypes.

SUMMARY OVERVIEW

Diseases: Phase 1—fever; Phase 2—ataxia, paresis, or paralysis of limbs, meningitis, encephalitis, meningoencephalitis, or polioencephalomyelitis; injury to thymus and spleen

Causative agent: tickborne encephalitis viruses (European, Siberian, and Far-East varieties)

Vectors: ticks, primarily *Ixodes ricinus*, *Ixodes persulcatus*, and *Haemaphysalis longicornis*

Common reservoirs: small mammals, deer, hares, and birds

Mode of transmission: humans—tick bites, blood transfusion, solid organ transplantation, consumption of raw milk; ticks—vertically, horizontally, transstadially, and cofeeding

Geographical distribution: Russia, Europe, and Asia

REFERENCES

1. Dobler G, Gniel D, Petermann R, Pfeffer M. Epidemiology and distribution of tick-borne encephalitis. *Wien Med Wochenschr.* 2012;162:230–238.
2. Caracciolo I, Bassetti M, Paladini G, et al. Persistent viremia and urine shedding of tick-borne encephalitis virus in an infected immunosuppressed patient from a new epidemic cluster in north-eastern Italy. *J Clin Virol.* 2015;69:48–51.
3. Jaenson TJT, Hjertqvist M, Bergström T, Lundkvis A. Why is tick-borne encephalitis increasing? A review of the key factors causing the increasing incidence of human TBE in Sweden. *Parasit Vectors.* 2012;5:184.
4. Süss J. Tick-borne encephalitis 2010: epidemiology, risk areas, and virus strains in Europe and Asia—an overview. *Ticks Tick Borne Dis.* 2011;2:2–15.
5. Soleng A, Edgar KS, Paulsen KM, et al. Distribution of *Ixodes ricinus* ticks and prevalence of tick-borne encephalitis virus among questing ticks in the Arctic Circle region of Northern Norway. *Ticks Tick Borne Dis.* 2018;9:97–103.
6. Velay A, Solis M, Kack-Kack W, et al. A new hot spot for tick-borne encephalitis (TBE): a marked increase of TBE cases in France in 2016. *Ticks Tick Borne Dis.* 2018;9:120–125.
7. Jääskeläinen A, Tonteri E, Pieninkeroinen A, et al. Siberian subtype tick-borne encephalitis virus in *Ixodes ricinus* in a newly emerged focus, Finland. *Ticks Tick Borne Dis.* 2016;7:216–223.
8. Dekker M, Laverman GD, de Vries A, Reimerink J, Geeraedts F. Emergence of tick-borne encephalitis (TBE) in the Netherlands. *Ticks Tick Borne Dis.* 2019;10:176–179.
9. Randolph SE. To what extent has climate change contributed to the recent epidemiology of tick-borne diseases? *Vet Parasitol.* 2010;167:92–94.
10. Lindqvist R, Upadhyay A, Överby AK. Tick-borne flaviviruses and the type 1 interferon response. *Viruses.* 2018;10:340.
11. Rotz LD, Khan AS, Lillibridge SR, Ostroff SM, Hughes JM. Public health assessment of potential biological terrorism agents. *Emerg Infect Dis.* 2002;8:225–230.
12. Sumilo D, Bormane A, Asokliene L, et al. Socio-economic factors in the differential upsurge of tick-borne encephalitis in Central and Eastern Europe. *Rev Med Virol.* 2008;18:81–95.
13. Sun R-X, Lai S-J, Yang Y, et al. Mapping the distribution of tick-borne encephalitis in mainland China. *Ticks Tick Borne Dis.* 2017;8:631–639.
14. Cuber P, Andreassen A, Vainio K, et al. Risk of exposure to ticks (Ixodidae) and the prevalence of tick-borne encephalitis virus (TBEV) in ticks in southern Poland. *Ticks Tick Borne Dis.* 2015;6:356–363.
15. Kentaro Y, Yamazaki S, Mottate K, et al. Genetic and biological characterization of tick-borne encephalitis virus isolated from wild rodents in Southern Hokkaido, Japan in 2008. *Vector Borne Zoonotic Dis.* 2013;13(6):406–414.
16. Liu JG, Li SX, Ouyang ZY, Tam C, Chen XD. Ecological and socioeconomic effects of China's policies for ecosystem services. *PNAS.* 2008;105:9477–9482.

17. Tonteri E, Kipar A, Voutilainen L. The three subtypes of tick-borne encephalitis virus induce encephalitis in a natural host, the bank vole (*Myodes glareolus*). *PLoS One.* 2012;8(12), e81214.

18. Hayasaka D, Nagata N, Fujii Y, et al. Mortality following peripheral infection with tick-borne encephalitis virus results from a combination of central nervous system pathology, systemic inflammatory and stress responses. *Virology.* 2009;390:139–150.

19. Dumpis U, Crook D, Oksi J. Tick-borne encephalitis. *Clin Infect Dis.* 1999;28(4):882–890.

20. Gelpi E, Preusser M, Garzuly F, Holzmann H, Heinz FX, Budka H. Visualization of Central European tick-borne encephalitis infection in fatal human cases. *J Neuropathol Exp Neurol.* 2005;64:506–512.

21. Gelpi E, Preusser M, Laggner U, et al. Inflammatory response in human tick-borne encephalitis: analysis of postmortem brain tissue. *J Neurovirol.* 2006;12:322–327.

22. Růžek D, Dobler G, Mantke OD. Tick-borne encephalitis: pathogenesis and clinical implications. *Travel Med Infect Dis.* 2010;8:223–232.

23. Haglund M, Gunther G. Tick-borne encephalitis—pathogenesis, clinical course and long-term follow-up. *Vaccine.* 2003;21(suppl. 1):S1–S18.

24. Lindqvist R, Kurhade C, Gilthorpe JD, Överby AK. Cell-type- and region-specific restriction of neurotropic flavivirus infection by viperin. *J Neuroinflammation.* 2018;15:80.

25. Duniewicz M. Clinical picture of Central European tick-borne encephalitis. *Munch Med Wochenschr.* 1976;118:1609–1612.

26. Kaiser R. The clinical and epidemiological profile of tick-borne encephalitis in Southern Germany 1994–1998: a prospective study of 656 patients. *Brain.* 1999;122:2067–2078.

27. Mickiene A, Laiskonis A, Gunther G, Vene S, Lundquist A, Lindquist L. Tick-borne encephalitis in an area of high endemicity in Lithuania: disease severity and long-term prognosis. *Clin Infect Dis.* 2002;35:650–658.

28. Seitelberger F, Jellinger K. Neuropathology of tick-borne encephalitis (with comparative studies of arbovirus encephalitis and of poliomyelitis). *Neuropathol Pol.* 1996;4:366–400.

29. Beer S, Brune N, Kesselring J. Detection of anterior horn lesions by MRI in Central European tick-borne encephalomyelitis. *J Neurol.* 1999;246:1169–1171.

30. Schellinger PD, Schmutzhard E, Fiebach JB, Pfausler B, Maier H, Schwab S. Poliomyelitic-like illness in Central European encephalitis. *Neurology.* 2000;55:299–302.

31. Stragapede L, Dinoto A, Cheli M, Manganotti P. Epilepsia partialis continua following a Western variant tick-borne encephalitis. *J Neurovirol.* 2018;24(6):773–775.

32. Růžek D, Vancová M, Tesařová M, Ahantarig A, Kopecky J, Grubhoffer L. Morphological changes in human neural cells following tick-borne encephalitis virus infection. *J Gen Virol.* 2009;90:1649–1658.

33. Puchhammer-Stockl E, Kunz C, Mandl CW, Heinz FX. Identification of tick-borne encephalitis virus ribonucleic acid in tick suspensions and in clinical specimens by a reverse transcription-nested polymerase chain reaction assay. *Clin Diagn Virol.* 1995;4:321–326.

34. Kupča AM, Essbauer S, Zoeller G, et al. Isolation and molecular characterization of a tick-borne encephalitis virus strain from a new tick-borne encephalitis focus with severe cases in Bavaria, Germany. *Ticks Tick Borne Dis.* 2010;1:44–51.

35. Arnez M, Avsic-Zupanc T. Tick-borne encephalitis in children: an update on epidemiology and diagnosis. *Expert Rev Anti-Infect Ther.* 2009;7:251–1260.

36. Kunze U, Asokliene L, Bektimirov T, et al. Tick-borne encephalitis in childhood—consensus 2004. *Wien Med Wochenschr.* 2004;154:242–245.

37. Yoshii K, Song JY, Park S-B, Yang J, Schmitt H-J. Tick-borne encephalitis in Japan, Republic of Korea and China. *Emerg Microbes Infect.* 2017;6, e82.

38. Luat LX, Tun MMN, Buerano CC, Aoki K, Morita K, Hayasaka D. Pathologic potential of variant clones of the Oshima strain of Far-Eastern subtype tick-borne encephalitis virus. *Trop Med Health.* 2014;42(1):15–23.

39. Goto A, Hayasaka D, Yoshii K, Mizutani T, Kariwa H, Takashima I. A BHK-21 cell culture-adapted tick-borne encephalitis virus mutant is attenuated for neuroinvasiveness. *Vaccine.* 2003;21(25–26):4043–4051.

40. Belikov SI, Kondratov IG, Potapova UV, Leonova GN. The relationship between the structure of the tick-borne encephalitis virus strains and their pathogenic properties. *PLoS One.* 2014;9(4), e94946.

41. Yoshii K, Sunden Y, Yokozawa K, et al. A critical determinant of neurological disease associated with highly pathogenic tick-borne flavivirus in mice. *J Virol.* 2014;88(10):5406–5420.

42. Werme K, Wigerius M, Johansson M. Tick-borne encephalitis virus NS5 associates with membrane protein Scribble and impairs interferon-stimulated JAK-STAT signaling. *Cell Microbiol.* 2008;10:696–712.

43. Melik W, Ellencrona K, Wigerius M, Hedstrom C, Elvang A, Johansson M. Two PDZ binding motifs within NS5 have roles in tick-borne encephalitis virus replication. *Virus Res.* 2012;169:54–62.

44. Wigerius M, Melik W, Elväng A, Johansson M. Rac1 and Scribble are targets for the arrest of neurite outgrowth by the virus NS5. *Mol Cell Neurosci.* 2010;44:260–271.

45. Sakai M, Muto M, Hirano M, Kariwa H, Yoshii K. Virulence of tick-borne encephalitis virus is associated with intact conformational viral RNA structures in the variable region of the 3′-UTR. *Virus Res.* 2015;203:36–40.

46. Formanová P, Cerny J, Bolfikova BC, et al. Full genome sequences and molecular characterization of tick-borne encephalitis virus strains isolated from human patients. *Ticks Tick Borne Dis.* 2015;6(1):38–46.

47. Leonova GN, Belikov S, Kondratov IG, Takashima I. Comprehensive assessment of the genetics and virulence of tick-borne encephalitis virus strains isolated from patients with inapparent and clinical forms of the infection in the Russian Far East. *Virology.* 2013;443:89–98.

48. Mandl CW, Holzmann H, Meixner T, et al. Spontaneous and engineered deletions in the 3'-noncoding region of tick-borne encephalitis virus: construction of highly attenuated mutants of a flavivirus. *J Virol.* 1998;72(3):2132–2140.

49. Chiba N, Iwasaki T, Mizutani T, Kariwa H, Kurata T, Takashima I. Pathogenicity of tick-borne encephalitis virus isolated in Hokkaido, Japan in mouse model. *Vaccine.* 1999;17(7-8):779–787.

50. Růžek D, Salát J, Singh SK, Kopecky J. Breakdown of the blood-brain barrier during tick-borne encephalitis in mice is not dependent on CD8+ T-cells. *PLoS One.* 2011;6(5), e20472.

51. Marsala SZ, Pistacchi M, Gioulis M, Mel R, Marchini C, Francavilla E. Neurological complications of tick borne encephalitis: the experience of 89 patients studied and literature review. *Neurol Sci.* 2014;35:15–21.

52. Palus M, Vancova M, Sirmarova J, Elsterova J, Perner J, Ruzek D. Tick-borne encephalitis virus infects human brain microvascular endothelial cells without compromising blood-brain barrier integrity. *Virology.* 2017;507:110–122.

53. Suidan GL, McDole JR, Chen Y, Pirko I, Johnson AJ. Induction of blood:brain barrier tight junction protein alterations by CD8 T cells. *PLoS One.* 2008;3, e3037.

54. Grygorczuk S, Zajkowska J, Swierzbinska R, Pancewicz S, Kondrusik M, Hermanowska-Szpakowicz T. Concentration of the beta-chemokine CCL5 (RANTES) in cerebrospinal fluid in patients with tick-borne encephalitis. *Neurol Neurochir Pol.* 2006;40(2):106–111.

55. Atrasheuskaya AV, Fredeking TM, Ignatyev GM. Changes in immune parameters and their correction in human cases of tick-borne encephalitis. *Clin Exp Immunol.* 2003;131:148–154.

56. Palus M, Zampachová E, Elsterová J, Růžek D. Serum matrix metalloproteinase-9 and tissue inhibitor of metalloproteinase-1 levels in patients with tick-borne encephalitis. *J Inf Secur.* 2014;68(2):165–169.

57. Kang X, Li Y, Wei J, et al. Elevation of matrix metalloproteinase-9 level in cerebrospinal fluid of tick-borne encephalitis patients is associated with IgG extravasation and disease severity. *PLoS One.* 2013;8(11), e77427.

58. Ignatieva EV, Igoshin AV, Yudin NS. A database of human genes and a gene network involved in response to tick-borne encephalitis virus infection. *BMC Evol Biol.* 2017;17(suppl. 2):259.

59. Barkhash AV, Perelygin AA, Babenko VN, et al. Variability in the 2'-5'-oligoadenylate synthetase gene cluster is associated with human predisposition to tick-borne encephalitis virus-induced disease. *J Infect Dis.* 2010;202:1813–1818.

60. Barkhash AV, Perelygin AA, Babenko VN, Brinton MA, Voevoda MI. Single nucleotide polymorphism in the promoter region of the *CD209* gene is associated with human predisposition to severe forms of tick-borne encephalitis. *Antivir Res.* 2012;93:64–68.

61. Barkhash AV, Voevoda MI, Romaschenko AG. Association of single nucleotide polymorphism rs3775291 in the coding region of the TLR3 gene with predisposition to tick-borne encephalitis in a Russian population. *Antivir Res.* 2013;99:136–138.

62. Barkhash AV, Babenko VN, Voevoda MI, Romaschenko AG. Association of IL28B and IL10 gene polymorphism with predisposition to tick-borne encephalitis in a Russian population. *Ticks Tick Borne Dis.* 2016;7:808–812.

63. Barkhash AV, Yurchenko AA, Yudin NS, et al. A matrix metalloproteinase 9 (MMP9) gene single nucleotide polymorphism is associated with predisposition to tick-borne encephalitis virus-induced severe central nervous system disease. *Ticks Tick Borne Dis.* 2018;9:763–767.

64. Kindberg E, Mickiene A, Ax C, et al. A deletion in the chemokine receptor 5 (CCR5) gene is associated with tick-borne encephalitis. *J Infect Dis.* 2008;197:266–269.

65. Kindberg E, Vene S, Mickiene A, Lundkvist A, Lindquist L, Svensson L. A functional toll-like receptor 3 gene (TLR3) may be a risk factor for tick-borne encephalitis virus (TBEV) infection. *J Infect Dis.* 2011;203:523–528.

66. Palus M, Bílý T, Elsterová J, et al. Infection and injury of human astrocytes by tick-borne encephalitis virus. *J Gen Virol.* 2014;95:2411–2426.

67. Moniuszko-Malinowska A, Penza P, Czupryna P, et al. Assessment of HMGB-1 concentration in tick-borne encephalitis and neuroborreliosis. *Int J Infect Dis.* 2018;70:131–136.

68. Ecker M, Allison SL, Meixner T, Heinz FX. Sequence analysis and genetic classification of tick-borne encephalitis viruses from Europe and Asia. *J Gen Virol.* 1999;80:179–185.

69. Nagy A, Nagy O, Tarcsai K, Farkas A, Takács M. First detection of tick-borne encephalitis virus RNA in clinical specimens of acutely ill patients in Hungary. *Ticks Tick Borne Dis.* 2018;9:485–489.

70. Kovalev SY, Kovalev TA. Reconsidering the classification of tick-borne encephalitis virus within the Siberian subtype gives new insights into its evolutionary history. *Infect Genet Evol.* 2017;55:159–165.

71. Dai X, Shang G, Lu S, Yang J, Xu J. A new subtype of Eastern tick-borne encephalitis virus discovered in Qinghai-Tibet Plateau, China. *Emerg Microbes Infect.* 2018;7:74.

72. Heyman P, Cochez C, Hofhuis A, et al. A clear and present danger: tick-borne diseases in Europe. *Expert Rev Anti-Infect Ther.* 2010;3(1):33–50.

73. Daniel M, Danielová V, Fialová A, Malý M, Kříž B, Nuttall PA. Increased relative risk of tick-borne encephalitis in warmer weather. *Front Cell Infect Microbiol.* 2018;8, Article90.

74. Korenberg EI, Kovalevskii YV. Variation in parameters affecting risk of human disease due to TBE virus. *Folia Parasitol.* 1994;42:307–312.

75. Korenberg EI. Seasonal population dynamics of *Ixodes* ticks and tick-borne encephalitis virus. *Exp Appl Acarol.* 2000;24:665–681.

76. Sakai M, Yoshii K, Sunden Y, Yokozawa K, Hirano M, Kariwa H. Variable region of the 3′UTR is a critical virulence factor in the Far-Eastern subtype of tick-borne encephalitis virus in a mouse model. *J Gen Virol.* 2014;95(Pt 4):823–835.

77. Mel'nikova OV, Adel'shin RV, Korzun VM, Trushina YN, Andaev EI. Tick-borne encephalitis virus isolates from natural foci of the Irkutsk region: clarification of the genotype landscape. *Vopr Virusol.* 2016;61(5):229–234.

78. Gritsun TS, Frolova TV, Zhankov AI, et al. Characterization of a Siberian virus isolated from a patient with progressive chronic tick-borne encephalitis. *J Virol.* 2003;77(1):25–36.

79. Gritsun TS, Nuttall PA, Gould EA. Tick-borne flaviviruses. *Adv Virus Res.* 2003;61:317–371.

80. Ponomareva EP, Mikryukova TP, Gori AV, et al. Detection of Far-Eastern subtype of tick-borne encephalitis viral RNA in ticks collected in the Republic of Moldova. *J Vector Borne Dis.* 2015;52:334–336.

81. Yurchenko OO, Dubina DO, Vynograd NO, Gonzalez J-P. Partial characterization of tick-borne encephalitis virus isolates from ticks of Southern Ukraine. *Vector Borne Zoonotic Dis.* 2017;17(8):550–557.

82. Pukhovskaya NM, Morozova OV, Vysochina NP. Tick-borne encephalitis virus in arthropod vectors in the Far East of Russia. *Ticks Tick Borne Dis.* 2018;9:824–833.

83. Moutailler S, Moro CV, Vaumourin E, et al. Co-infection of ticks: the rule rather than the exception. *PLoS Negl Trop Dis.* 2016;10(3), e0004539.

84. Hayasaka D, Suzuki Y, Kariwa H, et al. Phylogenetic and virulence analysis of tick-borne encephalitis viruses from Japan and Far-Eastern Russia. *J Gen Virol.* 1999;80:3127–3135.

85. Waldenström J, Lundkvist Å, Falk KI, et al. Migrating birds and tick-borne encephalitis virus. *Emerg Infect Dis.* 2007;13:1215–1218.

86. Kovalev SY, Kokorev VS, Belyaeva IV. Distribution of Far-Eastern tick-borne encephalitis virus subtype strains in the former Soviet Union. *J Gen Virol.* 2010;91:2941–2946.

87. Suzuki Y. Multiple transmissions of tick-borne encephalitis virus between Japan and Russia. *Genes Genet Syst.* 2007;82:187–195.

88. Frimmel S, Krienke A, Riebold D, et al. Tick-borne encephalitis virus habitats in north east Germany: reemergence of TBEV in ticks after 15 years of inactivity. *Bio Med Res Int.* 2010;, 308371.

89. Jaenson TGT, Petersson EH, Jaenson DGE, et al. The importance of wildlife in the ecology and epidemiology of the TBE virus in Sweden: incidence of human TBE correlates with abundance of deer and hares. *Parasit Vectors.* 2018;11:477.

90. Mikryukova TP, Moskvitina MS, Kononova YV, et al. Surveillance of tick-borne encephalitis virus in wild birds and ticks in Tomsk City and its suburbs (Western Siberia). *Ticks Tick Borne Dis.* 2014;5:145–151.

91. Chausov EV, Ternovoi VA, Protopopova EV, et al. Genetic diversity of Ixodid tick-borne pathogens in Tomsk City and suburbs. *Parazitologiia.* 2009;43:374–388.

92. Chausov EV, Ternovoi VA, Protopopova EV, et al. Variability of the tick-borne encephalitis virus genome in the 5′ noncoding region derived from ticks *Ixodes persulcatus* and *Ixodes pavlovskyi* in Western Siberia. *Vector Borne Zoonotic Dis.* 2010;10:365–375.

93. Romanenko VN, Kondrat'eva LM. The infection of Ixodid ticks collected from humans with tick-borne encephalitis virus in Tomsk City and its suburbs. *Parazitologiia.* 2011;45:3–10.

94. Bolotin EI, Kolonin GV, Kiselev AN, Matiushina OA. Distribution and ecology of *Ixodes pavlovskyi* (Ixodidae) in Sykhote-Alin. *Parazitologiia.* 1977;11:225–229.

95. Livanova NN, Tikunova NV, Livanov SG, Fomenko NV. Identification of species of ticks *Ixodes persulcatus* and *Ixodes pavlovskyi* (Ixodidae) on the basis of the results of the analysis fragment gene COI (cytochrome oxidase). *Parazitologiia.* 2012;46:340–349.

96. Iurchenko OA, Vinograd NA, Dubina DA. Molecular genetic characteristics of tick-borne encephalitis virus in the Crimea. *Vopr Virusol.* 2012;57:40–43.

97. Knap N, Avšič-Županc T. Factors affecting the ecology of tick-borne encephalitis in Slovenia. *Epidemiol Infect.* 2015;143:2059–2067.

98. Knap N, Avšič-Županc T. Correlation of TBE incidence with red deer and roe deer abundance in Slovenia. *PLoS One.* 2013;8, e66380.

99. Hubalek Z, Rudolf I. Tick-borne viruses in Europe. *Parasitol Res.* 2012;111:9–36.

100. Labuda M, Randolph SE. Survival strategy of tick-borne encephalitis virus: cellular basis and environmental determinants. *Zentralbl Bakteriol.* 1999;289:513–524.

101. Bakhvalova VN, Potapova OF, Panov VV, Morozova OV. Vertical transmission of tick-borne encephalitis virus between generations of adapted reservoir small rodents. *Virus Res.* 2009;140:172–178.

102. Labuda M, Kozuch O, Zuffová E, Elecková E, Hails RS, Nuttall PA. Tick-borne encephalitis virus transmission between ticks co-feeding on specific immune natural rodent hosts. *Virology.* 1997;235:138–143.

103. Jore S, Vanwambeke SO, Viljugrein H, et al. Climate and environmental change drives *Ixodes ricinus* geographical expansion at the Northern Range Margin. *Parasit Vectors.* 2014;7:11.

104. Klaus C, Beer M, Saier R, et al. Goats and sheep as sentinels for tick-borne encephalitis (TBE) virus-epidemiological studies in areas endemic and non-endemic for TBE virus in Germany. *Ticks Tick Borne Dis.* 2012;3(1):27–37.

105. Gresíková M, Sekeyová M, Stúpalová S, Necas S. Sheep milk-borne epidemic of tick-borne encephalitis in Slovakia. *Intervirology.* 1975;5(1-2):57–61.

106. Balling A, Plessow U, Beer M, Pfeffer M. Prevalence of antibodies against tick-borne encephalitis virus in wild game from Saxony, Germany. *Ticks Tick Borne Dis.* 2014;5:805–809.

107. Randolph SE, Asokliene L, Avsic-Zupanc T, et al. Variable spikes in tick-borne encephalitis incidence in 2006 independent of variable tick abundance but related to weather. *Parasit Vectors.* 2009;1:44.

108. Jaenson TGT, Lindgrenm E. The range of *Ixodes ricinus* and the risk of contracting Lyme borreliosis will increase northwards when the vegetation period becomes longer. *Ticks Tick Borne Dis.* 2011;2:44–49.

109. Fialová A, Cimburek Z, Iezzi G, Kopecký J. *Ixodes ricinus* tick saliva modulates tick-borne encephalitis virus infection of dendritic cells. *Microbes Infect.* 2010;12:580–585.

110. Dörrbecker B, Dobler G, Spiegel M, Hufert FT. Tick-borne encephalitis virus and the immune response of the mammalian host. *Travel Med Infect Dis.* 2010;8:213–222.

111. Kubes M, Fuchsberger N, Labuda M, Zuffova E, Nuttall PA. Salivary gland extracts of partially fed *Dermacentor reticulatus* ticks decrease natural killer cell activity *in vitro*. *Immunology.* 1994;82(1):113–116.

112. Hajnicka V, Kocakova P, Slovak M, Labuda M, Fuchsberger N, Nuttall PA. Inhibition of the antiviral action of interferon by tick salivary gland extract. *Parasite Immunol.* 2000;22(4):201–206.

113. Lieskovská J, Páleníková J, Langhansová H, Chmelař J, Kopecký J. Saliva of *Ixodes ricinus* enhances TBE virus replication in dendritic cells by modulation of pro-survival Akt pathway. *Virology.* 2018;514:98–105.

114. Lubick KJ, Robertson SJ, McNally KL, et al. Flavivirus antagonism of type I interferon signaling reveals prolidase as a regulator of IFNAR1 surface expression. *Cell Host Microbe.* 2015;18:61–74.

115. Skallova A, Iezzi G, Ampenberger F, Kopf M, Kopecky J. Tick saliva inhibits dendritic cell migration, maturation, and function while promoting development of Th2 responses. *J Immunol.* 2008;180(9):6186–6192.

116. Chambers TJ, Diamond MS. Pathogenesis of flavivirus encephalitis. *Adv Virus Res.* 2003;60:273–342.

117. Johnston LJ, Halliday GM, King NJ. Langerhans cells migrate to local lymph nodes following cutaneous infection with an arbovirus. *J Investig Dermatol.* 2000;114:560–568.

118. Kroschewski H, Allison SL, Heinz FX, Mandl CW. Role of heparan sulfate for attachment and entry of tick-borne encephalitis virus. *Virology.* 2003;308:92–100.

119. Phillpotts R, Stephenson J, Porterfield J. Antibody-dependent enhancement of tick-borne encephalitis virus infectivity. *J Gen Virol.* 1985;66:1831–1837.

120. Haslwanter D, Blaas D, Heinz FX, Stiasny K. A novel mechanism of antibody-mediated enhancement of flavivirus infection. *PLoS Pathog.* 2017;13, e1006643.

121. Pulkkinen LIA, Butcher SJ, Anastasina M. Tick-borne encephalitis virus: a structural view. *Viruses.* 2018;10:350.

122. Holzmann H, Stiasny K, Ecker M, Kunz C, Heinz FX. Characterization of monoclonal antibody-escape mutants of tick-borne encephalitis virus with reduced neuroinvasiveness in mice. *J Gen Virol.* 1997;78:31–37.

123. Kopecky J, Grubhoffer L, Kovar V, Jindrak L, Vokurkova D. A putative host cell receptor for tick-borne encephalitis virus identified by anti-idiotypic antibodies and virus affinoblotting. *Intervirology.* 1999;42:9–16.

124. Maldov DG, Karganova GG, Timofeev AV. Tick-borne encephalitis virus interaction with the target cells. *Arch Virol.* 1992;127:321–325.

125. Protopopova EV, Konavalova SN, Loktev VB. Isolation of a cellular receptor for tick-borne encephalitis virus using anti-idiotypic antibodies. *Vopr Virusol.* 1997;42:264–268.

126. Mandl CW. Steps of the tick-borne encephalitis virus replication cycle that affect neuropathogenesis. *Virus Res.* 2005;111:161–174.

127. Pletnev AG, Bray M, Lai CJ. Chimeric tick-borne encephalitis and dengue type 4 viruses: effects of mutations on neurovirulence in mice. *J Virol.* 1993;67:4956–4963.

128. Lindqvist R, Mundt F, Gilthorpe JD, et al. Fast type I interferon response protects astrocytes from flavivirus infection and virus-induced cytopathic effects. *J Neuroinflammation.* 2016;13:277.

129. Potokar M, Jorgačevski MJ, Avšič-Županc T, Zorec R. Tick-borne encephalitis virus infects rat astrocytes but does not affect their viability. *PLoS One.* 2014;9(1), e86219.

130. Hirano M, Muto M, Sakai M, et al. Dendritic transport of tick-borne flavivirus RNA by neuronal granules affects development of neurological disease. *PNAS.* 2017;114:9960–9965.

131. Kellman EM, Offerdahl DK, Melik W, Bloom ME. Viral determinants of virulence in tick-borne flaviviruses. *Viruses.* 2018;10:329.

132. Bílý T, Palus M, Eyer L, Elsterová J, Vancová M, Růžek D. Electron tomography analysis of tick-borne encephalitis virus infection in human neurons. *Sci Rep.* 2015;5:10745.

133. Hirano M, Yoshii K, Sakai M, Hasebe R, Ichii O, Kariwa H. Tick-borne flaviviruses alter membrane structure and replicate in dendrites of primary mouse neuronal cultures. *J Gen Virol.* 2014;95:849–861.

134. Gillespie LK, Hoenen A, Morgan G, Mackenzie JM. The endoplasmic reticulum provides the membrane platform for biogenesis of the flavivirus replication complex. *J Virol.* 2010;84:10438–10447.

135. Labuda M, Danielova V, Jones LD, Nuttall PA. Amplification of tick-borne encephalitis virus infection during co-feeding of ticks. *Med Vet Entomol.* 1993;7:339–342.

136. Miori L, Maiuri P, Hoenninger VM, Mandl CW, Marcello A. Spatial and temporal organization of tick-borne encephalitis flavivirus replicated RNA in living cells. *Virology.* 2008;379:64–77.

137. Carletti T, Zakaria MK, Marcello S. The host cell response to tick-borne encephalitis virus. *BBRC.* 2017;492:533–540.

138. Süss J, Klaus C, Diller R, Schrader C, Wohanka N, Abel U. TBE incidence versus virus prevalence and increased prevalence of the TBE virus in *Ixodes ricinus* removed from humans. *Int J Med Microbiol.* 2006;296(S1):63–68.

139. Lipowski D, Popiel M, Perlejewski K, et al. A cluster of fatal tick-borne encephalitis virus infection in organ transplant setting. *J Infect Dis.* 2017;215:896–901.

140. Markovinovic L, Kosanovic Licina ML, Tesic V, et al. An outbreak of tick-borne encephalitis associated with raw goat milk and cheese consumption, Croatia, 2015. *Infection.* 2016;44:661–665.

141. Brockmann SO, Oehme R, Buckenmaier T, et al. A cluster of two human cases of tick-borne encephalitis (TBE) transmitted by unpasteurised goat milk and cheese in Germany, May 2016. *Euro Surveill.* 2018;23(15):17–00336.

142. Holzmann H, Aberle SW, Stiasny K, et al. Tick-borne encephalitis from eating goat cheese in a mountain region of Austria. *Emerg Infect Dis.* 2009;15(10):1671–1673.

143. Balogh Z, Ferenczi E, Szeles K, et al. Tick-borne encephalitis outbreak in Hungary due to consumption of raw goat milk. *J Virol Methods.* 2010;163:481–485.

144. Gresiková M. Excretion of tick-borne encephalitis virus in the milk of subcutaneously infected cows. *Acta Virol.* 1958;2:188–192.

145. Gresiková M. Recovery of the tick-borne encephalitis virus from the blood and milk of subcutaneously infected sheep. *Acta Virol.* 1958;2:113–119.

146. Jeren T, Vince A. Cytologic and immunoenzymatic findings in CSF from patients with tick-borne encephalitis. *Acta Cytol.* 1998;42:330–334.

147. Růžek D, Salát J, Palus M, et al. CD8$^+$ T-cells mediate immunopathology in tick-borne encephalitis. *Virology.* 2009;384:1–6.

148. Grygorczuk S, Czupryna P, Pancewicz S, et al. Intrathecal expression of IL-5 and humoral response in patients with tick-borne encephalitis. *Ticks Tick Borne Dis.* 2018;9:896–911.

149. Holzmann H. Diagnosis of tick-borne encephalitis. *Vaccine.* 2003;21:S36–S40.

150. Palus M, Vojtíšková J, Salát J, et al. Mice with different susceptibility to tick-borne encephalitis virus infection show selective neutralizing antibody response and inflammatory reaction on the central nervous system. *J Neuroinflammation.* 2013;10:77.

151. Elsterova J, Palus M, Sirmarova J, Kopecky J, Niller HH, Ruzek D. Tick-borne encephalitis virus neutralization by high dose intravenous immunoglobulin. *Ticks Tick Borne Dis.* 2017;8:253–258.

152. Czupryna P, Moniuszko A, Pancewicz SA, Grygorczuk S, Kondrusik M, Zajkowska J. Tick-borne encephalitis in Poland in years 1993–2008—epidemiology and clinical presentation. A retrospective study of 687 patients. *Eur J Neurol.* 2011;18:673–679.

153. McAuley AJ, Sawatsky B, Ksiazek T, et al. Cross-neutralisation of viruses of the tick-borne encephalitis complex following tick-borne encephalitis vaccination and/or infection. *NPJ Vaccines.* 2017;2:5.

154. Kaiser R, Holzmann H. Laboratory findings in tick-borne encephalitis—correlation with clinical outcome. *Infection.* 2000;28:78–84.

155. Toporkova MG, Aleshin SE, Ozherelkov SV, Nadezhdina MV, Stephenson JR, Timofeev AV. Serum levels of interleukin 6 in recently hospitalized tick-borne encephalitis patients correlate with age, but not with disease outcome. *Clin Exp Immunol.* 2008;152:517–521.

156. Günther G, Haglund M, Lindquist L, Skoldenberg B, Forsgren M. Intrathecal IgM, IgA and IgG antibody response in tick-borne encephalitis. Long-term follow-up related to clinical course and outcome. *Clin Diagn Virol.* 1997;8:17–29.

157. Blom K, Cuapio A, Sandberg JT, et al. Cell-mediated immune responses and immunopathogenesis of human tick-borne encephalitis virus-infection. *Front Immunol.* 2018;9, 2174.

158. Blom K, Braun M, Pakalniene J, et al. NK cell responses to human tick-borne encephalitis virus infection. *J Immunol.* 2016;197:2762–2771.

159. Shilov YI, Ryzhaenkov VG. Alterations in the proliferative response of peripheral lymphocytes in tick-borne encephalitis. *Dokl Biol Sci.* 2000;375:553–555.

160. Lepej SZ, Misić-Majerus L, Jeren T, et al. Chemokines CXCL10 and CXCL11 in the cerebrospinal fluid of patients with tick-borne encephalitis. *Acta Neurol Scand.* 2007;115:109–114.

161. Tomazic J, Ihan A. Flow cytometric analysis of lymphocytes in cerebrospinal fluid in patients with tick-borne encephalitis. *Acta Neurol Scand.* 1997;95:29–33.

162. Andrews DM, Matthews VB, Sammels LM, Carrello AC, McMinn PC. The severity of Murray Valley encephalitis in mice is linked to neutrophil infiltration and inducible nitric oxide synthase activity in the central nervous system. *J Virol.* 1999;73:8781–8790.

163. Wang Y, Lobigs M, Lee E, Müllbacher A. CD8$^+$ T cells mediate recovery and immunopathology in West Nile virus encephalitis. *J Virol.* 2003;77:13323–13334.

164. Pirogova NP, Novitskii VV, Mikhailova OV. Cytogenetic disorders in peripheral blood lymphocytes of patients with febrile form of tick-borne encephalitis. *Bull Exp Biol Med.* 2004;137:61–63.

165. Plekhova NG, Somova LM, Drobot EI, Krylova NV, Leonova GN. Changes in the metabolic activity of macrophages under the influence of tick-borne encephalitis virus. *Biochemistry (Mosc).* 2007;72(2):199–207.

166. Weber E, Finsterbusch K, Lindquist R, et al. Type I interferon protects mice from fatal neurotropic infection with Langat virus by systemic and local antiviral responses. *J Virol.* 2014;88(21):12202–12212.

167. Överby AK, Popov VL, Niedrig M, Weber F. Tick-borne encephalitis virus delays interferon induction and hides its double-stranded RNA in intracellular membrane vesicles. *J Virol.* 2010;84:8470–8483.

168. Kurhade C, Zegenhagen L, Weber E, et al. Type I interferon response in olfactory bulb, the site of tick-borne flavivirus accumulation, is primarily regulated by IPS-1. *J Neuroinflammation.* 2016;13:22.

169. Albornoz A, Carletti T, Corazza G, Marcello A. The stress granule component TIA-1 binds tick-borne encephalitis virus RNA and is recruited to perinuclear sites of viral replication to inhibit viral translation. *J Virol.* 2014;88(12):6611–6622.

170. Yu C, Achazi K, Niedrig M. Tick-borne encephalitis virus triggers inositol-requiring enzyme 1 (IRE1) and transcription factor 6 (ATF6) pathways of unfolded protein response. *Virus Res.* 2013;178:471–477.

171. Yoshii K, Moritoh K, Nagata N, et al. Susceptibility to flavivirus-specific antiviral response of Oas1b affects the neurovirulence of the Far-Eastern subtype of tick-borne encephalitis virus. *Arch Virol.* 2013;158:1039–1046.

172. Taylor RT, Lubick KJ, Robertson SJ, et al. Trim79alpha, an interferon-stimulated gene product, restricts tick-borne encephalitis virus replication by degrading the viral RNA polymerase. *Cell Host Microbe.* 2011;10:185–196.

173. Upadhyay AS, Vonderstein K, Pichlmair A, et al. Viperin is an iron-sulfur protein that inhibits genome synthesis of tick-borne encephalitis virus via radical SAM domain activity. *Cell Microbiol.* 2014;16(6):834–848.

174. Panayiotou C, Lindqvist R, Kurhade C. Viperin restricts Zika virus and tick-borne encephalitis virus replication by targeting NS3 for proteasomal degradation. *J Virol.* 2018;92(7):e02054-17.

175. Vonderstein K, Nilsson E, Hubel P, et al. Viperin targets flavivirus virulence by inducing assembly of non-infectious capsid particles. *J Virol.* 2017;92(1):e01751-17.

176. Selinger M, Wilkie GS, Tong, et al. Analysis of tick-borne encephalitis virus-induced host responses in human cells of neuronal origin and interferon-mediated protection. *J Gen Virol.* 2017;98:2043–2060.

177. Överby AK, Weber F. Hiding from intracellular pattern recognition receptors, a passive strategy of flavivirus immune evasion. *Virulence.* 2011;2:238–240.

178. Miorin L, Albornoz A, Baba MM, D'Agaro P, Marcello A. Formation of membrane-defined compartments by tick-borne encephalitis virus contributes to the early delay in interferon signaling. *Virus Res.* 2012;163:660–666.

179. Best SM, Morris KL, Shannon JG, et al. Inhibition of interferon-stimulated JAK-STAT signaling by a tick-borne flavivirus and identification of NS5 as an interferon antagonist. *J Virol.* 2005;79:12828–12839.

180. Zajkowska J, Moniuszko-Malinowska A, Pancewicz SA, et al. Evaluation of CXCL10, CXCL11, CXCL12 and CXCL13 chemokines in serum and cerebrospinal fluid in patients with tick borne encephalitis (TBE). *Adv Med Sci.* 2011;56:311–317.

181. Zhang X, Zheng Z, Liu X, et al. Tick-borne encephalitis virus induces chemokine RANTES expression via activation of IRF-3 pathway. *J Neuroinflammation.* 2016;13:209.

182. Mickiene A, Pakalniene J, Nordgren J, et al. Polymorphisms in chemokine receptor 5 and toll-like receptor 3 genes are risk factors for clinical tick-borne encephalitis in the Lithuanian population. *PLoS One.* 2014;9, e106798.

183. Günther G, Haglund M, Lindquist L, Sköldenberg B, Fosgren M. Intrathecal production of neopterin and beta 2 microglobulin in tick-borne encephalitis (TBE) compared to meningoencephalitis of other etiology. *Scand J Infect Dis.* 1996;28:1318.

184. Pirogova NP, Mikhailova OV, Karpova MR. Features of the phagocytic activity of peripheral blood leukocytes in patients with tick-borne encephalitis. *Bull Exper Biol Med.* 2002;(suppl. 1):82–85.

185. Schnettler E, Tykalova H, Watson M, et al. Induction and suppression of tick cell antiviral RNAi responses by tick-borne flaviviruses. *Nucleic Acids Res.* 2014;42:9436–9446.

186. Roby JA, Pijlman GP, Wilusz J, Khromykh AA. Noncoding subgenomic flavivirus RNA: multiple functions in West Nile virus pathogenesis and modulation of host responses. *Viruses.* 2014;6:404–427.

187. Palus M, Sohrabi Y, Broman KW, et al. A novel locus on mouse chromosome 7 that influences survival after infection with tick-borne encephalitis virus. *BMC Neurosci.* 2018;19:39.

188. Lundkvist K, Vene S, Golovljova I, et al. Characterization of tick-borne encephalitis virus from Latvia: evidence for co-circulation of three distinct subtypes. *J Med Virol.* 2001;65:730–735.

189. Morozova OB, Bakhvalova VN, Potapov OF, et al. Evaluation of immune response and protective effect of four vaccines against the tick-borne encephalitis virus. *Vaccine.* 2014;32:3101–3106.

190. Chernokhaeva LL, Rogova YV, Kozlovskaya LL, et al. Experimental evaluation of the protective efficacy of tick-borne encephalitis (TBE) vaccines based on European and Far-Eastern TBEV strains in mice and *in vitro*. *Front Microbiol.* 2018;9, 1487.

191. Chidumayo NN, Yoshii K, Kariwa H. Evaluation of the European tick-borne encephalitis vaccine against Omsk hemorrhagic fever virus. *Microbiol Immunol.* 2014;58:112–118.

192. Chernokhaeva LL, Rogova YV, Vorovitch MF, Romanova LI, Kozlovskaya LI, Maikova GB. Protective immunity spectrum induced by immunization with a vaccine from the TBEV strain Sofjin. *Vaccine.* 2016;34:2354–2361.

193. Domnich A, Panatto D, Arbuzova EK, et al. Immunogenicity against Far Eastern and Siberian subtypes of tick-borne encephalitis (TBE) virus elicited by the currently available vaccines based on the European subtype: systematic review and meta-analysis. *Hum Vaccin Immunother.* 2014;10:2819–2833.

194. Orlinger KK, Hofmeister Y, Fritz R, et al. A tick-borne encephalitis virus vaccine based on the European prototype strain induces broadly reactive cross-neutralizing antibodies in humans. *J Infect Dis.* 2011;203:1556–1564.

195. Duehr J, Lee S, Singh G, et al. Tick-borne encephalitis virus vaccine-induced human antibodies mediate negligible enhancement of Zika virus infection in vitro and in a mouse model. *mSphere.* 2018;3(1):e00011-18.

196. Sanina N, Chopenko N, Mazeika A, et al. Immunogenicity and protective activity of a chimeric protein based on the domain III of the tick-borne encephalitis virus E protein and the OmpF porin of *Yersinia pseudotuberculosis* incorporated into the TI-complex. *Int J Mol Sci.* 2018;19(10):E2988.

197. Pripuzova NS, Gmyl LV, Romanova LI, et al. Exploring of primate models of tick-borne flaviviruses infection for evaluation of vaccines and drugs efficacy. *PLoS One.* 2013;8, e61094.

198. Aberle H, Schwaiger J, Aberle SW, et al. Human CD4[+] T helper cell responses after tick-borne encephalitis vaccination and infection. *PLoS One.* 2015;10(10), e0140545.

199. Schwaiger J, Aberle JH, Stiasny K, et al. Specificities of human CD4[+] T cell responses to an inactivated flavivirus vaccine and infection: correlation with structure and epitope prediction. *J Virol.* 2014;88:7828–7842.

200. Ershova AS, Gra OA, Lyaschuk AM, et al. Recombinant domains III of tick-borne encephalitis virus envelope protein in combination with dextran and CPGs induce immune response and partial protectiveness against TBE virus infection in mice. *Infect Dis Ther.* 2016;16:544.

201. Heiss BL, Maximova OA, Pletnev AG. Insertion of microRNA targets into the flavivirus genome alters its highly neurovirulent phenotype. *J Virol.* 2011;85(4):1464–1472.

202. Bukin YS, Dzhioev P, Tkachev S, et al. A comparative analysis on the physicochemical properties of tick-borne encephalitis virus envelope protein residues that affect its antigenic properties. *Virus Res.* 2017;238:124–132.

203. Eyer L, Valdés JJ, Gil VA, et al. Nucleoside inhibitors of tick-borne encephalitis virus. *Antimicrob Agents Chemother.* 2015;59:5483–5493.

204. Eyer L, Kondo H, Zouharova D, et al. Escape of tick-borne flavivirus from 2′-C-methylated nucleoside antivirals is mediated by a single conservative mutation in NS5 that has a dramatic effect on viral fitness. *J Virol.* 2017;91:e01028–17.

205. Krylova NV, Leonova GN, Maystrovskaya OS, Popov AM, Artyukov AA. Mechanisms of antiviral activity of the polyphenol complex from seagrass of the *Zosteraceae* family against tick-borne encephalitis virus. *Bull Exp Biol Med.* 2018;165(1):61–63.

206. Eyer L, Zouharová D, Širmarová J, et al. Antiviral activity of the adenosine analogue BCX4430 against West Nile virus and tick-borne flaviviruses. *Antivir Res.* 2017;142:63–67.

CHAPTER 10

Louping-Ill Virus

INTRODUCTION AND HISTORY

The name of louping-ill virus (LIV) is derived from the old Scot word "to loup" ("leap"), in reference to an uncoordinated gait and tendency to jump seen in afflicted animals. Shepherds in the early 19th century knew that affected sheep came from certain upland heather pastures and that animals from disease-free pastures that were imported into the infected pastures were also at risk of developing the disease.[1] LIV was first isolated from sheep in 1930.[2] Symptoms of this disease were known to be due to a "filterable agent" and could be experimentally reproduced in sheep and pigs.[3] Injection of the virus into mice and monkeys also resulted in clinical disease with the type of lesions typical of viral encephalomyelitis.[1,4]

The first report of a LIV infection in humans was in 1934 in a laboratory worker.[5] Over a decade later, the first three known incidences of naturally acquired disease in humans were reported.[6,7] The first two cases occurred in a farmer and in a man involved in sheep-dipping. The third case involved a previously healthy shepherd boy 17 years of age. At the time of diagnosis, louping-ill was widespread in his flock and had led to the death of many lambs. Sheep ticks, *Ixodes ricinus*, were abundant in the sheep and many, including half-buried ticks, were also found on the patient. Louping-ill is prevalent among sheep in the spring due to the increase in the activity of *I. ricinus*.[8] Early louping-ill symptoms in the young shepherd included neck pain along the sternomastoid muscles.[7] About a week later, while tending the flock, he vomited several times, fell asleep for hours, and had difficulty walking. Within the next few days, he developed a high fever, a sore neck with Kernig's sign, back pain, dizziness, drowsiness, and inability to pass urine. He soon became semicomatose, restless, and irrational with short-term memory loss and slurred speech. His muscle tone was generally increased; however, the cranial nerves were normal and nystagmus was not present. Cerebral spinal fluid contained leukocytes, primary lymphocytes, but no bacteria. Within days, his condition rapidly improved and he recovered almost completely.[7]

Louping-ill has been present in Scotland and northern England as well as in Northern Ireland for at least 100 years. It is found in sheep grazing on upland heather and rough grass and is associated with ticks and red grouse kept as game birds on Scottish sporting estates. Louping-ill was detected in 16 dead or moribund red grouse in Scotland in the 1960s and 1970s.[9–11]

THE DISEASE

Louping-Ill Pathology in Agricultural Animals

Louping-ill has been best characterized in sheep due to its relative rarity in humans. Infected sheep develop fever and weakness, progressing to meningoencephalitis with cerebellar ataxia, generalized tremor, jumping, vigorous kicking, salivation, and clamping of jaws. This may be followed by paralysis, coma, and death.[12] In one study of experimentally infected sheep ($n = 8$) and lambs ($n = 4$) inoculated intracranially with LIV, all animals developed severe neurological symptoms, progressing from slight ataxia to complete flaccid paralysis 6–18 h later.[13] High levels of viremia were also seen, ending prior to the onset of severe neurological symptoms in all of the sheep, but viruses were still detectable at death in the four lambs. Two of 12 animals inoculated with a 10-fold higher viral dose subcutaneously were killed when moribund and four of the remaining animals developed nonfatal neurological symptoms.[14] Hemagglutination-inhibiting (HI) antibodies were present in the serum of all animals inoculated subcutaneously, but were absent in those inoculated intracranially. Antibodies were detected in sheep significantly earlier than in lambs.[14]

In a separate study by the same research group, 33 sheep were inoculated subcutaneously with LIV. Of these, 12.1% died and an additional 54.5% were killed with severe neurological symptoms. These animals became moribund between days 6 and 11 postinfection. Ataxia rapidly progressed to complete flaccid paralysis within 3–5 h. The surviving sheep did not develop the symptoms of encephalomyelitis, although two of them became chronically debilitated. The maximum levels of viremia were seen on days 3–4, but, as in their previous study of sheep inoculated intracranially, viremia rapidly declined until none of these adult animals remained viremic at the time of death or development of severe nervous symptoms.[14] The extent of viremia reflected the severity of the subsequent pathology. The subsequent decrease in viral titer was linked to the appearance of circulating HI antibody and the rise of

Zika and Other Neglected and Emerging Flaviviruses. https://doi.org/10.1016/B978-0-323-82501-6.00014-1

neutralizing antibody activity. Antibodies appeared sooner and rose to higher levels in surviving vs susceptible animals and appear to be the major protective factor in survivors, although small amounts of interferon were also present. Unlike the situation in many other viral infections, the immune response protected the animals, rather than leading to pathogenic inflammatory responses.[13]

Neuropathological lesions in sheep infected with LIV either naturally or experimentally are characteristic of nonsuppurative meningoencephalomyelitis with focal microgliosis and neuronal necrosis with neuronophagia. Lesions in lambs are localized and are often distributed along with neuronal processes, suggesting that LIV may be disseminated along axonal pathways.[15] Necrosis is most common in the Purkinje cells of the cerebellum and the medulla and spinal cord. Mononuclear, and some polymorphonuclear, cells may be present in these parts of the central nervous system (CNS). Histiocytes within the areas of gliosis contain LIV antigen and may contribute to viral clearance.[15] The perivascular cuffs contain plasmacytes and sometimes polymorphonuclear cells.[16–18] Coinfection with LIV and the bacterium *Anaplasma phagocytophilum* or an acute infection with *Toxoplasma gondii*, a neurotropic protist, increases louping-ill pathology and is accompanied by a reduced antibody response.[1,19,20]

Naturally occurring, fatal cases of louping-ill have been found in cattle in Dartmoor, England, since 2001.[21] When six calves were experimentally inoculated subcutaneously with LIV, all developed short-term low-intensity viremia that subsided when HI serum antibody was detected. One calf developed severe meningoencephalitis and mild neurological changes were seen in one other animal.[22] Due to the low virus levels, calves do not appear to play a role in the transmission of LIV to ticks or result in the infection of other vertebrates. This may or may not be the case for adult cattle.

Naturally occurring LIV-associated neurological disease was found in a Scottish colt, which subsequently recovered within 2 weeks, and in a cluster of seven naturally infected horses in Devon, England.[23,24] The animals' ages ranged from 7 months to 20 years and included several breeds. All of the LIV-infected English horses developed some degree of ataxia, with some having a nearly complete inability to stand or move. Other symptoms included muscle tremors of the neck and facial area, anorexia, depression, mania, and avoidance of bright daylight. All of the infected horses lived on the edge of a moorland region that contained LIV-infected sheep. Upon testing 68 other, apparently healthy, horses living within a two-mile radius, an additional

five seropositive animals were found, two of which had previously demonstrated neurological symptoms. Four LIV-infected free-range horses in Ireland also developed encephalitis, resulting in the death of two of the animals.[25] LIV was isolated from both the brain and spinal cord of one horse. Experimental infection of horses results in fever, moderate viremia for 2–3 days (one-thousandth of the level present in sheep), and antibody production. Age was not a factor in LIV infection of horses. Based on these findings, horses may have the potential to serve as amplifying hosts for LIV.[26]

Louping-ill has also been reported in an alpaca on the edge of Dartmoor. It presented with posterior weakness, progressing to recumbence when under stress, and tremors of the head and neck. While the farm did not have a recorded history of tick-associated disease, it is surrounded by common moorland grazing areas and neighboring farms had reported louping-ill in both cattle and sheep within the previous 2 years.[27] Louping-ill in this alpaca is similar to that previously reported in a llama on the Island of Lewis.[28]

Louping-Ill Pathology in Birds

Experimental infection in the tarsal pad of red grouse results in a high rate of mortality and sufficient viremia to infect tick vectors. Symptoms in infected grouse include depression, anorexia, muscular weakness, and regurgitation of crop contents on handling. In this study, within 2 weeks, 78.4% of the birds died ($n=37$). Louping-ill additionally impairs breeding success in red grouse, according to a 1978 study that found that the number of chicks per brood was only 0.6 in areas with high tick abundance compared to 5.5 per brood in low-tick areas. Similarly, in high-tick regions, 84% of adult grouse had anti-LIV antibody ($n=61$), while only 1 of 10 grouse was seropositive in low-tick regions. Infected chicks (15.4% of 162 tested) also weighed significantly less than similarly aged uninfected birds.[29,30] Viremia in adult grouse peaks at day 4 of infection and its decline is associated with the presence of high titers of HI antibody. The magnitude and the duration of viremia in those birds that die are greater than those seen in surviving grouse and also than those found in sheep. Grouse are the only wild animal species that regularly develop sufficient levels of looping-ill viremia after experimental infection to be able to infect the tick vectors.[31]

The presentation of encephalitis in experimentally infected grouse differs from that in sheep, being more rostral, with less prominent motor neuron necrosis.[1] It should be noted, however, that the routes of inoculation differ among studies in grouse and other animals.

In grouse, mild foci of nonsuppurative meningitis are seen in the more anterior regions of the brain, over the cerebrum and optic lobes, on days 5–7 postinfection, while nonsuppurative encephalitis is seen on day 8. During the next week, the disease increases in severity and becomes more generalized. The early inflammatory response consists of pericapillary and perivenular cuffs of two types of unclassified, dividing mononuclear cells in the meninges and underlying brain tissue. Lymphocytic infiltrates were only seen in 1 of 32 infected birds. Degenerate neurons were rare and primarily localized in the anterior brainstem and basal ganglia. A similar disease is seen following experimental infection of the moorland willow grouse and the tundra ptarmigan.[32] Subclinical infection with low levels of viremia occurs upon infection of several species of woodland birds, including black grouse, capercaillie (a species of woodland grouse), and the ring-necked pheasant.[1] It appears, therefore, that LIV first became established in the forests and woodlands, where the avian species developed immunity. LIV appears to have much more recently moved into the upland grazing areas due to the introduction of sheep into these regions. The red and willow grouse, therefore, have yet to develop an effective resistance to LIV infection.[32]

Louping-III Pathology in Rodents

Intraperitoneal infection of mice with LIV leads to 100% mortality, but only when using high levels of virus. Antiserum against LIV prevents clinical manifestation, infection, and mortality in mice inoculated with either LIV or TBEV.[33] Inoculation of mice with cerebrospinal fluid (CSF) from a louping-ill patient causes disease in a small number of animals, some of which subsequently leap wildly about their cages. After several passages in mice, rodents that were inoculated intracranially develop symptoms and lesions typical of those seen in murine louping-ill. The virus initially circulates in the blood, but not the CNS. Later, the virus is absent from the blood as a HI antibody response develops and, although the animals appear to be well, the virus is present in the brain and CSF. These mice then develop encephalitis since insufficient levels of circulating antibody pass through the blood–brain barrier.[7]

Although experimental infection of field voles, bank voles, and wood mice induces anti-LIV antibody production, it fails to produce a sufficient level of viremia to support transmission to ticks.[34–36] In Scotland, field-caught small mammals carry few ticks and these are uninfected larvae. Additionally, none of these mammals are LIV-infected or have seroconverted.[35] Very low levels of viremia are also found in brown rats.[37] It is

thus unlikely that rodents play a significant role in LIV maintenance or transmission in nature.

Louping-III Pathology in Nonhuman Primates

Rhesus macaques, patas monkeys, and vervet monkeys are resistant to LIV inoculated subcutaneously with LIV. They do not develop clinical signs and, only rarely, brain lesions. These monkeys do, however, become viremic and some develop antibodies. Following intranasal or intracranial inoculation, however, all monkeys develop lesions characteristic of acute encephalitis, whether or not they are symptomatic.[33] Small levels of LIV are present after day 9 postinfection, followed by very high levels between days 14 and 16 that decrease slowly. Lesions in the CNS consist of very large meningeal cellular exudates, multilayered perivascular cuffs containing lymphocyte-like cells, and diffuse and focal microglial infiltration accompanied by neuronal degeneration.[38] Eosinophilic necrosis, disappearance of neurons, and spongy degeneration occur in Purkinje cells and large neurons in the dentate nucleus of the cerebellum. In severe cases, microglial infiltration occurs together with very high degrees of proliferation and hypertrophy of astrocytes. The anterior spinal cord columns, the reticular formations and spinal nuclei of the medulla, the substantia nigra of the midbrain, and the medial nucleus of the thalamus are also damaged.[33]

Louping-III Pathology in Humans

Louping-ill in humans is biphasic, beginning with an acute, febrile illness that occurs about a week after the initial symptoms. It clinically resembles acute poliomyelitis caused by other viral infections of the CNS[39,40] and is characterized by acute encephalitis of short duration and localized involvement of the basal ganglia, midbrain, and cerebellum, accompanied by cerebellar ataxia.[7] Reported symptoms include headache, photophobia, multiple rounds of vomiting, and severe, persistent pain around the subcostal margin. Hand weakness and back weakness and stiffness may be present, in addition to severe paralysis of the lower-motor-neuron type in both arms and legs.[40] Abdominal reflexes disappear along with a slight reduction of the triceps jerk. Lumbar puncture produces clear and colorless fluid with 55 mg protein/100 mL CSF in the absence or presence of cells. In the latter case, the cells are predominantly lymphocytes in some patients, while in others, neutrophils predominate.[7,40] Recovery may be prolonged, but is usually complete. Mild to moderate confirmed cases of louping-ill have occurred in laboratory workers after an accidental cut or puncture of the skin of the hand or finger with material containing LIV.[41] Laboratory-acquired symptoms include lymphadenopathy, fever and chills, double vision, incoordination, vomiting and severe diarrhea, anorexia, and delirium.

Cellular Pathology and Louping-Ill

On a cellular level, severe changes occur in the mitochondria of neurons of the pyriform cortex and pons of young LIV-infected rodents, including the formation of mitochondrial inclusion bodies. Most neurons in the pyriform cortex develop pathological changes in many of their cellular structures, including the mitochondria, endoplasmic reticulum, Golgi apparatus, and cytoplasmic matrix.[38] The number and the length of cristae in the enlarged mitochondria increase, with the formation of convolutions. Some swollen mitochondria appear to be very large, multilocular bodies whose free spaces are filled with dense particles. In other mitochondria, the proliferating cristae form a convoluted mass of tubules and membranes. Globular cytoplasmic bodies arise from the outer mitochondrial membrane. Dark, round, dense bodies are present beside degenerating mitochondria. Additionally, many granular structures are found that appear similar to lysosomes.[38] Within the endoplasmic reticulum, extended canals, vesicles, and cisternae also form. Prior to viral maturation, large cytoplasmic masses of ribosome-like particles are also visible. Mature virus particles are found within vesicles of the distended and hypertrophied Golgi apparatus and in inclusion bodies that appear similar to mitochondria. These cellular changes are similar to those seen in the brains of LIV-infected sheep as well as in cells infected by other flaviviruses.[38]

THE VIRUS

LIV Transmission and Hosts

Ticks have long been known to be important for the acquisition of louping-ill disease.[1,42–44] The transmission of LIV was later found to usually occur via the bite of *I. ricinus* sheep ticks. LIV can be recovered from ticks feeding on the affected sheep and/or ticks that had fed on ill sheep as nymphs.[8] The virus is found in the Far-Western part of the TBEV complex range and is primarily found in the United Kingdom (northern England, Scotland, and Wales) and Ireland, as well as a reported case in Norway.[4,6] Localization of louping-ill cases closely follows the range of *I. ricinus*, particularly in the upland grazing areas.[45] Spring lambing in these areas coincides with the peak seasonal activity of LIV's sheep tick vector.[12]

In addition to the transmission via tick bite, consumption of infected goat or sheep milk or dairy products also allows the transmission of LIV to humans and other animals. In one study, LIV was present in the blood and milk of seven goats inoculated with LIV subcutaneously. While only one goat developed transient illness, approximately one-third of 13 kids suckling these goats became infected and markedly symptomatic. One kid died and two others were killed *in extremis.*[46] The virus is also excreted into ewe's milk.[47] The presence of LIV in unpasteurized milk could represent a public health hazard.

Sheep, red grouse, and mountain hares (*Lepus timidus*) are the most ecologically important hosts for LIV transmission.[30,48–50] While clinical louping-ill occasionally occurs in farmed red deer, roe deer, and Cantabrian chamois, wild cervids are not believed to serve as LIV reservoirs.[48] Similarly, experimentally infected rabbits produced anti-LIV antibodies, but the level of viremia is believed to be insufficient to allow the transmission to ticks.[35] Sheep and ticks, however, are sufficient to maintain an enzootic cycle of LIV, since sheep host *I. ricinus* larvae, nymphs, and adults.[35,51] While transstadial transmission of LIV does occur, transovarial transmission has not been reported in *I. ricinus.*[36]

While red grouse do not host adult *I. ricinus*, they do host larvae and nymphs and can maintain LIV in the absence of sheep or mountain hares in locales that also have viremic or nonviremic adult tick hosts, such as red deer.[48] Although infected red deer do not themselves become viremic or transmit LIV to ticks, they do host adult *I. ricinus*. Since red grouse are rarely found in the absence of other tick or LIV hosts, they may thus serve an important role in maintaining enzootic cycles of LIV.[48] Given a high enough level of such nonviremic hosts, LIV can persist in areas in the absence of viremic hosts.[36,52] The presence of too many nonviremic hosts may, however, create a "dilution effect" in which tick bites are "wasted," leading to decreased viral presence.[53]

The prevalence of LIV-infected red grouse chicks increased from 9% in the first week of life to levels as high as 37% at week 4, coinciding with seasonal rises in questing tick numbers.[29–54] Interestingly, 73%–98% of grouse LIV infections result from young birds eating ticks, including *I. ricinus* adults.[48] Preening may also result in grouse ingestion of adult ticks in which virus titer and prevalence are greater than in biting nymphs.[36]

Mountain hares host *I. ricinus* larvae, nymphs, and adults[54] and allow efficient nonviremic, cofeeding transmission between infected adult ticks and uninfected nymphs that are cofeeding in close proximity on the same naïve hare. The greatest amount of such non-viremic transmission occurs when the recipient nymphs feed to repletion on hares 3–7 days after the attachment of infected adult ticks.[55] No such tick-to-tick LIV transmission is seen in ticks feeding on red deer or rabbits, even when the deer had low-level viremia. TBEV is also transmitted by cofeeding on an uninfected vertebrate host.[56] In fact, nonviremic hosts may allow LIV transmission for longer periods of time than viremic hosts and cofeeding may be one of the principal mechanisms for virus persistence in an area.[52] Transmission via cofeeding is enhanced by tick saliva[57] but is decreased to 4% in ticks feeding on virus-immune hares.[55] In regions without deer and where all sheep have been vaccinated against LIV and treated frequently with acaricides, culling of mountain hares to extremely low densities has reduced LIV seroprevalence in red grouse to very low levels.[30] This method has been used for tick and LIV control.[48]

The distribution of LIV is very patchy. LIV may be absent from areas with high densities of reservoir hosts, and LIV-free sheep-grazing regions may be immediately adjacent to regions with high LIV prevalence.[48] This may be partially due to the presence of at least three types of LIV transmission cycles that involve ticks. The first cycle uses sheep as the sole mammalian LIV host and occurs in Wales, some parts of England, and crofting areas on the west coast of Scotland and the Scottish islands. The second cycle involves red grouse, mountain hares, and red deer and is found in the Highlands of Scotland. In order to protect the economically valuable red grouse game birds from potentially fatal LIV infection, sheep are either removed from the region, are treated with acaricides, or vaccinated against LIV. The third cycle involves a mixture of sheep and red grouse in northern England or sheep, red grouse, red deer, and mountain hares in parts of the Scottish Highlands.[48] These different transmission cycles may contribute to the presence of various subtypes of LIV in different regions of the United Kingdom, as described later.

Louping-III, Russian Spring–Summer Encephalitis, and Tickborne Encephalitis Viruses

Complement-fixation and neutralization tests have demonstrated that LIV is antigenically very closely related to the other flaviviruses responsible for Far-Eastern tickborne encephalitis (TBEV-FE), formerly known as Russian spring–summer encephalitis, but not to tested mosquito-borne encephalitis viruses, such as Japanese encephalitis virus, WNV, and St. Louis encephalitis virus.[58,59] Interestingly, intraperitoneal, but not intracerebral, cross-resistance tests support a close relationship between LIV and TBEV-FE.[59] In addition to many clinical and epidemiological similarities between LIV and TBEV-FE, neutralization assays indicate that these viruses are serologically nearly identical to each other and to viral isolates from meningoencephalitis outbreaks in Czechoslovakia and Austria, while differing serologically from mosquito-borne flaviviruses. Serum from an individual with laboratory-acquired LIV infection tested positive for TBEV-FE by complement fixation and neutralization tests, providing further evidence for the similarity of these viruses.[58] Studies of antigenic reactivity using monoclonal antibodies indicate that LIV is also closely related to isolates of another, Western, subtype of TBEV, present in Slovenia, Czechoslovakia, and western Russia (TBEV-Eur).[60] A separate study of antigenic reactivity using a different panel of monoclonal antibodies prepared against the prototype LIV demonstrated antigenic heterogeneity of LIV isolates.[61] Furthermore, most people vaccinated against TBEV produce antibodies that cross-neutralize LIV with similar titers against both of these tickborne flaviviruses.[62]

Given the similarities discussed previously, it has been suggested that LIV, TBEV-FE, and TBEV-Eur are the subtypes of TBEV.[61,63,64] HI assays, however, detect no reaction between convalescent serum against the reference strain of TBEV and LIV,[65] suggesting that LIV is not a subtype of TBEV. The ranges of LIV and TBEV-FE differ greatly as well, with the latter being endemic in Russia; northern, western, and southwestern regions of China; and Japan.[66,67] Moreover, unlike louping-ill, TBE is common in people and survivors often display residual paralyses.[6] *The Ninth Report of the International Committee on Taxonomy of Viruses* also regards LIV and TBEV to be distinctly different species.[68]

LIV is also closely related to the Spanish goat encephalitis virus[69] that struck 17 members of a herd of the nearly extinct Bermeya goats in 2011. The affected goats developed severe to fatal disease.[70] Goats vaccinated against LIV, however, are completely protected against subcutaneous challenge with the goat virus.[69]

Subtypes of LIV

LIVs have been divided by different researchers into different groups. One method of grouping results in four geographically separate lineages in the British Isles and is based on the molecular phylogeny of the E protein gene. Genotype 1 is present in Scotland and England, genotype 2 is present in Scotland, genotype 3 is present in Wales, and genotype 4 is present in Ireland.[71] LIV is very rarely found outside of the British Isles, however, based on antigenic and molecular assays, a Norwegian isolate was found to belong to the Scottish and English genotype 1.[71,72]

The Ninth Report of the International Committee on Taxonomy of Viruses, however, divides LIVs differently into the following five subtypes: British subtype (LIV-Brit), Irish subtype (LIV-Ir), Spanish subtype, Turkish sheep encephalitis virus subtype, and Greek goat encephalitis virus subtype.[73–75] Several differences have been found among these subtypes, including a lower degree of virulence in several of the LIV-Brit strains when compared to LIV-Ir strains.[71]

THE IMMUNE RESPONSE
Anti-LIV Antibodies

In areas where louping-ill is endemic, adult sheep rarely become clinically ill, since active immunity may be acquired while they were yet lambs and subsequently reinforced by repeated infections.[76] Lambs receive maternal anti-LIV HI antibody in colostrum. Since these antibodies are able to block experimental subcutaneous infection, young lambs may be protected from natural infection with LIV as well.[77] The half-life of colostrum antibodies is approximately 2 weeks. Other antibodies also play a vital role in long-term immunity. While complement-fixing anti-LIV antibodies are present in sheep serum 2–6 weeks after experimental infection, they are transient, lasting less than 21 weeks in almost half of the infected animals. Neutralizing antibodies, however, appear 1–4 weeks postinfection and their levels remain stable.[76] The production of these antibodies corresponds to the end of viremia.[78]

Despite the close antigenic relationship between LIV and TBEV, while anti-TBEV antibodies protect against neurological disease in sheep challenged subcutaneously with TBEV, it is not when they are challenged with LIV. LIV-related viremia and disease severity are, nevertheless, decreased in the presence of anti-TBEV antibodies.[78] In the LIV-challenged sheep, febrile infection is accompanied by transient viremia and increased blood levels of IFN-α. This is soon followed by neuroinvasion and upregulation of interferon-inducible genes and chemokines, including IL-1β, Mx1, IFN-γ, and CXCL10.[78] Detection of LIV in the CNS is associated with detectable levels of T cells, which outnumber B cells in this locale. Chemokine-induced infiltration of T cells into the CNS may contribute to pathology and death. LIV has successfully adapted to replicate in sheep cells and disseminates widely and rapidly, while TBEV is controlled early after infection by the sheep humoral immune response, preventing its dissemination to the CNS. This occurs in the absence of detectable type I IFN and immunopathology.[78]

Soon after the infection of sheep, LIV replication occurs in the lymph nodes and spleen, leading to viremia before the infection of neurons and the consequent neuropathology.[79] Since LIV is neurotropic, its antigens are restricted to necrotic neurons and their cell processes and are not found on glial cells or the vascular endothelium, as is seen during infection of some to the other neurotropic flaviviruses.[4,15,16,80] The site of perivascular inflammation in the brain contains plasmacytes, as well as anti-LIV IgM or IgG. In sheep inoculated subcutaneously, high concentrations of LIV E protein-specific HI antibodies are present in the CSF of all animals,[81] similar to the cases of louping-ill in humans.[5,7,82] The ratio of LIV-specific IgM to IgG is similar in the serum and CSF. Antibodies in the CNS are produced locally and the presence of greater levels of IgM than IgG in this site is associated with acute disease, while the presence of only IgG, indicative of prior infection, is associated with survival.[81] In addition to antibodies, elevated leukocyte levels are present in the CSF of humans[5,7,82] and monkeys[83] with louping-ill.

Sheep surviving subcutaneous infection with LIV have high levels of HI antibodies in the CSF and are at least temporarily resistant to intracranial challenge.[84] Following either passive or active immunization of sheep, LIV levels in nervous tissues and CSF decrease, but without a corresponding increase in their survival upon intracranial challenge, despite the presence of circulating HI IgG in all immunized animals.[84] LIV-specific HI antibodies, however, are not found in the CSF in the majority of the immunized animals. Interestingly, meningitis is more severe in the vaccinated group. Severe perivascular inflammation is present in immunized animals as well, while absent in nonimmunized control sheep. Neuronophagia of necrotic neurons by macrophages also occurs in immunized animals.

LIV-Specific Vaccines

In 1931 and 1934, trials of an anti-LIV vaccine were conducted in thousands of sheep. The vaccine was effective; however, it also transmitted the protein agent of the lethal prion disease, scrapie, to some of the vaccinated animals. The vaccine contained brain, spinal cord, and spleen tissue from LIV-inoculated sheep. It was formalin-inactivated, which eliminated viable virus, but not prions. Eventually, research into the linkage between the LIV vaccine and scrapie laid the foundations for study of other prion-related spongiform encephalopathies in humans and cattle.[1]

More recent vaccine strategies have employed recombinant viral vectors. One such construct used vaccinia virus expressing the LIV premembrane/truncated envelope protein (PrM/TrE).[85] This construct induced LIV-specific neutralizing antibodies that protect 89.4% of mice after challenge ($n = 19$), compared to only 20% survival in the absence of the premembrane region from the vaccine.

Another recombinant vaccine composed of the LIV prM/E gene incorporated into a Semliki Forest virus (SFV) vector was developed that correctly processed and released E protein from transfected cells.[86] Antibodies, primarily IgG2a, were produced by mice immunized with this recombinant vaccine, indicating an active Th1 response that also stimulated T cell proliferation. Mice vaccinated intraperitoneally were significantly protected from normally lethal LIV intraperitoneal challenge. No serious CNS pathology was present in vaccinated mice surviving challenge with a highly virulent strain of LIV.[86] SFV vectors incorporating the LIV NS1 protein were also protective when given intraperitoneally, but not intranasally, despite the production of anti-LIV IgA in the latter group. Recombinant SFV vectors are particularly promising since they are suicidal, only undergoing one round of replication in infected cells. Such recombinant vaccines also provide better protection than naked DNA or chemically inactivated LIV vaccines.[87] Only recombinant vaccine fully protects mice against neuronal degeneration and encephalitis after challenge with all but the most virulent strain of LIV, despite the development of humoral immunity by all three tested vaccine types.[87]

Several studies have found that passive immunization potentiates inflammation during infection with other flaviviruses, including Venezuelan equine encephalomyelitis virus and the normally nonpathogenic Langat virus.[88,89] Caution, therefore, is advisable in LIV vaccine development. Additionally, using ELISA or viral neutralizing assays to determine the prevalence of TBEV in sentinel sheep or goat sera should take into consideration the ability of anti-LIV antibodies to cross-react with TBEV in these tests and may lead to false-positive findings.[90]

OTHER METHODS OF DISEASE PREVENTION

While there is currently no licensed vaccine for humans, there are licensed vaccines for use in some other viral hosts. Efforts to protect economically valuable, LIV-vulnerable animals, such as sheep and red grouse, include treating sheep with acaricides and repeated vaccination against LIV. The commercially available vaccine used to protect animals contains an inactivated virus mixed with liquid paraffin/montanide as an adjuvant. One subcutaneous injection provides protection for 2 years.[45,91] Consistent vaccination, in the presence or absence of acaricide treatment, decreases the proportion of seropositive sheep in an area of northern England in which sheep and red grouse are the only LIV transmission hosts present.[50,92] Three acaricide treatments were significantly more effective than two treatments although these treatments are ineffective by themselves. After 5 years, LIV infection was eliminated in only one-third of the farms, perhaps due to transmission by wild animal populations, including mountain hares and grouse. By contrast, area farms not following a constant vaccination program had variable results or an increase in infection rates. Louping-ill shows great spatial variation, so that areas with high seroprevalence are adjacent to those with low seroprevalence, thus preventive measures utilized in one farm may not affect neighboring farms.[92]

Red grouse residing in areas with high or low LIV prevalence may be treated by several methods, including placing slow-release acaricidal wing tags on hens that rub onto chicks during brooding or a one-off pour-on acaricide directly onto the chicks. While both methods greatly reduce tick burden on chicks, only the latter has been found to reduce LIV seroprevalence and increase grouse survival.[93] Since deer also serve as hosts for the LIV tick vector, deer management strategies are also employed, including culling or using fencing to exclude deer from key areas. These strategies decrease both deer and *I. ricinus* abundance.[94] Lowering deer density has drawbacks, however, due to the intrinsic popularity of deer, as well as deer hunting. While treating deer with acaricides has yet to be tried to control louping-ill, it has been used in the Eastern United States to control Lyme borreliosis. Areas where white-tailed deer are treated using rollers at feeding stations have a substantial reduction in *Ixodes scapularis* nymphs and density of infected nymphs per deer.[95] Trials of such an approach to decrease tick infestation of deer may be useful in preventing louping-ill in Great Britain as well, especially given the loss of valuable animals to this disease and the rarity of severe disease in humans.

TREATMENT

The broad-spectrum antiviral compound imino-C-nucleoside BCX4430 is active against a wide range of RNA viruses, including TBEV and some mosquito-borne flaviviruses, such as DENV-2, ZIKV, YFV, and JEV. It also is active in preventing louping-ill, although at three- to eightfold higher concentrations than are needed to protect against TBEV.[96] Perhaps other antiflaviviral drugs will also be found to either prevent louping-ill or reduce disease severity.

SUMMARY OVERVIEW

Diseases: severe neurological disease, progressing from slight ataxia to complete flaccid paralysis and death
Causative agent: louping-ill virus
Type of agent: tick-borne encephalitis virus complex
Vector: sheep tick (*Ixodes ricinus*)
Common reservoirs: sheep, red grouse, mountain hares
Mode of transmission: tick bite
Geographical distribution: primarily the United Kingdom and Ireland
Year of emergence: 1930 in sheep, 1934 in humans

REFERENCES

1. Buxton D, Reid HW. 120 years of louping-ill research: an historical perspective from the archive of the Journal of Comparative Pathology. *J Comp Pathol.* 2017;157:270–275.
2. Pool WA, Brownlee A, Wilson RD. The etiology of 'louping-ill'. *J Comp Pathol Ther.* 1930;43:253.
3. Gordon WS, Brownlee A, Wilson RD, MacLeod J. Studies in louping-ill: an encephalomyelitis of sheep. *J Comp Pathol Ther.* 1932;45:106–140.
4. Hurst WE. The transmission of 'louping-ill' to the mouse and the monkey: histology of the experimental disease. *J Comp Pathol Ther.* 1931;44:231–245.
5. Rivers TM, Schwentker FF. Louping ill in man. *J Exp Med.* 1934;59:669.
6. Davison G, Neubauer C, Hurst EW. Meningo-encephalitis in man due to the louping-ill virus. *Lancet.* 1948;ii:453–457.
7. Brewis EG, Neubauer C, Hurst EW. Another case of louping-ill in man; isolation of the virus. *Lancet.* 1949;1(6556):689–691.
8. MacLeod J, Gordon WS. Studies in louping-ill, an encephalomyelitis of sheep. II. Transmission by the sheep tick, *Ixodes ricinus. J Comp Pathol Ther.* 1932;45:240–252.
9. Williams H, Thorburn H, Ziffo GS. Isolation of louping-ill virus from the red grouse. *Nature.* 1963;200:193–194.
10. Watt JA, Brotherston JG, Campbell J. Louping-ill in red grouse. *Vet Rec.* 1963;75:1151.
11. Reid HW, Boyce JB. Louping-ill virus in red grouse in Scotland. *Vet Rec.* 1974;95:150.
12. Hubálek Z, Rudolf I. Tick-borne viruses in Europe. *Parasitol Res.* 2012;111:9–36.
13. Reid HW, Doherty PC. Experimental louping-ill in sheep and lambs. I. Viraemia and the antibody response. *J Comp Pathol.* 1971;81:291–298.
14. Reid HW, Doherty PC. Louping-ill encephalomyelitis in the sheep. I. The relationship of viraemia and the antibody response to susceptibility. *J Comp Pathol.* 1971;81:521–529.
15. Sheahan BJ, Moore M, Atkins GJ. The pathogenicity of louping ill virus for mice and lambs. *J Comp Pathol.* 2002;126:137–146.
16. Brownlee A, Wilson RD. Studies in the histopathology of louping-ill. *J Comp Pathol Ther.* 1932;45:67–92.
17. Doherty PC, Reid HW. Experimental louping-ill in sheep and lambs. II. Neuropathology. *J Comp Pathol.* 1971;81:331–337.
18. Doherty PC, Reid HW. Louping-ill encephalomyelitis in the sheep. II. Distribution of virus and lesions in nervous tissue. *J Comp Pathol.* 1971;81:531–536.
19. Reid HW, Buxton D, Pow I, Brodie TA, Holmes PH, Urquhart GM. Response of sheep to experimental concurrent infection with tick-borne fever (*Cytoecetes phagocytophila*) and louping-ill virus. *Res Vet Sci.* 1986;41:56–62.
20. Reid HW, Buxton D, Gardiner AC, Pow I, Finlayson J, MacLean MJ. Immunosuppression in toxoplasmosis: studies in lambs and sheep infected with louping-ill virus. *J Comp Pathol.* 1982;92:181–190.
21. Twomey DF, Cranwell MP, Reid HW, Tan JFV. Louping ill on Dartmoor. *Vet Rec.* 2001;149:687.
22. Reid HW, Buxton D, Finlayson IP. Experimental louping-ill virus infection of cattle. *Vet Rec.* 1981;108(23):497–498.
23. Fletcher JM. Louping-ill in the horse. *Vet Rec.* 1937;49:17–18.
24. Hyde J, Nettleton P, Marriott L, Willoughby K. Louping ill in horses. *Vet Rec.* 2007;160(15):532.
25. Timoney PJ, Donnelly WJ, Clements LO, Fenlon M. Encephalitis caused by louping ill virus in a group of horses in Ireland. *Equine Vet J.* 1976;8:113–117.
26. Timoney PJ. Susceptibility of the horse to experimental inoculation with louping ill virus. *J Comp Pathol.* 1980;90:73–86.
27. Cranwell MP, Josephson M, Willoughby K, Marriott L. Louping ill in an alpaca. *Vet Rec.* 2008;162(1):28.
28. MacAldowie C, Patterson IAP, Nettleton PF, Low H, Buxton D. Louping ill in llamas (*Lama glama*) in the Hebrides. *Vet Rec.* 2005;156:420–421.
29. Reid HW, Duncan JS, Phillips JDB, Moss R, Watson A. Studies on louping-ill virus (flavivirus group) in wild red grouse (*Lagopus lagopus scoticus*). *J Hyg.* 1978;81:321–329.
30. Laurenson MK, Norman RA, Gilbert L, Reid HW, Hudson PJ. Identifying disease reservoirs in complex systems: mountain hares as reservoirs of ticks and louping-ill virus, pathogens of red grouse. *J Anim Ecol.* 2003;72:177–185.
31. Reid HW. Experimental infection of red grouse with louping-ill virus (flavivirus group). I. The viraemia and antibody response. *J Comp Pathol.* 1975;85(2):223–229.
32. Reid HW, Moss R, Pow I, Buxton D. The response of three grouse species (*Tetrao urogallus, Lagopus mutus, Lagopus lagopus*) to louping-ill virus. *J Comp Pathol.* 1980;90:257–263.
33. Zlotnik I, Grant DP, Carter GB. Experimental infection of monkeys with viruses of the tick-borne encephalitis complex: degenerative cerebellar lesions following inapparent forms of the disease or recovery from clinical encephalitis. *Br J Exp Pathol.* 1976;57:200.

34. Seamer J, Zlotnik I. Louping-ill and Semliki Forest virus infections in the short-tailed vole *Microtus agrestis* (L.). *Br J Exp Pathol.* 1970;51:385–393.

35. Gilbert L, Jones LD, Hudson PJ, Gould EA, Reid HW. Role of small mammals in the persistence of louping-ill virus: field survey and tick co-feeding studies. *Med Vet Entomol.* 2000;14:277–282.

36. Hudson PJ, Norman R, Laurenson MK, et al. Persistence and transmission of tick-borne viruses: *Ixodes ricinus* and louping-ill virus in red grouse populations. *Parasitology.* 1995;111(suppl):S49–S58.

37. Reid HW. *Vectors in Biology.* Academic Press; 1984.

38. Zlotnik I, Harris WJ. The changes in cell organelles of neurons in the brains of adult mice and hamsters during Semliki forest virus and louping ill encephalitis. *Br J Exp Pathol.* 1970;51:37–42.

39. Lawson JH, Manderson WG, Hurst EW. Louping-ill meningo-encephalitis. A further case and a serological survey. *Lancet.* 1949;2(6581):697–699.

40. Likar M, Dane DS. An illness resembling acute poliomyelitis caused by a virus of the Russian spring-summer encephalitis/louping ill group in Northern Ireland. *Lancet.* 1958;1(7018):456–458.

41. Reid HW, Gibbs CA, Burrells C, Dougherty PC. Laboratory infections with louping-ill virus. *Lancet.* 1972;1(7750):592–593.

42. Hogg J. The Ettrick shepherd. In: *The Shepherd's Guide;* 1807. Facsimile published by the British Veterinary Association; 1807.

43. M'Fadyean J. Louping-ill in sheep. *J Comp Pathol Ther.* 1994;7:207–219.

44. M'Fadyean J. The etiology of louping-ill. *J Comp Pathol Ther.* 1990;3:145–154.

45. Jeffries CL, Mansfield KL, Phipps LP, et al. Louping ill virus: an endemic tick-borne disease of Great Britain. *J Gen Virol.* 2014;95:1005–1014.

46. Reid HW, Buxton D, Pow I, Finlayson J. Transmission of louping-ill virus in goat milk. *Vet Rec.* 1984;114(7):163–165.

47. Reid HW, Pow I. Excretion of louping-ill virus in ewes' milk. *Vet Rec.* 1985;117(18):470.

48. Gilbert L. Louping ill virus in the UK: a review of the hosts, transmission and ecological consequences of control. *Exp Appl Acarol.* 2016;68:363–374.

49. Gilbert L, Norman R, Laurenson KM, Reid HW, Hudson PJ. Disease persistence and apparent competition in a three-host community: an empirical and analytical study of large scale wild populations. *J Anim Ecol.* 2001;70:1053–1061.

50. Newborn D, Baines D. Enhanced control of sheep ticks in upland sheep flocks: repercussions for red grouse co-hosts. *Med Vet Entomol.* 2012;26:63–69.

51. Ogden NH, Hailes RS, Nuttal PA. Interstadial variation in the attachment sites of *Ixodes ricinus* ticks on sheep. *Exp Appl Acarol.* 1998;22:227–232.

52. Norman R, Ross D, Laurenson MK, Hudson PJ. The role of non-viraemic transmission on the persistence and dynamics of a tick borne virus—louping ill in red grouse (*Lagopus lagopus scoticus*) and mountain hares (*Lepus timidus*). *J Math Biol.* 2004;48:119–134.

53. Norman R, Bowers RG, Begon M, Hudson PJ. Persistence of tick-borne virus in the presence of multiple host species: ticks act as reservoirs and result in parasite mediated competition. *J Theor Biol.* 1999;200:111–118.

54. Hudson P, Gould E, Laurenson K, et al. The epidemiology of louping-ill, a tick borne infection of red grouse (*Lagopus lagopus scoticus*). *Parassitologia.* 1997;39(4):319–323.

55. Jones L, Gaunt M, Hails R, et al. Amplification of louping-ill virus infection during co-feeding of ticks on mountain hares (*Lepus timidus*). *Med Vet Entomol.* 1997;11:172–176.

56. Labuda M, Jones LD, Williams T, Danielova V, Nuttall PA. Efficient transmission of tick-borne encephalitis virus between cofeeding ticks. *J Med Entomol.* 1993;30:295–299.

57. Jones LD, Kaufman WR, Nuttall PA. Modification of the skin feeding site by tick saliva mediates virus transmission. *Experientia.* 1992;48(8):779–782.

58. Casals J, Webster LT. Close relation between Russian spring-summer encephalitis and louping-ill viruses. *Science.* 1943;97(2515):246–248.

59. Casals J, Webster LT. Relationship of the virus of louping ill in sheep and the virus of Russian spring-summer encephalitis in man. *J Exp Med.* 1994;79(1):45–63.

60. Stephenson R, Lee JM, Wilton-Smith PD. Antigenic variation among members of the tick-borne encephalitis complex. *J Gen Virol.* 1984;65:81–89.

61. Hubálek Z, Pow I, Reid HW, Hussain MH. Antigenic similarity of Central European encephalitis and louping-ill viruses. *Acta Virol.* 1995;39(5–6):251–256.

62. Mansfield KL, Horton DL, Johnson N, et al. Flavivirus-induced antibody cross-reactivity. *J Gen Virol.* 2011;92:2821–2829.

63. Pond WL, Warren J. The Russian spring-summer encephalitis and louping ill group of viruses; relationship of European and Asiatic strains of Russian spring-summer encephalitis viruses and louping ill virus. *J Infect Dis.* 1953;93:294–300.

64. Pond WL, Russ SB. Serological aspects of virus meningo-encephalitis; a study of the reactions of two viruses isolated during the 1953 epidemics in Slovenia and Austria. *Bull World Health Organ.* 1955;12:591–594.

65. Gresíkova M, Sekeyová M. Antigenic variation of the viruses belonging to the tick-borne encephalitis complex as revealed by human convalescent serum and monoclonal antibodies. *Acta Virol.* 1987;31(2):152–157.

66. Lu Z, Broker M, Liang G. Tick-borne encephalitis in mainland China. *Vector Borne Zoonotic Dis.* 2008;8:713–720.

67. Takashima I, Morita K, Chiba M, et al. A case of tick-borne encephalitis in Japan and isolation of the virus. *J Clin Microbiol.* 1997;35:1943–1947.

68. Pletnev A, Gould E, Heinz FX. *Virus Taxonomy: Ninth Report of the International Committee on Taxonomy of Viruses.* Elsevier; 2011.

69. Salinas LM, Casais R, Marín JFG, et al. Vaccination against louping ill virus protects goats from experimental challenge with Spanish goat encephalitis virus. *J Comp Pathol.* 2017;156:409–418.

70. Balseiro A, Royo LJ, Martínez CP. Louping ill in goats, Spain, 2011. *Emerg Infect Dis.* 2012;18(6):976–978.

71. Gao GF, Zanotto PM, Holmes EC, Reid HW, Gould EA. Molecular variation, evolution and geographical distribution of louping ill virus. *Acta Virol.* 1997;41(5):259–268.

72. Gao GF, Jiang WR, Hussain MH, et al. Sequencing and antigenic studies of a Norwegian virus isolated from encephalomyelitic sheep confirm the existence of louping ill virus outside Great Britain and Ireland. *J Gen Virol.* 1993;74:109–114.

73. King AMQ, Adams MJ, Carstens EB, Lefkowitz EJ. *Ninth Report of the International Committee on Taxonomy of Viruses.* Elsevier; 2012.

74. Grard G, Moureau G, Charrel RN, et al. Genetic characterization of tick-borne flaviviruses: new insights into evolution, pathogenetic determinants and taxonomy. *Virology.* 2007;361:80–92.

75. Mansfield KL, Morales AB, Johnson N, et al. Identification and characterization of a novel tick-borne flavivirus subtype in goats (*Capra hircus*) in Spain. *J Gen Virol.* 2015;96:1676–1681.

76. Williams H, Thorburn H. The serological response of sheep to infection with louping-ill virus. *J Hyg.* 1961;59:437–447.

77. Reid HW, Boyce JB. The effect of colostrum-derived antibody on louping-ill virus infection in lambs. *J Hyg (Lond).* 1986;77:349–354.

78. Mansfield KL, Johnson N, Banyard AC, et al. Innate and adaptive immune responses to tick-borne flavivirus infection in sheep. *Vet Microbiol.* 2016;185:20–28.

79. Doherty PC, Smith W, Reid HW. Louping-ill encephalomyelitis in the sheep. V. Histopathogenesis of the fatal disease. *J Comp Pathol.* 1972;82:337–344.

80. Doherty PC, Reid HW, Smith W. Louping-ill encephalomyelitis in the sheep. IV. Nature of the perivascular inflammatory response. *J Comp Pathol.* 1991;81:545–549.

81. Reid HW, Doherty PC, Dawson AM. Louping-ill encephalomyelitis in the sheep. III. Immunoglobulins in cerebrospinal fluid. *J Comp Pathol.* 1991;81:537–543.

82. Webb HE, Connolly JH, Kane FF, O'Reilly KJ, Simpson DIH. Laboratory infections with louping-ill with associated encephalitis. *Lancet.* 1968;2(7562):255–258.

83. Galloway IA, Perdrau JR. Louping-ill in monkeys. Infection by the nose. *J Hyg (Lond).* 1935;35:339–346.

84. Doherty PC, Vantsis JT. Louping-ill encephalomyelitis in the sheep. VII. Influence of immune status on neuropathology. *J Comp Pathol.* 1973;83:481–491.

85. Venugopal K, Shiu SYW, Gould EA. Recombinant vaccinia virus expressing PrM and E glycoproteins of louping ill virus: induction of partial homologous and heterologous protection in mice. *Res Vet Sci.* 1994;57:188–193.

86. Fleeton MN, Sheahan BJ, Gould EA, Atkins GJ, Liljeström P. Recombinant Semliki Forest virus particles encoding the prME or NS1 proteins of louping ill virus protect mice from lethal challenge. *J Gen Virol.* 1999;80:1189–1198.

87. Fleeton MN, Liljeström P, Sheahan BJ, Atkins NJ. Recombinant Semliki Forest virus particles expressing louping ill virus antigens induce a better protective response than plasmid-based DNA vaccines or an inactivated whole particle vaccine. *J Gen Virol.* 2000;81:749–758.

88. Berge TO, Gleiser CA, Gochenour Jr WS, Miesse ML, Tigertt WD. Studies on the virus of Venezuelan equine encephalomyelitis. II. Modification by specific immune serum of response of central nervous system of mice. *J Immunol.* 1961;87:509.

89. Webb HE, Wight DG, Wiernik G, Platt GS, Smith CE. Langat virus encephalitis in mice. II. The effect of irradiation. *J Hyg (Lond).* 1968;66(3):355–364.

90. Klaus C, Ziegler U, Kalthoff D, Hoffmann B, Beer M. Tick-borne encephalitis virus (TBEV)—findings on cross reactivity and longevity of TBEV antibodies in animal sera. *BMC Vet Res.* 2014;10:78.

91. Shaw B, Reid HW. Immune responses of sheep to louping-ill virus vaccine. *Vet Rec.* 1981;109:529–531.

92. Laurenson MK, McKendrick IJ, Reid HW, Challenor R, Mathewson GK. Prevalence, spatial distribution and the effect of control measures on louping-ill virus in the Forest of Bowland, Lancashire. *Epidemiol Infect.* 2007;135:963–973.

93. Laurenson MK, Hudson PJ, McGuire K, Thirgood SJ, Reid HW. Efficacy of acaricidal tags and pour on as prophylaxis against ticks and louping-ill in red grouse. *Med Vet Entomol.* 1997;11:389–393.

94. Gilbert L, Maffey GL, Ramsay SL, Hester AJ. The effect of deer management on the abundance of *Ixodes ricinus* in Scotland. *Ecol Appl.* 2012;22:658–667.

95. Brei B, Brownstein JS, George JE, et al. Evaluation of the United States Department of Agriculture Northeast Area-Wide Tick Control Project by meta-analysis. *Vector Borne Zoonotic Dis.* 2009;9:423–430.

96. Eyer L, Zouharová D, Sirmarová J, et al. Antiviral activity of the adenosine analogue BCX4430 against West Nile virus and tick-borne flaviviruses. *Antiviral Res.* 2017;142:63–67.

CHAPTER 11

Powassan Virus

INTRODUCTION

The two lineages of Powassan virus (POWV) are the causative agents for Powassan neuroinvasive disease. A POWV Lineage 1 was initially isolated in 1958 in Powassan, Ontario, Canada, from the brain of a young boy who died of encephalitis.[1] This virus bears some serological relationship to the Far Eastern tickborne encephalitis virus (TBEV-FE), formerly known as Russian spring–summer encephalitis (RSSE) virus. Both are members of the TBEV complex but are distinct species. Tickborne encephalitic flaviviruses appear to have evolved from nonencephalitic viruses that migrated eastward and northeastward from Africa into Asia and southern Pacific islands. They then migrated northward to Far East Asia before spreading westward across Eurasia into Western Europe over the last 2000–4000 years. Only the Powassan virus is known to have made its way to North America.[2]

POWV is found primarily in Canada and the United States and, to a far lesser extent, in Russia. It is the only pathogenic tickborne flavivirus that is known to infect humans in North America.[2] Antibodies to POWV have also been detected in Mexico.[3] On the Eastern Seaboard, POWV is found from Virginia to Nova Scotia and inland in New York, Pennsylvania, and Quebec. In the interior of the United States, it has been reported in the North Central states (Michigan, Wisconsin, and Minnesota) and western and Pacific coast states (Colorado, New Mexico, and California). It is also found across Canada (Ontario, Quebec, Alberta, and British Columbia) and in other very cold regions, such as Alaska and Siberia.[4–6] In Siberia, voles host the virus, while in New Mexico, infection occurs in pinion mice and deer mice. The pinion mice have a higher prevalence rate than is seen in deer mice.[6]

In addition to expanding its geographical range over time, prevalence of POWV is increasing in both its tick vectors and vertebrate hosts. Infections typically occur from May to September and are often associated with known tick exposure.[7] Between 1999 and 2005, the average yearly number of human POWV cases was 1.3 in the United States, compared to 0.7 cases per year during the 40 preceding years.[8] Furthermore, from 1958 to 1998, 27 cases were reported, while from 1999 to 2016, there were 98 known cases, reflecting an increase of 671% over 18 years.[5] Similarly, the numbers of infected deer are increasing.[9] Significantly, infected snowshoe hares, wild murine rodents, and horses have displayed neurological disease manifestations.[5]

POWV is a rarely reported cause of encephalitis in the United States. In the northeastern part of the country, POWV Lineage II is transmitted to humans by *Ixodes scapularis* ticks. POWV is serologically indistinguishable from deer tick virus (DTV) and both POWV and DTV use the same tick vector. In addition, they have an 84% nucleoside sequence identity. It has thus been suggested that they represent different lineages of the same encephalitis virus.[4,10–12]

HISTORY

Since its discovery in 1958, over 100 human cases of Powassan virus encephalitis have been reported in North America.[1,13] Although the first reported discovery of POWV in humans occurred in Canada, later studies found the virus in a tick pool collected in 1952 in Colorado, in the western United States.[14,15] POWV was first isolated in Russia in 1972 from *Haemaphysalis longicornis* ticks[16,17] and, in 1978, from the blood of a healthy woman following a tick bite. At that time, the examination of sera from Russia detected an antibody against TBEV in 69.2% of the tested encephalitis patients ($n = 117$), an antibody against POWV in 4.3% of the patients, and antibodies against both viruses in 4.3% of the encephalitis patients.[18] Subsequent seroepidemiological studies and viral isolations revealed that POWV is present in ticks, rodents, and humans.[18–20] Comparative analysis of the complete viral genome sequences determined that a 2006 Russian strain of POWV from an infected human was 99.8% similar to the strain isolated in Canada in 1958.[21] As many as 3.2% of the people living in the northern Ontario region of Canada are seropositive, despite low numbers of reported cases of POWV-associated encephalitis, indicating that POWV is not usually infectious to humans or that infection is rarely pathogenic.[20] POWV-associated disease may also be misdiagnosed. Reported disease incidence is increasing, whether due to increased numbers of people infected by one of the POWV lineages or increased surveillance and detection. From 2006 through 2016, 99 cases of this viral disease were reported from 12 states in the United States. Of these, 89 cases were neuroinvasive. The states with the highest disease incidence were Minnesota (0.468 cases per 100,000 population), Wisconsin (0.333), Maine (0.226), and Massachusetts (0.197). Of concern, the highest numbers of cases were reported in 2011 ($n = 16$), 2013 ($n = 15$), and 2016 ($n = 22$).[22]

POWV Lineage I are present in the Great Lakes region of North America, but more recently, cases of POWV Lineage II have been reported in the northeastern part of the United States. Lineage II was first isolated from *I. scapularis* ticks in 1997.[23] The recent increase in human cases of Powassan encephalitis may be due, at least partially, to the emergence of this lineage in new areas, especially in the Hudson Valley of New York State. Hudson Valley reported 14 Powassan encephalitis cases from 2004 to 2012 and 4 more cases in 2013, accounting for 72% of the patients with POWV encephalitis. *I. scapularis* are responsible for more than 75% of the human tick bites in this region, while no bites were attributable to *Ixodes cookei*, strongly suggesting that most of the encephalitis cases in that area are due to POWV Lineage II, rather than to Lineage I.[24,25] Lineage II, but not Lineage I, viruses were only found in *I. scapularis* and up to 6% of the tested adult ticks were infected by POWV Lineage II.[24,25] A study of Pennsylvania ticks from 2013 to 2015 found that 66.9% were adult *I. scapularis* ($n = 2973$ ticks) and that the statewide POWV infection rate was 0.05%.[26] Studies in New York and Connecticut have detected Lineage II virus in 3% of the tested ticks. In contrast, as many as 55% of the ticks were positive for *Borrelia burgdorferi*, the spirochete that is the causative agent of Lyme disease.[27,28] Additionally, the reported prevalence of POWV-infected deer in Connecticut, Vermont, and Maine has increased from less than 25% before 1996 up to 80%–90% in 2005–09. This increase in the infection rate of deer was accompanied by a similar increase in Powassan encephalitis in humans of the region. Deer from Connecticut tend to have more exposure to Lineage II virus than animals from Vermont or Maine, which may be related to having greater more *I. scapularis* ticks, which are more prevalent in southern, than northern, New England.[9]

THE DISEASE

POWV infection may be asymptomatic,[29] but usually results in severe encephalitis in humans. The neuroinvasive and nonneuroinvasive forms of illness were added to the nationally notifiable disease list in 2001

and 2004, respectively.[22] Symptoms of the infection are generally similar to those found in eastern equine encephalitis and TBE.[7,30] Symptoms of POWV infection, however, include cerebellovestibular lesions, differentiating it from TBE.[20] Infected mice may also develop a poliomyelitis-like syndrome with viral antigen and mononuclear cell infiltration present in the anterior horn of the spinal column.[31,32] In 2014, 80% of the reported cases in the United States were neuroinvasive.[33] Symptoms include fever, joint pain, headache, vomiting, unilateral weakness, confusion, seizures, and, in one case, classical erythema migrans,[26] in addition to encephalitis and meningitis. Approximately 70% of the POWV neuroinvasive diseases reported are encephalitis, 20% are meningoencephalitis, and 10% are meningitis.[13] Ataxia, dysarthria, nystagmus, and ophthalmoplegia may also be present.[8] Death is rare and occurs in approximately 10% of the cases with encephalitis.[34] However, about 50% of the neurological sequelae are chronic, including many cases of hemiplegia, paralysis of the shoulder muscles, and severe headache.[13] In addition to the CNS, the viral antigen is also present in the cortical and pericortical sections of the spleen as well as in the perivascular region of the liver.[31]

In a study of 13 patients with POWV encephalitis, the areas of the CNS primarily affected were the vertebral cortex and basal ganglia (54% of the cases), the brain stem (31%), cerebellum and thalamus (23%), and the meninges (15%), with 69% affecting only the left portion of the brain. All of the patients who died were over the age of 60 years. Infection is more common in this group of adults and children.[25]

A 2013–15 report studied eight encephalitis patients in Massachusetts and New Hampshire, most of whom had previously been healthy. Their ages ranged from 21 to 82 years.[7] Before this study, only two cases of POWV encephalitis had been reported in Massachusetts and one in New Hampshire.[35] Early symptoms include fever, headache, and altered consciousness. Pleocytosis of lymphocytes or neutrophils was present in all eight cases. This was accompanied by elevated levels of protein in the CSF; however, CSF glucose levels were normal. In all but one case, magnetic resonance imaging (MRI) detected deep foci of increased T2/fluid-attenuation inversion recovery signal intensity.[7] MRI abnormalities may be present in the left putamen and bilateral caudate nuclei and were sometimes accompanied by asymmetric bilateral thalamic involvement and microhemorrhages scattered about the cerebral and cerebellar white matter.[36,37] Imaging abnormalities demonstrate infection of the deep gray matter, primarily in the basal ganglia, but also in the cerebral cortex, thalami, brain stem, and cerebellum.[8] A fatal case additionally had hyperintensities throughout the superior cerebellum, left pons, and bilateral basal ganglia as well as other changes in the parietal or temporal lobes.[35] Diffusion restriction in patients is associated with poor outcome.[7]

Due to the relative lack of awareness and the necessity of using specialized laboratory tests to confirm the diagnosis, the prevalence of POWV-associated encephalitis may be underreported. POWV infection should be included in the differential diagnosis of all encephalitis cases in the northern United States, especially the northeast.[38] An especially important finding is that POWV infection can kill fetuses of infected, immunocompetent mice and is additionally able to replicate in second-trimester human maternal and fetal tissue explants.[39]

THE VIRUSES

POWV Lineages I and II are found in different regions of the United States.[12] I. cookei is the major vector for Lineage I, while Lineage II is transmitted primarily by I. scapularis ticks. The two lineages are not able to be distinguished serologically and their E protein cross-reacts with several epitopes found in other flaviviruses, including TBEV, Japanese encephalitis virus (JEV), and West Nile virus (WNV).[21] Additionally, from 1972 to 2006, Russian strains of POWV isolated from humans and several species of ticks had very high homology, suggesting little genetic variation over time. Lineage II viruses are similar to, but distinct from Lineage I viruses, having 84% pairwise similarity in the tested portion of the viral E gene.[23] The two lineages are only accurately differentiated by genetic sequence analysis.[25]

Due to the relatively high mutation rate of RNA viruses, intrahost genetic diversity is seen in many viruses, including the mosquito-borne flaviviruses DENV and WNV, which exist as true quasispecies. This is not the case for the tickborne POWV, in which the proportion of nonsynonymous to synonymous mutations varies very little between the intrahost viral populations ($pN = 0.944$) and the experimental controls ($pN = 1$), indicating that POWV does not appear to exist as a quasispecies.[40] By contrast, strong purifying POWV selection occurs between hosts.

In the Great Lakes region of North America, Lineage I viruses primarily cycle between North American woodchucks and I. cookei, one-host ticks that are distantly related to Ixodes dammini. Since I. cookei is more restricted to mammal burrows than I. scapularis and is highly specific for woodchucks and rodents, they rarely feed on humans, except in Maine, and POWV

encephalitis is uncommon.[29,41] Opossums, skunks, and raccoons are also reservoirs for I. cookei nymphs. In Ontario, red squirrels and chipmunks may serve as POWV reservoirs as well. Red squirrels are commonly infected with Ixodes marxi.[4,42] Anti-POWV antibodies have additionally been reported in other wild rodents, such as pinyon mice and deer mice in New Mexico, northern red-backed voles in Siberia and Alaska, and southern red-backed voles in southern Alaska.[6] Blood and tissues from trapped wild mammals and dogs from southern Ontario during the summers of 2015 and 2016, however, were negative for POWV by reverse-transcriptase-polymerase chain reaction (RT-PCR) ($n = 724$) and only a single pool of I. cookei ($n = 53$) was RT-PCR positive. This region of Canada thus appears to have only had low levels of POWV in mammals during that time period.[43]

In the laboratory, I. dammini are competent vectors of I. cookei-derived POWV.[44] POWV has also been isolated from both soft- and hard-bodied ticks, including I. marxi, Ixodes spinipalpus, Ixodes persulcatus, Dermacentor andersoni, Dermacentor silvarum, and H. longicornis.[13] In North America, several different POWV transmission cycles have been suggested: (a) arboreal squirrels and chipmunks and I. marxi in the eastern region, (b) medium-sized rodents and carnivores and I. cookei in eastern and mid-western regions, and (c) small- and medium-sized mammals and I. spinipalpus in the northwestern region.[45] In Far Eastern Russia, however, POWV has been isolated from mosquitoes (Aedes togoi and Anopheles hrycanus).[46]

POWV Lineage II has a different geologic preference than Lineage I, with foci of transmission in Massachusetts, Connecticut, Wisconsin, and Minnesota and a historical presence in Colorado and West Virginia.[24] Lineage II RNA or infectious virus has been isolated from pools of ticks (53 positive pools; $n = 870$) and people in New York State. In some regions of the northeastern and north-central United States, Lineage II virus prevalence in adult deer ticks is high, but reports of human infection are uncommon.[47,48] This suggests either that Lineage II does not readily infect humans, either intrinsically or because of its vector's feeding preferences, or that human infection is not usually pathogenic[32].

In addition to POWV Lineage II, I. scapularis are very common vectors of other human tickborne infections in the northeastern United States, including bacteria and protozoa (B. burgdorferi, Babesia microti, and Anaplasma phagocytophilum). A study conducted in the Upper Midwest of the United States found that 85.7% of the patients with serologic evidence of acute POWV infection were also IgM-positive for *B. burgdorferi*,[49] indicating probable concurrent and recent infection with the latter. Another study of adult *I. scapularis* from a Lyme disease-endemic region of New York found that two POWV Lineage II-positive ticks (*n* = 7) were coinfected with *B. burgdorferi* and one tick, with *A. phagocytophilum*.[50] This, together with the findings mentioned earlier of a high rate of coinfection with Lineage II POWV and neuropathogenic tickborne bacteria in humans, suggests that it may be prudent to test both humans and ticks that are seropositive for POWV Lineage II for a possible coinfection with one of several other microbial disease agents to obtain a clearer picture of the underlying source(s) of the observed disease. Coinfection thus complicates the identification of the etiologic agent for infectious neurological disease, since the illness could be due to either one of the microbes or immunopathological interactions between Lineage II viruses and *B. burgdorferi*.

POWV Lineage II is transmitted to their vertebrate hosts within 15 min after tick attachment, much more rapidly than is the case for other microbes transmitted by this tick, which typically occurs 12–48 h after attachment.[51] *I. scapularis* develops from egg to larva to nymph and to adult with a blood meal between each. All developmental stages are able to transmit virus orally to uninfected hosts irrespective of the stage in which the ticks were initially infected by the virus.[44] Transstadial transmission efficiency between larvae and nymphs is 22% and viral titer increases about 100-fold during molting.[51]

White-tailed deer serve as the principal host for POWV Lineage II and white-footed mice, as its principal reservoir host.[52] Neutralizing antibodies to Lineage II viruses have been detected in birds in British Columbia, Canada, demonstrating their exposure to infected ticks.[1] Some of the following passerine birds in the United States also have anti-POWV neutralizing antibody (0.55%; *n* = 727): a veery, a gray catbird, a northern cardinal, and an eastern towhee. By contrast, POWV Lineage I was not found in any of the tested vertebrates or ticks in that location.[24] This study also found that POWV incidence is higher in adult ticks collected from areas east of the Hudson River.

Although the major vector for POWV Lineage II is *I. scapularis*, it has also been isolated from the brain tissue of mice inoculated with homogenates from tick salivary glands of the eastern North American *I. dammini* tick. The risk of infection peaks during June and July. *I. scapularis* are small ticks, whose adults are approximately the size of a sesame seed and nymphs, are about the size of a poppy seed.[34] These ticks prefer wooded areas or areas with large amounts of brush. They parasitize hosts at or near the ground level, attaching as their human or animal host walks by.[34] An infection rate of 0%–3.9% has been reported in *I. scapularis* ticks in Connecticut,[28] 0%–3.84% in New York State,[24,27] and 0.05% in Pennsylvania in adult ticks derived from hunter-harvested white-tailed deer in the fall. The latter figure is likely to be an underestimate due to the age of the ticks and the season of the year.[26]

In addition to POWV, white-footed mice are important natural reservoirs for several other severe or life-threatening zoonotic diseases of humans, including those caused by the microbes listed previously (Lyme disease, human granulocytic anaplasmosis, babesiosis, and ehrlichiosis), as well as hard tickborne relapsing fever.[53] While mice may be unable to clear some of the microbes responsible for these diseases, mice experience only limited pathology and have partial resistance to them.

POWV Lineage II is less infectious than other members of the TBE complex. When Lineage II-inoculated suckling or adult mice live in the same cage with noninoculated mice, the latter do not become infected, indicating that the aerosol transmission of virus between mice rarely occurs, if at all.[23] Experimental infection leads to fulminant meningoencephalitis in all infected horses.[54] Small numbers of dogs develop a febrile illness following high-dose inoculation with POWV, but naturally infected dogs are asymptomatic.[55] Cats, pigs, and goats were also asymptomatic after the experimental infection with the virus, but POWV is present in the milk of the latter.[56,57] Hamsters, monkeys, chickens, rabbits, and horses have been used to study POWV-associated pathogenesis, in addition to neurological studies using nonhuman primates.[4,13,58]

THE IMMUNE RESPONSE

Tick salivary factors secreted into the feeding pool of the mammalian host's skin contain many bioactive molecules, including immunomodulators.[59,60] The bite-site lesions from even uninfected *I. scapularis* nymphs result in a rapid, proinflammatory response, followed by the localization of innate immune cells to the area within 12 h.[61] Additionally, in POWV-infected young mice, viral load in tick salivary glands increases early after attachment and feeding.[62] Furthermore, when some strains of mice are co-inoculated with POWV and tick saliva in the footpad, all of the animals receiving a high-dose viral inoculum die, following increased virus dissemination and more rapid disease progression when compared to virally inoculated mice that did not receive the saliva, in which all mice survive the infection. Mice receiving only a low viral dose in the absence of salivary gland extract develop no clinical signs of infection and no mice die. However, all mice receiving tick saliva as well as a low dose of virus (similar to levels found in an infected tick bite) experience neuroinvasion, paralysis, and death.[63] Tick saliva, therefore, appears to create a cutaneous microenvironment that aids POWV establishment and disease development. This phenomenon, known as saliva-activated transmission, also occurs during the infection with several other viruses and bacteria, including TBEV, Thogotovirus, *Francisella tularensis*, and several *Borrelia* species.[63] In the presence of saliva extract, the draining popliteal lymph nodes of infected ticks upregulate the expression of proinflammatory cytokines, such as IL-1β, IL-6, and TNF-α, at early times post infection. Levels of these cytokines then decrease later in the course of infection. Tick saliva extracts also increase the levels of IL-4 and the anti-inflammatory IL-10 cytokine during both early and late infection. By days 7–8 of infection, both inflammatory cytokines and the chemokines CCL7 and CCL11 are significantly upregulated.[63]

Three hours after POWV-infected tick attachment and feeding, skin biopsies reveal that 40 host genes are upregulated and 11 are downregulated in comparison with animals bitten by uninfected ticks.[64] Alteration of gene expression contributes to a complex proinflammatory environment where proinflammatory genes related to granulocyte recruitment, migration, and accumulation (IL-1β, IL-6, IL-36A, and CCR3), as well as toll-like receptor 4 (TLR4), are upregulated.[64] IL-36A upregulates IL-6 production and regulates numbers of mononuclear phagocytes and neutrophils at the site of infection. CCR3 induces chemotaxis of lymphocytes and eosinophils into the tick bite site. TLR4 aids in viral recognition by phagocytic cells and induces the production of additional proinflammatory cytokines. The production of a free nitrogen species, nitric oxide, is induced as well at this time via activation of the inducible nitric oxide synthetase enzyme.[64] At this time, histopathology reveals the presence of a rapid, robust, localized cellular infiltrate in the feeding site, which contains neutrophils and a smaller number of macrophages, particularly in the deep subdermal region, extending down into the underlying skeletal muscle. Such an infiltrate is not present at the feeding site of uninfected ticks.[65] Macrophages and fibroblasts in the vicinity contain the POWV E protein. By 6h, uninfected as well as POWV-infected mice contain scattered neutrophil and mononuclear cell infiltrates that are smaller than those seen 3h previously.[65] Most proinflammatory genes are

also downregulated at 6h post infection as well, including IL-1β, IL-18, IFN-γ, and TNF-α. Interestingly, both IL-2 and IL-4 expression is downregulated at 3 and 6h.[64] At 12h post infection, mononuclear cells, neutrophils, and fibroblasts are present in the submuscular layer of uninfected and infected skin sections and some lymphocytes, but not plasma cells, are present at 24h.[65]

In mice infected via the hind footpad, POWV infects skin fibroblasts and macrophages, the latter cell type being its primary target in the spleen.[31] Interestingly, in the CNS, the major site of POWV infection, neurons are the virus' primary target in humans and mice, although oligodendrites are also able to host POWV.[8,31,66]

While laboratory mice (*Mus musculus*) are useful in studying flavivirus-associated encephalitis, the natural rodent reservoir of POWV Lineage II, *Peromyscus* whitefooted mice, responds very differently. Unlike the laboratory C57BL/6 or BALB/c mice strains, *Peromyscus leucopus* mice do not develop encephalitis or die.[23,67] Early during infection, relatively equivalent levels of viral RNA are found in cells from both *P. leucopus* and laboratory mice in vitro, suggesting that these viruses are able to enter *P. leucopus* cells efficiently. Moreover, following intracranial infection, 4-week-old wildcaught *P. leucopus* mice seroconvert and develop a low viral load with limited spread and replication in the olfactory bulb and ventricles. While all tested young *P. leucopus* mice infected in this manner develop mild lymphocytic perivascular cuffing and microgliosis in the CNS from 5 to 15 days post infection, they remain asymptomatic and the inflammation spontaneously resolves within a month. In contrast, similar infection of 4-week-old C57BL/6 and BALB/c laboratory mice produces widespread viral replication in the brain and is 60% or 100% lethal in these mice species, respectively, by day 5 of infection. *P. leucopus*, therefore, provides a more natural and useful animal model for the exploration of successful host-resistant strategies.[67] Using this model, 42 and 232 genes were found to be differentially expressed in infected animals after 1 and 7 days, respectively. These genes are associated with IFN signaling.[68] In vitro, resistance to POWV's and other flavivirus' replication in *P. leucopus* primary fibroblasts relies upon type I IFN and is dependent upon the IFN-α receptor and signal transducer and activator of transcription 1 (STAT1).[69]

Necrotizing inflammation has been seen in the brains of the patients with severe Lineage II-associated disease, particularly in the motor neurons of the brain stem, anterior horns of the spinal cord, cerebellum, basal ganglia, and thalamus, and to a lesser extent in the white matter.[8,31] Large numbers of CD4+

T lymphocytes are found in the leptomeninges and perivascular spaces, while CD8[+] T killer cells are seen in the brain parenchyma next to dying neurons, suggesting a pathogenic immune response. Brain microglia activation is also present.[31]

VACCINATION AND TREATMENT

Among viruses of the TBEV complex, there exits only one licensed human vaccine and it is for TBEV itself. While vaccine sera successfully neutralize most of the tested viruses from the TBEV complex, in only 63% of the cases did the sera neutralize POWV with a titer of 60, demonstrating minimal efficacy of the TBEV vaccine in the prevention of POWV infection.[70]

As is the case for many other flaviviruses, there is no specific drug regimen to treat the POWV-associated disease. Patients with severe illness may need general supportive care in hospitals as well as respiratory support. In a study of hospitalized patients, 50% required endotracheal intubation and mechanical ventilation, while 36% required tracheostomy and placement of a gastric feeding tube.[25] Treatment attempts that include the administration of steroids, intravenous immunoglobulin, and ribavirin/interferon have produced mixed results.[25,71] In a study of Lineage II-associated encephalitis, all five patients treated with corticosteroids survived, while 71% of the patients not receiving corticosteroids died $(n = 13)$.[25]

SUMMARY OVERVIEW

Diseases: encephalitis/meningitis and poliomyelitis-like syndrome
Causative agents: Powassan viruses Lineages I and II
Type of agent: member of the tickborne encephalitis complex
Vectors: primarily *Ixodes cookei* and *I. scapularis*
Common reservoirs: primarily white-footed mouse and other small rodents; woodchucks, opossums, skunks
Mode of transmission: tick bite
Geographical distribution: North America; Russia
Year of emergence: 1958 (North America); the late 1970s (Russia)

REFERENCES

1. McLean DM, Bergman SK, Goddard EJ, Graham EA, Purvin-Good KW. North-south distribution of arbovirus reservoirs in British Columbia, 1970. *Can J Public Health.* 1971;62:120–124.

2. Lindqvist R, Upadhyay A, Överby AK. Tick-borne flaviviruses and the type I interferon response. *Viruses.* 2018;10:340.

3. Reeves WC, Mariotte CO, Johnson HN, Scrivani RE. Encuesta serological sobre los virus transmitidos por artropodos en la zona de Hermosillo, Mexico. *Reimpreso Bol Oficina Sanit Panam.* 1962;52:228–229.

4. Hermance ME, Thangamani S. Powassan virus: an emerging arbovirus of public health concern in North America. *Vector Borne Zoonotic Dis.* 2017;17:453–462.

5. Fatmi SS, Zehra R, Carpenter DO. Powassan virus—a new reemerging tick-borne disease. *Front Public Health.* 2017;5, Art342.

6. Deardorff ER, Nofchissey RA, Cook JA, et al. Powassan virus in mammals, Alaska and New Mexico, USA, and Russia, 2004-2007. *Emerg Infect Dis.* 2013;19(20):12–16.

7. Piantadosi A, Rubin DB, McQuillen DP, et al. Emerging cases of Powassan virus encephalitis in New England: clinical presentation, imaging, and review of the literature. *Clin Infect Dis.* 2016;62:707–713.

8. Doughty CT, Yawetz S, Lyons J. Emerging causes of arbovirus encephalitis in North America: Powassan, chikungunya, and Zika viruses. *Curr Neurol Neurosci Rep.* 2017;17:12.

9. Nofchissey RA, Deardorff ER, Blevins TM, et al. Seroprevalence of Powassan virus in New England deer, 1979-2010. *Am J Trop Med Hyg.* 2013;88:1159–1162.

10. Beasley DW, Suderman MT, Holbrook MR, Barrett AD. Nucleotide sequencing and serological evidence that the recently recognized deer tick virus is a genotype of Powassan virus. *Virus Res.* 2001;79:81–89.

11. Kuno G, Artsob H, Karabatsos N, Tsuchiya KR, Chang GJ. Genomic sequencing of deer tick virus and phylogeny of Powassan-related viruses of North America. *Am J Trop Med Hyg.* 2001;65:671–676.

12. Ebel GD, Spielman A, Telford SR. Phylogeny of North American Powassan virus. *J Gen Virol.* 2001;82:1657–1665.

13. Dobler G. Zoonotic tick-borne flaviviruses. *Vet Microbiol.* 2010;140:221–228.

14. Goldfield M, Austin SM, Black HC, Taylor BF, Altman R. A nonfatal human case of Powassan virus encephalitis. *Am J Trop Med Hyg.* 1973;22:78–81.

15. Thomas LA, Kennedy RC, Eklund CM. Isolation of a virus closely related to Powassan virus from *Dermacentor andersoni* collected along North Cache la Poudre virus, Colorado. *Proc Soc Exp Biol Med.* 1973;104:355–360.

16. L'vov DK, Leonova GN, Gromashevskiĭ VL, Belikova NP, Berezina LK. Isolation of the Powassan virus from *Haemaphysalis neumanni* Dönitz 1905 ticks in the Maritime Territory. *Vopr Virusol.* 1974;5:538–541.

17. L'vov DK, Leonova GN, Gromashevsky VL, et al. Powassan virus isolation from ticks, *Haemaphysalis neumanni* Donitz 1905, in Primor'ye region. *Vopr Virusol.* 1974;19:538–541.

18. Leonova GN, Isachkova LM, Baranov NI, Krugliak SP. Role of Powassan virus in the etiological structure of tick-borne encephalitis in the Primorsky Krai. *Vopr Virusol.* 1980;2:173–176.

19. Krugliak SP, Leonova GN. The significance of *Ixodes* ticks in the southern Far East in the circulation of Powassan virus. *Vopr Virusol.* 1989;34:358–362.

20. McLean DM, McQueen EJ, Petite HE, MacPherson LW, Scholten TH, Ronald K. Powassan virus: field investigations in northern Ontario, 1959 to 1961. *Can Med Assoc J.* 1962;86:971–974.

21. Leonova GN, Kondratov IG, Ternovoi VA, et al. Characterization of Powassan viruses from Far Eastern Russia. *Arch Virol.* 2009;154:811–820.

22. Krow-Lucal ER, Lindsey NP, Fischer M, Hills SL. Powassan virus disease in the United States, 2006–2016. *Vector Borne Zoonotic Dis.* 2018;18:286–290.

23. Telford III SR, Armstrong PM, Katavolos P, et al. A new tick-borne encephalitis-like virus infecting New England deer ticks, *Ixodes dammini. Emerg Infect Dis.* 1997;3:165–170.

24. Dupois II AP, Peters RJ, Prusinski MA, Falco RC, Ostfeld DS, Kramer LD. Isolation of deer tick virus (Powassan virus, Lineage II) from *Ixodes scapularis* and detection of antibody in vertebrate hosts sampled in the Hudson Valley, New York State. *Parasit Vectors.* 2013;6:185.

25. El Khoury MY, Camargo JF, White JL, et al. Potential role of deer tick virus in Powassan encephalitis cases in Lyme disease-endemic areas of New York, USA. *Emerg Infect Dis.* 2013;19:1926–1933.

26. Campagnolo ER, Tewari D, Farone TS, Livengood JL, Mason KL. Evidence of Powassan/deer tick virus in adult black-legged ticks (*Ixodes scapularis*) recovered from hunter-harvested white-tailed deer (*Odocoileus virginianus*) in Pennsylvania: a public health perspective. *Zoonoses Public Health.* 2018;65:589–594.

27. Aliota MT, Dupuis AP, Wilczek MP, Peters RJ, Ostfeld RS, Kramer LD. The prevalence of zoonotic tick-borne pathogens in *Ixodes scapularis* collected in the Hudson Valley, New York State. *Vector Borne Zoonotic Dis.* 2014;14:1–6.

28. Anderson JF, Armstrong PM. Prevalence and genetic characterization of Powassan virus strains infecting *Ixodes scapularis* in Connecticut. *Am J Trop Med Hyg.* 2012;87:754–759.

29. Artsob H. Powassan encephalitis. In: Monath TP, ed. *The Arboviruses: Epidemiology and Ecology.* vol IV. CRC Press; 1989:29–49.

30. Deibel R, Flanagan TD, Smith V. Central nervous system infections. Etiologic and epidemiologic observations in New York State. *N Y State J Med.* 1977;77:1398–1404.

31. Santos I, Hermance ME, Gelman BB, Thangamani S. Spinal cord ventral horns and lymphoid organ involvement in Powassan virus infection in a mouse model. *Viruses.* 2016;8:220.

32. Tavakoli NP, Wang H, Dupuis M, et al. Brief report: fatal case of deer tick virus encephalitis. *N Engl J Med.* 2016;360:2099–2107.

33. Center for Disease Control and Prevention. *ArboNET Map Viewer;* 2016. Accessed September 22, 2016. http://disease-maps.usgs.gov/mapviewer.

34. Minnesota Department of Health. *Powassan Virus Disease;* 2020. Accessed July 8, 2020. www.health.state.mn.us/diseases.powassan/index.html.

35. Lindsey NP, Lehman J, Staples JE, Fischer M. West Nile virus and other arboviral diseases—United States, 2013. *MMWR.* 2014;63:521–526.

36. Choi E, Taylor R. A case of Powassan viral hemorrhagic encephalitis involving bilateral thalami. *Clin Neurol Neurosurg.* 2012;114:172–175.

37. Hicar M, Edwards K, Bloch K. Powassan virus infection presenting as acute disseminated encephalomyelitis in Tennessee. *Pediatr Infect Dis J.* 2011;30:86–88.

38. Center for Disease Control and Prevention. *Lifecycle of Blacklegged Ticks;* 2018. Accessed March 21, 2018. https://www.cdc.gov/lyme/transmission/blacklegged.html.

39. Platt DJ, Smith AM, Arora N, Diamond MS, Coyne CB, Miner JJ. Zika virus-related neurotropic flaviviruses infect human placental explants and cause fetal demise in mice. *Sci Transl Med.* 2018;10, eaao7090.

40. Brackney DE, Brown IK, Nofchissey RA, Fitzpatrick KA, Ebel GD. Homogeneity of Powassan virus populations in naturally infected *Ixodes scapularis. Virology.* 2010;402:366–371.

41. Ebel GD. Update on Powassan virus: emergence of a North American tick-borne flavivirus. *Annu Rev Entomol.* 2010;55:95–110.

42. McLean DM, Larke RP. Powassan and Silverwater viruses: ecology of two Ontario arboviruses. *Can Med Assoc J.* 1963;88:182–185.

43. Smith K, Oesterle PT, Jardine CM, et al. Powassan virus and other arthropod-borne viruses in wildlife and ticks in Ontario, Canada. *Am J Trop Med Hyg.* 2018;99:458–465.

44. Costero A, Grayson MA. Experimental transmission of Powassan virus (Flaviviridae) by *Ixodes scapularis* ticks (Acari:Ixodidae). *Am J Trop Med Hyg.* 1996;55:536–546.

45. Main Jr AJ. The epizootology of some tick-borne arboviral diseases. *J N Y Entomol Soc.* 1977;85:209–211.

46. Karabatsos N. *International Catalogue of Arboviruses.* 3rd ed. American Society of Tropical Medicine and Hygiene; 1985.

47. Ebel GD, Foppa I, Spielman A, Telford III SR. A focus of deer tick virus transmission in the North-Central United States. *Emerg Infect Dis.* 1999;5:570–574.

48. Ebel GD, Campbell EN, Goethert HK, Spielman A, Telford III SR. Enzootic transmission of deer tick virus in New England and Wisconsin sites. *Am J Trop Med Hyg.* 2000;63:36–42.

49. Frost HM, Schotthoefer AM, Thomm M, et al. Serologic evidence of Powassan virus infection in patients with suspected Lyme disease. *Emerg Infect Dis.* 2017;23:1384–1388.

50. Tokarz R, Jain K, Bennett A, Briese T, Lipkin WI. Assessment of polymicrobial infections in ticks in New York State. *Vector Borne Zoonotic Dis.* 2010;10:217–221.

51. Ebel GD, Kramer LD. Short report: duration of tick attachment required for transmission of Powassan virus by deer ticks. *Am J Trop Med Hyg.* 2004;71:268–271.

52. Stafford KC, Williams SC. *Deer, Ticks and Lyme Disease. Deer Management as a Strategy for the Reduction of Lyme Disease.* The Connecticut Agricultural Experiment Station; 2014. Accessed July 7, 2020.

53. Barbour AG. Infection resistance and tolerance in *Peromyscus* spp., natural reservoirs of microbes that are virulent for humans. *Semin Cell Dev Biol.* 2017;61:115–122.

54. Little PB, Thorsen J, Moore W, Weninger M. Powassan virus encephalitis: a review and experimental studies in the horse and rabbit. *Vet Pathol.* 1985;22:500–507.

55. Furumoto HH. Susceptibility of dogs for St. Louis encephalitis and some other selected arthropod-borne viruses. *Am J Vet Res.* 1969;30:1371–1380.

56. Kokernot RH, Radivojevic B, Anderson RJ. Susceptibility of wild and domestic mammals to four arboviruses. *Am J Vet Res.* 1969;30:2197–2203.

57. Woodall JP, Roz A. Experimental milk-borne transmission of Powassan virus in the goat. *Am J Trop Med Hyg.* 1997;26:190–192.

58. Frolova MP, Isachkova LM, Shestopalova NM, Pogodina VV. Experimental encephalitis in monkeys caused by the Powassan virus. *Neurosci Behav Physiol.* 1985;15:62–69.

59. Wikel S. Ticks and tick-borne pathogens at the cutaneous interface: host defenses, tick countermeasures, and a suitable environment for pathogen establishment. *Front Microbiol.* 2013;4:337.

60. Kazimírová M, Štibrániová I. Tick salivary compounds: their role in modulation of host defenses and pathogen transmission. *Front Cell Infect Microbiol.* 2013;3:43.

61. Heinze D, Carmical R, Aronson J, Thangamani S. Early immunologic events at the tick-host interface. *PLoS One.* 2012;7, e47301.

62. Alekseev A, Chunikhin S. The experimental transmission of the tick-borne encephalitis virus by Ixodid ticks (the mechanisms, time periods, species and sex differences). *Parazitologiia.* 1990;24:177–185.

63. Hermance ME, Thangamani S. Tick saliva enhances Powassan virus transmission to the host, influencing its dissemination and the course of disease. *J Virol.* 1990;89:7852–7860.

64. Hermance ME, Thangamani S. Proinflammatory cytokines and chemokines at the skin interface during Powassan virus transmission. *J Invest Dermatol.* 2014;134:2280–2283.

65. Hermance ME, Santos RI, Kelly BC, Valbuena G, Thangamani S. Immune cell targets of infection at the tick-skin interface during Powassan virus transmission. *PLoS One.* 2016;11, e0155889.

66. Gholam BI, Puksa S, Proviast JP. Powassan encephalitis: a case report with neuropathology and literature review. *Can Med Assoc J.* 1999;161:419–422.

67. Mlera L, Meade-White K, Saturday G, Scott D, Bloom ME. Modeling Powassan virus infection in *Peromyscus leucopus*, a natural host. *PLoS Negl Trop Dis.* 2017;11, e0005346.

68. Mlera L, Meade-White K, Dahlstrom E, et al. *Peromyscus leucopus* mouse brain transcriptome response to Powassan virus infection. *J Neurovirol.* 2018;24:75–87.

69. Izuogu AO, McNally KL, Harris SE, et al. Interferon signaling in *Peromyscus leucopus* confers a potent and specific restriction to vector-borne flaviviruses. *PLoS One.* 2017;12, e0179781.

70. McAuley AJ, Sawatsky B, Ksiazek T, et al. Cross-neutralisation of viruses of the tick-borne encephalitis complex following tick-borne encephalitis vaccination and/or infection. *NPJ Vaccines.* 2017;2:5.

71. Patel KM, Johnson J, Zacharioudakis IM, Boxerman JL, Flanigan TP, Reece RM. First confirmed case of Powassan neuroinvasive disease in Rhode Island. *IDCases.* 2018;12:84–87.

CHAPTER 12

Kyasanur Forest Disease and Alkhurma Hemorrhagic Fever Viruses

INTRODUCTION

Alkhurma hemorrhagic fever virus (AHFV) is present in Saudi Arabia and surrounding regions. It has 89%–92% homology with Kyasanur Forest disease virus (KFDV), found primarily in India.[1] Genome sequencing has revealed that AHFV and KFDV are very similar in polyprotein properties, C and E proteins, RNA–RNA interaction sequences, NS3 and NS5 polymerase, as well as 5′ untranslated region structures. AHFV is now classified as a variant of KFDV.[2] The first complete genomic sequence of AHFV indicates that it has the longest polyprotein of all tick-borne flaviviruses.[1,3] Later sequencing of an AHFV isolate from Najran found 99% homology with previous isolates, having the most significant variations in the C protein and NS4a genes, as well as in the length of the 3′UTR.[4] A 2019 study, however, reveals a much greater genetic diversity among AHFVs isolated from different hosts and geographical regions than was previously realized, especially in the E protein gene region.[5]

AHFV has greater genetic diversity in virus isolates from ticks than in human isolates. Analysis of full-length genome sequences suggests a divergence of AHFV and KFDV 700 years ago, so the range of these and other AHFV/KFDV-like viruses may be greater than currently known. Such hemorrhagic fever viruses might also be present between Saudi Arabia and India.[6] Indeed, close relatives to AHFV and KFDV, Karshi and Farm Royal viruses, are present in Uzbekistan and Afghanistan, respectively.[7] Dispersal of an AHFV and KFDV ancestral virus may have occurred by camels and their ticks traveling along the Silk Road that linked Europe to China several centuries ago.[6]

HISTORY

Kyasanur Forest Disease (KFD)

KFD (monkey fever) was first noted during die-offs of nonhuman primates, the black-faced langur (*Presbytis entellus*) and the red-faced bonnet monkey (*Macaca radiata*), and a human outbreak in the Kyasanur forest region of the Karnataka State of southwest India in 1957.[6,8,9] Monkeys are very susceptible to severe illness and death. Upon the animal's death, infected ticks drop to the forest floor, creating viral hotspots in which humans may become infected. KFDV resides in evergreen, semievergreen, and neighboring, moist, deciduous forests.[2] Several outbreaks in humans and sporadic cases have led to 400–500 reported cases yearly during the past five decades.[10] Disease was restricted to five districts in a region of the Western Ghats, Karnataka State until 2011,[11,12] when it emerged in other areas of Karnataka and into Tamil Nadu and Kerala States, which run parallel to the western coast of peninsular India, as well as Goa and Maharashtra between 2012 and 2017.[13–18] The disease is continuing to move into new areas of these states as well as Gujarat State and parts of West Bengal State.[12,19] Serological evidence of KFDV infection is also present in the Andaman Islands.[20–22] KFDV was isolated from a febrile patient in Yunnan, China, as well and was named "Nanjianyin virus."[23] This isolate, however, most likely represented a laboratory artifact since it is virtually identical at the nucleoside level with the 1957 reference strain from India, which is often used in other reference laboratories, including those in China.[2]

In an outbreak of KFD in humans and monkeys in the Kerala State in 2015, 91% of the people were older than 15 years. Most of the patients belonged to two tribes, both of which depended on the forest for their livelihood. Many members of these groups engage in trench digging and fire line work or trap monkeys for game meat. The major vectors of KFDV, *Haemaphysalis spinigera* and *Haemaphysalis turturis* ticks, are abundant in the affected areas.[21] Monkeys are infected by the bite of infected ticks, leading to enzootic die-offs.[8,24] A substantial increase in numbers and proportions of infected monkeys has occurred over the course of the past few decades.[25]

A large outbreak of KFD occurred in the Sindhudurg district of the Maharashtra State of India in 2016, with 130 human cases of laboratory confirmed disease using either PCR or IgM ELISA, in addition to an infected monkey and tick pool. Females comprised 59% of the confirmed cases, and the greatest

Zika and Other Neglected and Emerging Flaviviruses. https://doi.org/10.1016/B978-0-323-82501-6.00009-8

proportion of the patients was 14–50 years old.[18,26] The fatality rate among these cases was 2.3%. Almost all of the cases (93.1%) had visited Western Ghats forest, a hotspot of disease, including migrant workers in cashew nut or coconut farms and people who collect firewood, dry leaves, and grass.[25,26] The former group of migrant workers is believed to have spread the virus into new locales in the Goa State.[25] Anti-KFDV IgG antibodies were also detected among the healthy population of the region, indicative of prior KFDV infection.[26] Seroprevalance rates of 9.7% ($n = 745$) and 9.1% ($n = 165$) were recorded in the affected area and two neighboring villages, respectively. A clinical to subclinical ratio of 6:1 was found in the KFD-affected areas.[26] Not surprisingly, the Kattunayakan community, which is completely dependent on the forest for their livelihood, was the most affected during this outbreak. None of the area's Paniyas, landless farm laborers who rarely visit the forest, were affected.[21]

Changes in the forest ecosystem may play a large role in the spread of KFDV, as forests are converted to agricultural land, with accompanying timber extraction and road development.[27] KFDV is found naturally in the wild in an enzootic cycle that involves ticks; small mammals, such as rodents and shrews; ground birds; and monkeys in these forested areas.[28] Humans are dead-end hosts. Trees are being replaced by shrubs, providing suitable environments for small mammals, especially rodents, and birds. These serve as hosts for tick larvae and nymphs, which occupy the microclimate under the leaves and within the bushes.[29] Wildlife, including nonhuman primates in the remaining forest patches, uses the new agricultural crops as a food source, bringing them into closer contact with humans.[30] Regions containing waterlogged crops, such as rice paddies, have increased humidity, which helps to maintain a year-long tick life cycle.[31]

Alkhurma Hemorrhagic Fever (AHF)

AHF was first detected in 1995 in western Saudi Arabia along the coast of the Red Sea. It led to the death of a 32-year-old butcher exposed to sheep surmised to having been infected with AHFV.[32] Five other butchers were also infected in late 1995. In 2001–2003, the disease reemerged and spread to other areas of the country, including Mecca, and southward to the border of Yemen.[33–35] It is also present in Djibouti and southern Egypt, bordering the Red Sea, and in Sudan. Visitors to Egypt who had contact with healthy camels brought the virus into Europe, causing a number of imported cases in Italy.[36–39] A study conducted between 2012 and 2016 found a lower incidence rate in Saudi citizens than in foreigners or expatriate workers,[40] suggesting that Saudis may be partially immune, perhaps due to a prior, asymptomatic, or mild infection. Less than 100 human AHFV infections are typically reported annually.[41]

Massive movements of people and animals that occur during the yearly Hajj (pilgrimage) play a role in the acquisition and, perhaps, dispersal of AHFV.[34,42] During this time, 2–3 million people from all over the world meet in the holy city of Mecca in western Saudi Arabia to perform Hajj, which involves the slaughter of hundreds of thousands of livestock.[34]

Different patterns have been noted between the 2001–2003 AHFV outbreak in Mecca and disease in southern Saudi Arabia from 2003 to 2009. In the latter, the proportion of infected females was higher than that during the Mecca outbreak, disease was reported in children under the age of 10 years, infection occurred more commonly in family units, and the mortality was much lower (1.3% and 25%, respectively). Some of these differences may be due to the rural nature of life in the southern area of Saudi Arabia, where closely related families and extended family members often live together in large houses with sheep and goats kept in the backyards, where they are cared for by all family members. Milking and butchering of infected, but asymptomatic, animals are important means of acquiring disease from livestock.[35]

THE DISEASES

Fever, headache, and body ache are commonly observed among confirmed KFD or AHF patients along with myalgia, retro-orbital pain, sore throat, rash, cough, diarrhea and vomiting, anorexia, and hypotension. Blood may contain elevated liver enzymes. Severe or fatal cases may include hemorrhagic manifestations, such as epistaxis (bleeding from the nose), ecchymoses (bleeding under the skin), petechiae, vomiting blood, or neurological disease, including convulsions, coma, and encephalitis. Many flaviviruses cause hemorrhagic disease, while others cause neurological disease. In the case of KFDV, both hemorrhagic and neurological diseases may occur simultaneously.[32,34,42–44] Symptoms typically persist for 5 days. A second episode of fever may also occur.[18]

Despite their genetic similarities, some clinical findings differ in human cases of KFD and AHF, while other findings are similar.[45] Neurologic involvement is more commonly seen during AHF, while gastrointestinal hemorrhage is more commonly seen in people with fatal KFD.[12,32,33,35,46] Transient lymphopenia is a prominent feature of both diseases, perhaps as a result of an early type I IFN response that leads to upregulation of the following interferon-stimulated genes (ISGs): Mx1, 2′,5′-oligoadenylate synthase (OAS), ISG15; interferon response factor 7 (IRF7); signal transducer and activator of transcription-1 (STAT-1); and toll-like receptor-3 (TLR-3), as is seen in various mosquito-borne flavivirus diseases as well. Humans infected with either viral type also develop hypoalbuminemia and elevated blood urea nitrogen and liver transaminase.[45]

In immunocompetent mouse strains (C57BL/6, C3H, and A/J) inoculated subcutaneously with either KFDV or AHFV, KFDV infection is more likely to be lethal (90%–100% mortality rate vs 10%–50%, in KFD and AHF, respectively) and is associated with higher viral loads. The KFDV-infected mice have greater abnormalities in chemistry panels and pathology in the brain and gastrointestinal tract than AHFV-infected mice.[45] In the mouse model, both viruses disseminate to the spleen within 24 h after infection, with a lower viral load present in the AHFV-infected mice. KFDV replicates in the small intestine, and by day 6 postinfection, causes acute necrotizing disease. AHFV loads are lower in the intestine during this time period without evidence of gastrointestinal hemorrhage, although mice infected with either virus develop inflammation of enteric nerve plexi, associated with neuronal degeneration and depletion.[45] Unlike the situation in humans, however, mice did not become febrile or develop biphasic or delayed onset disease.

KHF Disease

KHF generally presents as a biphasic disease. It begins with a sudden onset of severe fever and headache, followed by back pain, severe pain in the extremities, prostration, bradycardia, lymphadenopathy, petechiae, and bleeding from the eyes, nose, mouth, or gastrointestinal tract with bloody stools and sputum.[47] This phase is followed by an afebrile period of 1–2 weeks. Afterward, mild meningoencephalitis and fever develop in 1%–20% of the patients with possible headache, mental disturbances, and tremors, in the absence of meningitis or encephalitis.[34,47] A small number of patients develop coma or bronchopneumonia before death. The case fatality rate of KFD has ranged from 2% to 10% in different outbreaks.[8,14,48] During reconvalescence, meningitis-like symptoms, such as vomiting, neck stiffness, mental disturbances, tremors, and extreme weakness of muscles, occur in some cases. Convulsion and loss of consciousness are also seen but are rare.[49] During the 2016 outbreak in Maharashtra, patients reported fever, headache, weakness, and myalgia (100%, 93.1%,

84.6%, and 83.1%, respectively).[26] Hemorrhagic manifestations are present in approximately one-third of laboratory-confirmed cases and may initially present as oral mucosal inflammation and nontender maculopapular eruptions on the soft and hard palates. Ocular manifestations, such as conjunctival congestion, are found in almost all cases; serous discharge in 63%, and retina and vitreous humor disorder in 13% of the patients. Persistent hematological symptoms are linked to poor prognosis. No specific skin lesions or rashes are found.[50] The KFDV genome contains eight mature miRNAs that regulate expression of two host genes, *ANGPT1* (encoding angiopoietin 1) and *TFRC* (encoding the transferrin receptor). These proteins play a role in the development of KFD-induced hemorrhagic fever and neurological disease.[51] Autopsies of patients with fatal KFD reveal a prominence of macrophages and lymphocytes in the liver and spleen, degeneration of the liver and kidneys and, sometimes, hemorrhagic pneumonia.[47,52,53]

KFD in infant mice includes gliosis and inflammation in the nervous system, necrosis with neural loss, and syncytium formation in the brain. Microscopic necrotic lesions and hepatocyte vacuolation are present in the liver, and epithelial cell necrosis is found in the small intestine. KFDV antigens are detectable in these organs.[54]

AHF Disease

AHF is associated with both hemorrhagic and neurological diseases, either of which may terminate in death. Inoculation of AHFV into newborn Wistar rats by the intracranial route results in tremors, irritability, convulsions, spasms that caused backward arching of the head, neck, and spine and spastic paresis. The spastic paresis begins in the hind limbs and progresses to the rest of the body. All tested animals (n = 16) in this study had high virus titers in the brain and died of meningoencephalitis within a week.[55] Examination of the livers of infected rats revealed patchy mixed inflammatory infiltrate in the portal tracts, similar to those seen in infection with Powassan virus, another flavivirus. The kidneys appear to be normal.

In humans, AHF, with a purported fatality rate of about 25% among symptomatic patients, is classified as a BioSafety Level 4 agent.[43] In the 2001 outbreak, 55% of hospitalized patients developed hemorrhagic manifestations, 35% developed neurological disease, and elevated levels of creatine phosphokinase were common.[33–35] Three other hemorrhagic fever viruses are also present in Saudi Arabia: Crimean-Congo hemorrhagic fever, dengue hemorrhagic fever, and Rift Valley fever viruses, complicating the diagnosis of AHF. Rift Valley hemorrhagic fever, however, has a far lower rate of hemorrhagic fever and death, while having higher rates of visual complications and severe hemolytic anemia.[34] The high death rate seen in AHF in symptomatic patients may not give a complete view of the fatality rate among those infected with AHFV since at least one study found many asymptomatic family members who had seroconverted, suggesting that the reported fatality rates may actually be closer to that of KFDV infection.[33] In a retrospective analysis of all laboratory-confirmed cases of AHF in Saudi Arabia from January 1, 2009 to December 31, 2011 (*n* = 233), the case fatality rate was 0.4%.[56] The low case fatality rate may possibly have resulted in changes in the pathogenicity of AHFV strains[57] or the development of herd immunity. More rapid and aggressive symptomatic management may also play a role in the observed decrease in case fatality rates. Intriguingly, the first and only reported case from the Taif region of Saudi Arabia was fatal and had been initially diagnosed as dengue, suggesting that other AHF cases from that region or other regions may also be misdiagnosed.[34,41] It also suggests the possibility that high mortality rates may occur when AHFV enters into new territories.

This retrospective study also revealed that disease incidence rose from 59 to 93 cases between 2009 and 2011 and that the virus had spread to other areas of Saudi Arabia.[56] This increase may in part be due to greater awareness of the disease, better surveillance, and improved diagnostic capabilities.[1] Approximately one-third of the known cases did not come into direct contact with animals or their products. Almost all of the cases reported gastrointestinal symptoms—a new development. These symptoms included anorexia, nausea, abdominal pain, and vomiting. Hemorrhagic manifestations, surprisingly, were found in less than 5% of the cases, while CNS involvement (disorientation, hallucination, and convulsions) were seen in less than 30% of the patients.[56] CNS manifestations and elevated levels of serum bilirubin levels are associated with high mortality rates.[34] One of Italian patients who had been infected following a trip to Egypt had intense muscle weakness and rhabdomyolysis.[34] He was also unable to walk or move his limbs for several days.

This retrospective study found that case numbers peak in July and December and that the lowest number of cases occur in February. Less than 5% of those infected were under the age of 15 years and over 45% were 25–45 years old (range = 3–85 years).[56] Approximately 40% of the cases had occupations related to the direct handling of animals, about 25% were housewives and

maids, and 23% were placed into a group comprised of white collar jobs, such as teachers, students, and government employees.[56]

THE VIRUSES

In addition to the some differences in disease manifestations, AHFV and KFDV have important ecological differences. Transmission of KFDV to humans generally occurs in a forested region of India, while transmission of AHFV to humans occurs in a semidesert environment.[1] KFDV is not found in secretions other than blood, but neither virus has been clearly shown to be transmitted via a human-to-human route.[17]

KFDV Characteristics

Human cases of KFD decrease with the beginning of the monsoon month in early June as the larval tick population increases under the forest litter and are subsequently activated as the litter dries.[29,58] Laboratory-confirmed cases of KFD are associated with either contact with ticks, primarily *Haemaphysalis* species, people entering the Shimoga forest region, people handling or incinerating sick or dead monkeys, and laboratory infections.[6] Hotspots may exist in forested regions, and may form a monkey-tick-human KFDV cycle.[28] The black-faced langur and the red-faced bonnet monkey are infected by the bite of infected ticks and, like humans, are highly susceptible to KFD, with a mortality rate of up to 85%.[28] Viral reservoirs include the Blanford's rat, the striped forest squirrel, and the house shrew, all of which develop high virus titers. They are infested by *Haemaphysalis* larvae, nymphs, and adult ticks.[59] The gray langur, shrews, ground-dwelling birds, flying squirrels, Malabar giant squirrels, white-tailed rats, white-bellied rats, and bats additionally carry KFDV.[31] High viral titers may also be attained following experimental infection of black-napped hares, porcupines, gerbils, and long-tailed tree mice.[2] All other tested wild or domestic animals (cattle, sheep, goats, dogs, and cats) have not developed clinical disease.[49] Cattle do, however, harbor all life stage forms of *H. spinigera* ticks and the presence of cattle is associated with increased tick larval density. Having cattle in cleared forest areas may thus increase tick density in areas frequented by humans.[2]

KFDV is transmitted primarily by the painless bite of *H. spinigera* hard ticks, especially the nymph stage and, to a lesser extent, to direct contact with infected rodents.[34] KFDV in ticks are able to be transmitted via transovarial and transstadial routes, which are important for viral maintenance in natural settings.[17] Other

Haemaphysalis species are also vectors for KFDV, including *H. turturis, H. uana kinneari, H. minuta, H. cuspidata, H. bispinosa, H. kyasanurensis, H. wellingtoni,* and *H. aculeate,*[28] as well as *Ixodes petauristae.*[2] These vector species are present in all geographical areas of India; however, KFH is only known to be present in outbreaks in the five districts of Karnataka, Tamil Nadu State, Kerala State, Goa State, and Maharashtra State.[14,18] Several other tick genera are also able to transmit KFDV, including *Argas, Dermacentor, Hyalomma, Ornithodoros,* and *Rhipicephalus* species, but have not been shown to actually play such a role in natural settings.[47,60]

After feeding, female ticks lay eggs, which hatch and transform to larvae under the foliage. They then drop onto their vertebrate hosts, particularly small mammals, and feed on them. Upon maturing into nymphs, the ticks drop from the host, which has moved while the nymphs were attached, thus increasing the foci of infection. The nymphs then climb to shrubs, settling at the apex of leaves as they await their next vertebrate host. KFD occurs in monkeys and forest dwellers since *Haemaphysalis* species ticks may be present anywhere the previous host has moved while grazing.

AHFV Characteristics

AHF is most frequent from March to July in western Saudi Arabia, corresponding to the peak of tick activity in early March.[33,61] Transmission to humans occurs via tick bites, as well as by direct contact with infected blood from viremic vertebrate hosts, including camels, sheep, and goats, especially sheep.[35,62] The district in which AHF was first reported is a holding site for these animals, which are imported from Africa and Australia prior to their transport to Saudi Arabia's southwestern provinces.[35] AHFV RNA has been detected in *Ornithodoros savignyi* soft ticks collected from camels in this seaport region where camels rest. These nocturnal ticks infect multiple hosts, commonly targeting humans and other animals resting under trees.[36] AHFV is also found in *Hyalomma dromedarii* hard ticks removed from camels in the same region.[63] Two of 546 tick pools collected from slaughtered cattle in Djibouti contained ALFV RNA. Both infected ticks were *Amblyomma lepidum,* an East African and Iranian tick, while all tested *H. dromedarii* were negative. Both cattle had been imported from Ethiopia.[38] Based upon serological studies, AHFV appears to be endemic in the far northwestern and eastern areas of Saudi Arabia as well, despite the fact that no human AHFV disease or infection has been reported.[64] Infected *O. savignyi* and *H. dromedarii* ticks reside in these regions, however. AHFV may be present, therefore, throughout the Arabian Peninsula.

AHFV RNA has recently been found in immature *Hyalomma rufipes* ticks taken from northward migratory birds in the North Mediterranean Basin.[65] This viral RNA was detected in 2010 in five fully engorged ticks (four nymphs, one larva) from three bird species that overwinter in sub-Saharan Africa and breed in Europe. A sedge warbler was infested by two AHFV-positive nymphs. Other AHFV RNA-positive ticks were found on a common redstart, a western yellow wagtail, and an eastern woodchat shrike in Greece and Turkey.[65] *H. rufipes* ticks are found throughout Africa and in the Arabian Peninsula along the Red Sea coast. It is a two-host tick in which both larva and nymphs ingest blood from the same host. The immature ticks typically infest birds or small mammals, while adults feed on larger mammals, including buffaloes and large birds, in addition to camels and cattle.[65] The latter two animals are implicated as reservoir hosts for AHFV. This is in keeping with the suggestion that AHFV originated in Africa and was brought into Saudi Arabia by migratory birds.[6]

Those at risk for infection by AHFV include herdsmen, live-animal retailers, women who prepare meat prior to cooking and feeding livestock, as well as those residing in neighborhoods with livestock or exposure to tick bites. In the 2001 outbreak in Saudi Arabia, 90% of those infected were female ($n = 20$) and none were under the age of 10 years.[34] Consumption of unpasteurized milk is also linked to AHFV infection.[33,35] Additionally, infection is found in pilgrims slaughtering sacrificial animals.[40]

Interestingly, while human AHFV cases have been associated with exposure to camels and sheep, the virus has not been isolated from these animals.[42] It has also been suggested that AHFV is transmitted by mosquito bites[34,44,66] and, while proof of this route of infection is lacking, AHFV is able to propagate in cultured mosquito cells.[55] A separate study performed in Saudi Arabia, however, found no statistically significant difference in mosquito exposure between patients and uninfected control subjects.[33] Additionally, unlike the tendency of tick-borne viruses to remain in stable foci, as is the case for AHFV, mosquito-borne viruses typically suddenly emerge and rapidly spread to new locales, resulting in large epidemics.[67] The "One Health" approach may help to better understand AHFV vectors and reservoir hosts and their role in transmission of AHFV to humans.[40]

THE IMMUNE RESPONSE

Relatively little is known about the protective or pathogenic roles of the immune response against KFDV. However, pretreatment with type I IFN decreases KFDV titer in an epithelial cell line in vitro. ISGs are present in the brains of KFDV-infected mice, demonstrating an activated IFN response in the CNS in vivo.[45,68] One such ISG, tripartite motif 79α (TRIM79α), is a potent inhibitor of KFDV replication.[69] Nevertheless, pre- or posttreatment with IFN-α2a does not eliminate KFDV in infected cultured cells primarily due to antagonism of type I IFN responses by the RNA polymerase region of the viral NS5 protein.[70] Inhibition of IFN responses by NS5 also occurs in a number of other flaviviruses.[71] However, a single treatment of cultured cells with either IFN-αWA or IFN-αK is more effective than IFN-α2a in reducing KFDV titers. Low IFN concentration limits cytopathic effect, but much higher amounts are required to inhibit virion release.[72]

In the first week after disease onset, titers of complement-fixing and hemagglutination-inhibiting antibodies start to increase. Neutralizing antibodies are subsequently produced during the second week. These antibodies primarily target the KFDV E protein and prevent viral attachment, entry, and replication within host cells.[73] The geographical spread of KFDV could be due to mutations that allow the newer strains to escape the immune response, specifically alterating the proposed B lymphocyte epitopes in the viral E protein, leading to the loss of effective antibodies. Nevertheless, examination of KFDV isolates from a 2014 outbreak in Karnataka State were 99% identical to older strains, and those mutations which did occur did not alter the B lymphocyte epitopes.[74] Interestingly, IgE serves as a disease cofactor, increasing the immunopathology of KFD.[53]

PREVENTION AND CONTROL

Karnataka state government initiated mass vaccination campaigns using formalin-inactivated tissue culture vaccine for people between the ages of 7 and 65 years living in areas with KFD activity in humans, monkeys, or ticks from August to November and in villages within a radius of 5 km.[17] The vaccine schedule is two doses initially and after 1 month to those aged 7–65 years, followed by a booster at 6–9 months. Vaccine efficacy, however, is low (62.4% and 82.9%, for the first two doses and the booster dose, respectively), indicating a short-lived immunity and the need for booster doses annually for 5 years.[50] This strategy, however, has been impeded by the limited availability of the booster vaccine. This was exemplified by the situation in Karnataka in 2011, in which the population did receive the initial two doses; however, no booster vaccination was given due to its unavailability. This was followed by an

upsurge of KFD cases the next year.[75] Vaccine coverage has also been found to be low, and some cases are present greater than 5 km away from villages that had been vaccinated the previous year. This vaccination strategy, therefore, may be only partially effective in preventing the spread of KFDV transmission.[76] Immunization against tick-borne encephalitis virus (TBEV), however, provides cross-neutralizing antibodies to both KFDV and AHFV, with 84% and 74% of the vaccines having detectable viral neutralization, respectively.[77]

Preventive measures include education, avoiding tick-exposure for both humans and cattle by fully clothing when entering the forest, washing the body and cloths in hot water after returning from the forest, applying tick repellants (such as N-diethyl-meta-toluamide (DEET) and dimethyl phthalate (DMP), avoiding cattle grazing in deep forests and scrubbing them weekly to remove ticks, and avoiding sleeping outside of the house. Covering the forest floor with gamma-hexachlorocyclohexane may aid in decreasing tick populations as well.[18,50] It should be noted that many of these preventive measures may not be practical. In some regions of India, rapid reporting of monkey deaths, safe disposal their carcasses, and dusting with wettable powder in and around the monkey death spots are used to decrease transmission.[21]

TREATMENT

Since there is no approved, effective treatment for AHF, patients are given supportive care. Numerous nucleoside analogs, including 2′-C-methylcytidine, 6-azauridine, 6-azauridine triacetate, and the adenosine analog NITD008 provide incomplete suppression of KFDV growth in culture.[68,78] The latter compound has lower potency against AHFV and KFDV than against TBEV and Omsk hemorrhagic fever virus in in vitro assays of its activity against tick-borne flavivirus diseases.

SUMMARY OVERVIEW: KYASANUR FOREST VIRUS

Diseases: severe neurological disease and hemorrhagic fever, sometimes in a single patient
Type of agent: tick-borne encephalitis virus complex
Vectors: Haemaphysalis spinigera and H. turturis ticks
Common reservoirs: the Blanford's rat, striped forest squirrel, and house shrew
Mode of transmission: tick bite, direct contact with infected primates
Geographical distribution: India
Year of emergence: 1957

SUMMARY OVERVIEW: ALKHURMA VIRUS

Diseases: severe neurological disease and hemorrhagic fever, sometimes in a single patient

Type of agent: tick-borne encephalitis virus complex

Vectors: Hyalomma rufipes and *Amblyomma lepidum* ticks

Common reservoirs: camels, cattle, and birds

Mode of transmission: tick bite, contact with infected camel or sheep blood or their milk

Geographical distribution: primarily Saudi Arabia; Djibouti; southern Egypt, bordering the Red Sea; and Sudan

Year of emergence: 1995

REFERENCES

1. Charrel RN, Zaki AM, Attoui H, et al. Complete coding sequence of the Alkhurma virus, a tick-borne flavivirus causing severe hemorrhagic fever in humans in Saudi Arabia. *Biochem Biophys Res Commun.* 2001;287:455–461.
2. Mehla R, Kumar SRP, Yadav P, et al. Recent ancestry of Kyasanur Forest disease virus. *Emerg Infect Dis.* 2009;15(9):1431–1437.
3. Palanisamy N, Akaberi D, Strand J, Lundkvist Å. Comparative genome analysis of Alkhumra hemorrhagic fever virus with Kyasanur Forest disease and tick-borne encephalitis viruses by the *in silico* approach. *Pathog Glob Health.* 2018;112(4):210–226.
4. Madani TA, Azhar EI, Abuelzein E-T, et al. Complete genome sequencing and genetic characterization of Alkhumra hemorrhagic fever virus isolated from Najran, Saudi Arabia. *Intervirology.* 2014;57:300–310.
5. Ul-Rahman A. Genetic diversity of Alkhurma hemorrhagic fever virus in Western Asia. *Infect Genet Evol.* 2019;70:80–83.
6. Dodd KA, Bird BH, Khristova ML, et al. Ancient ancestry of KFDV and AHFV revealed by complete genome analyses of viruses isolated from ticks and mammalian hosts. *PLoS Negl Trop Dis.* 2011;5(10), e1352.
7. Gould EA, Moss SR, Turner SL. Evolution and dispersal of encephalitic flaviviruses. *Arch Virol.* 2004;18(suppl):65–84.
8. Work TH, Trapido H. Kyasanur Forest disease: a new virus disease in India: summary of preliminary report of investigations of the VRC on the epidemic disease affecting forest villagers and wild monkeys of Shimoga District, Mysore State. *Indian J Med Sci.* 1957;11:41–42.
9. Bhatt PN, Work TH, Varma MG, et al. Isolation of Kyasanur Forest disease from infected humans and monkeys of Shimoga District, Mysore State. *Indian J Med Sci.* 1966;20:316–320.
10. Lani R, Moghaddam E, Haghani A, Chang LY, Abu Bakar S, Zandi K. Tick-borne viruses: a review from the perspective of therapeutic approaches. *Ticks Tick Borne Dis.* 2014;5:457–465.
11. Sreenivasan MA, Bhat HR, Rajagopalan PK. The epizootics of Kyasanur Forest disease in wild monkeys during 1964-1973. *Trans R Soc Trop Med Hyg.* 1986;80:810–814.
12. Pattnaik P. Kyasanur Forest disease: an epidemiological view in India. *Rev Med Virol.* 2006;16(3):151–165.
13. Mourya DT, Yadav PD, Sandhya VK, Reddy S. Spread of Kyasanur Forest disease, Bandipur Tiger Reserve, India, 2012-2013. *Emerg Infect Dis.* 2013;19:1540–1541.
14. Mourya DT, Yadav PD, Patil DY. Highly infectious tick borne viral diseases: Kyasanur Forest disease and Crimean-Congo hemorrhagic fever in India. *WHO South East Asia J Public Health.* 2014;3(1):8–21.
15. Yadav PD, Patil DY, Sandhya VK, Prakash KS, Surgihalli R, Mourya DT. Outbreak of Kyasanur Forest disease in Thirthahalli, Karnataka, India, 2014. *Int J Infect Dis.* 2014;26:132–134.
16. Tandale BV, Balakrishnan A, Yadav PD, Marja N, Mourya DT. New focus of Kyasanur Forest disease virus activity in a tribal area in Kerala, India, 2014. *Infect Dis Poverty.* 2015;4:13.
17. Murhekar MV, Kasabi GS, Mehendale SM, Mourya DT, Yadav PD, Tandale BD. On the transmission pattern of Kyasanur Forest disease (KFD) in India. *Infect Dis Poverty.* 2015;4:37.
18. Awate P, Yadav P, Patil D, et al. Outbreak of Kyasanur Forest disease (monkey fever) in Sindhudurg, Maharashtra State, India, 2016. *J Infect.* 2016;6:759–761.
19. Sarkar JK, Chatterjee SN. Survey of antibodies against arthropod-borne viruses in the human sera collected from Calcutta and other areas of West Bengal. *Indian J Med Res.* 1962;50:833–841.
20. Padbidri VS, Wairagkar NS, Joshi GD, et al. A serological survey of arboviral diseases among the human population of the Andaman and Nicobar Islands, India. *Southeast Asian J Trop Med Public Health.* 2002;33:794–800.
21. Sadanandane C, Elango A, Marja N, Sasidharan PV, Raju KHK, Jambulingam P. An outbreak of Kyasanur Forest disease in the Wayanad and Malappuram districts of Kerala, India. *Ticks Tick Borne Dis.* 2017;8:25–30.
22. Yadav PD, Sahay RR, Mourya DT. Detection of Kyasanur Forest disease in newer areas of Sindhudurg district of Maharashtra State. *Indian J Med Res.* 2018;148:453–455.
23. Wang J, Zhang H, Fu S, et al. Isolation of Kyasanur Forest disease virus from febrile patient, Yunnan, China. *Emerg Infect Dis.* 2009;5:326–328.
24. John JK, Kattoor JJ, Nair AR, Bharathan AP, Valsala R, Sadanandan GV. Kyasanur Forest disease: a status update. *Adv Anim Vet Sci.* 2014;2:329–336.
25. Patila DY, Yadava PD, Shetea AM, et al. Occupational exposure of cashew nut workers to Kyasanur Forest disease in Goa, India. *Int J Infect Dis.* 2017;61:67–69.
26. Gurav YK, Yadav PD, Gokhale MD, et al. Kyasanur Forest disease prevalence in Western Ghats proven and confirmed by recent outbreak in Maharashtra, India, 2016. *Vector Borne Zoonotic Dis.* 2018;18(3):164–172.
27. Walsh JF, Molyneux DH, Birley MH. Deforestation: effects on vector-borne disease. *J Parasitol.* 1993;106:55–65.
28. Mourya DT, Sapkal GN, Yadav D. Difference in vector ticks dropping rhythm governs the epidemiology of Crimean-Congo haemorrhagic fever & Kyasanur Forest disease in India. *Indian J Med Res.* 2016;144:633–635.

29. Ajesh K, Nagaraja BK, Sreejith K. Kyasanur Forest disease virus breaking the endemic barrier: an investigation into ecological effects on disease emergence and future outlook. *Zoonoses Public Health.* 2017;64:e73–e80.

30. Isabirye-Basuta GM, Lwanga JS. Primates populations and their interactions with changing habitats. *Int J Primatol.* 2008;29:35–48.

31. Boshell J. Kyasanur Forest disease: ecologic considerations. *Am J Trop Med Hyg.* 1969;18:67–80.

32. Zaki AM. Isolation of a flavivirus related to the tick-borne encephalitis complex from human cases in Saudi Arabia. *Trans R Soc Trop Med Hyg.* 1997;91:179–181.

33. Alzahrani AG, Al Shaiban MA, Al Mazroa MA, et al. Alkhurma hemorrhagic fever in humans, Najran, Saudi Arabia. *Emerg Infect Dis.* 2010;16(12):1882–1888.

34. Madani TA. Alkhumra virus infection, a new viral hemorrhagic fever in Saudi Arabia. *J Infect.* 2005;51:91–97.

35. Madani TA, Azhar EI, Abuelzein E-TME, et al. Alkhumra (Alkhurma) virus outbreak in Najran, Saudi Arabia: epidemiological, clinical, and laboratory characteristics. *J Infect.* 2011;62:67–76.

36. Carletti F, Castilletti C, Di Caro A, et al. Alkhurma hemorrhagic fever in travelers returning from Egypt, 2010. *Emerg Infect Dis.* 2010;16(12):1979–1982.

37. Ravanini P, Hasu E, Huhtamo E, et al. Rhabdomyolysis and severe muscular weakness in a traveler diagnosed with Alkhurma hemorrhagic fever virus infection. *J Clin Virol.* 2011;52:254–256.

38. Horton KC, Fahmy NT, Watany N. Crimean Congo hemorrhagic fever virus and Alkhurma (Alkhumra) virus in ticks in Djibouti. *Vector Borne Zoonotic Dis.* 2016;16(10):680–682.

39. Musso M, Galati V, Stella MC, Capone A. A case of Alkhumra virus infection. *J Clin Virol.* 2015;66:12–14.

40. Tambo E, El-Dessouky AG. Defeating re-emerging Alkhurma hemorrhagic fever virus outbreak in Saudi Arabia and worldwide. *PLoS Negl Trop Dis.* 2018;12(9), e0006707.

41. Memish ZA, Fagbo SF, Assiri AM, et al. Alkhurma viral hemorrhagic fever virus: proposed guideline for detection, prevention and control in Saudi Arabia. *PLoS Negl Trop Dis.* 2012;6(7), e1604.

42. Memish ZA, Charrel RN, Zaki AM, Fagbo SF. Alkhurma haemorrhagic fever—a viral haemorrhagic disease unique to the Arabian Peninsula. *Int J Antimicrob Agents.* 2010;36:S53–S57.

43. Charrel RN, Zaki AM, Fakeeh M, et al. Low diversity of Alkhurma hemorrhagic fever virus, Saudi Arabia, 1994-9. *Emerg Infect Dis.* 2015;11:683–688.

44. Charrel RN, Zaki AM, Fagbo S, de Lamballerie X. Alkhurma hemorrhagic fever virus is an emerging tick-borne flavivirus. *J Infect.* 2006;52:463–464.

45. Dodd KA, Bird BH, Jones MEB, Nichol ST, Spiropoulou CF. Kyasanur Forest disease virus infection in mice is associated with higher morbidity and mortality than infection with the closely related Alkhurma hemorrhagic fever virus. *PLoS One.* 2014;9(6), e100301.

46. Adhikari Prabha MR, Prabhu MG, Raghuveer CV, Bai M, Mala MA. Clinical study of 100 cases of Kyasanur Forest disease with clinicopathological correlation. *Indian J Med Sci.* 1993;47:124–130.

47. Holbrook MR. Kyasanur Forest disease. *Antiviral Res.* 2012;96:353–362.

48. Mourya DT, Yadav PD. Recent scenario of emergence of Kyasanur Forest disease in India and public health importance. *Curr Trop Med Rep.* 2016;3(1):7–13.

49. Dobler G. Zoonotic tick-borne flaviviruses. *Vet Microbiol.* 2010;140:221–228.

50. Munivenkatappa A, Sahay RR, Yadav PD, Viswanathan R, Mourya DT. Clinical and epidemiological significance of Kyasanur Forest disease. *Indian J Med Res.* 2018;148(2):145–150.

51. Saini S, Thakur CJ, Kumar V. Genome wide computational prediction of miRNAs in Kyasanur Forest disease virus and their targeted genes in human. *Mol Biol Res Commun.* 2020;9(2):83–91.

52. Iyer CG, Laxmana Rao R, Work TH, Narasimha Murthy DP. Kyasanur Forest disease VI. Pathological findings in three fatal human cases of Kyasanur Forest disease. *Indian J Med Sci.* 1959;13:1011–1022.

53. Pavri K. Clinical, clinicopathologic, and hematologic features of Kyasanur Forest disease. *Rev Infect Dis.* 1989;11(suppl. 4):S854–S859.

54. Basu A, Yadav P, Prasad S, et al. An early passage human isolate of Kyasanur Forest disease virus shows acute neuropathology in experimentally infected CD-1 mice. *Vector Borne Zoonotic Dis.* 2016;16(7):496–498.

55. Madani TA, Kao M, Abuelzein E-TME, et al. Propagation and titration of Alkhumra hemorrhagic fever virus in the brains of newborn Wistar rats. *J Virol Methods.* 2014;199:39–45.

56. Memish ZA, Fagbo SF, Ali AO, Al-Hakeem R, Elnagi FM, Bamgboye EA. Is the epidemiology of Alkhurma hemorrhagic fever changing? A three-year overview in Saudi Arabia. *PLoS One.* 2014;9(2), e85564.

57. Memish ZA, Balkhy HH, Francis C, Cunningham G, Hajeer AH, Almuneef MA. Alkhumra haemorrhagic fever: case report and infection control details. *Br J Biomed Sci.* 2005;62:37–39.

58. Trapido H, Rajagopalan PK, Work TH, Varma MGR. Kyasanur Forest disease. VIII. Isolation of Kyasanur Forest disease virus from naturally infected ticks of the genus *Haemaphysalis. Indian J Med Res.* 1959;47:133–138.

59. Parola P, Raoult D. Ticks and tick-borne bacterial diseases in humans: an emerging infectious threat. *Clin Infect Dis.* 2001;32:897–928.

60. Bhat HR, Naik SV, Ilkal MA, Banerjee K. Transmission of Kyasanur Forest disease virus by *Rhipicephalus haemaphysaloides* ticks. *Acta Virol.* 1978;22:241–244.

61. Pigott DC. Hemorrhagic fever viruses. *Crit Care Clin.* 2005;21:765–783.

62. Shibl A, Senok A, Memish Z. Infectious diseases in the Arabian Peninsula and Egypt. *Clin Microbiol Infect.* 2012;11:1068–1080.

63. Charrel RN, Fagbo S, Moureau G, Alqahtani MH, Temmam S, de Lamballerie X. Alkhurma hemorrhagic fever virus in *Ornithodoros savignyi* ticks. *Emerg Infect Dis.* 2007;13:153–155.

64. Memish ZA, Albarrak A, Almazroa MA, et al. Seroprevalence of Alkhurma and other hemorrhagic fever viruses, Saudi Arabia. *Emerg Infect Dis.* 2011;17(12):2316–2318.

65. Hoffman T, Lindeborg M, Barboutis C, et al. Alkhurma hemorrhagic fever virus RNA in *Hyalomma rufipes* ticks infesting migratory birds, Europe and Asia Minor. *Emerg Infect Dis.* 2018;24(5):879–882.

66. Madani TA, Kao M, Azhar EI, et al. Successful propagation of Alkhumra (misnamed as Alkhurma) virus in C6/36 mosquito cells. *Trans R Soc Trop Med Hyg.* 2011;106:180–185.

67. Lindqvist R, Upadhyay A, Överby AK. Tick-borne flaviviruses and the type I interferon response. *Viruses.* 2018;10:340.

68. Flint M, McMullan LK, Dodd KA, et al. Inhibitors of the tick-borne, hemorrhagic fever-associated flaviviruses. *Antimicrob Agents Chemother.* 2014;58:3206–3216.

69. Taylor RT, Lubick KJ, Robertson SJ, et al. TRIM79α, an interferon-stimulated gene product, restricts tick-borne encephalitis virus replication by degrading the viral RNA polymerase. *Cell Host Microbe.* 2011;10(3):185–196.

70. Cook BWM, Cutts TA, Court DA, Theriault S. The generation of a reverse genetics system for Kyasanur Forest disease virus and the ability to antagonize the induction of the antiviral state *in vitro. Virus Res.* 2012;163:431–438.

71. Laurent-Rolle M, Boer EF, Lubick KJ, et al. The NS5 protein of the virulent West Nile virus NY is a potent antagonist of type I interferon-mediated JAK-STAT signaling. *J Virol.* 2010;84(7):3503–3515.

72. Cook BWM, Ranadheera C, Nikiforuk AM, et al. Limited effects of type I interferons on Kyasanur forest disease virus in cell culture. *PLoS Negl Trop Dis.* 2016;10(8), e0004871.

73. Shah SZ, Jabbar B, Ahmed N, et al. Epidemiology, pathogenesis, and control of a tick-borne disease—Kyasanur Forest disease: current status and future directions. *Front Cell Infect Microbiol.* 2018;8, 149.

74. Shil P, Yadav PD, Patil AA, Balasubramanian R, Mourya DT. Bioinformatics characterization of envelope glycoprotein from Kyasanur Forest disease virus. *Indian J Med Res.* 2018;147:195–201.

75. Kasabi GS, Murhekar MV, Yadav PD, et al. Kyasanur Forest disease, India, 2011-2012. *Emerg Infect Dis.* 2013;19:278–281.

76. Kiran S, Pasi A, Kumar S, et al. Kyasanur Forest disease outbreak and vaccination strategy, Shimoga District, India, 2013-2014. *Emerg Infect Dis.* 2015;21(1):146–149.

77. McAuley AJ, Sawatsky B, Ksiazek T, et al. Cross-neutralisation of viruses of the tick-borne encephalitis complex following tick-borne encephalitis vaccination and/or infection. *NPJ Vaccines.* 2017;2:5.

78. Lo MK, Shi PY, Chen YL, Flint M, Spiropoulou CF. *In vitro* antiviral activity of adenosine analog NITD008 against tick-borne flaviviruses. *Antiviral Res.* 2016;130:46–49.

CHAPTER 13

Omsk Hemorrhagic Fever Virus

INTRODUCTION

Omsk hemorrhagic fever is an acute disease caused by the Omsk hemorrhagic fever virus (OHFV) and is prevalent in some areas of western Siberia. OHFV is one of the tickborne flaviviruses that is known to cause hemorrhagic fever, in league with Kyasanur forest disease virus (KFDV) in southern India and the Alkhurma hemorrhagic fever virus (AHFV) variant subset of KFDV in Saudi Arabia, as well as with some strains of the Far-Eastern subtype of tickborne encephalitis virus (FE-TBEV) in the Novosibirsk region of Russia. OHFV is closely related to FE-TBEV, having a similar morphology and mode of replication.[1] OHFV differs from the other tickborne encephalitis serocomplex viruses, however, in that *Dermacentor reticulatus* hard ticks are its primary vector. *D. reticulatus* is a member of the family Ixodidae that is found in wooded areas of Europe and western Asia. The other members of the tickborne encephalitis viral complex use *Ixodes* species ticks.[2] While many studies have been carried out on both OHFV and TBEV, many of the findings about OHFV were published in Russian-language journals and proceedings, leading to a relative dearth of information about OHFV in English-language reviews.

HISTORY

Sporadic cases of a novel, acute hemorrhagic fever disease were first reported in 1941 in the northern lake-steppe and forest-steppe and marsh areas of the Omsk region of Siberia in Russia. The causative virus, OHFV, was isolated in 1947. The Novosibirsk region has over 3000 lakes found at altitudes of 150–200 m above sea level. It has a continental climate with a long winter and a short, hot, wet summer in which most of rainfall occurs.[3] Two types of natural OHFV "pseudofoci" are present in western Siberia. In the first, active area, seroprevalence in humans is about 35% and includes children, while in the other potential area, it is less than 15% and does not appear to include anyone under the age of 14 years.[1,4,5] Following its discovery, more than 1000 cases of Omsk hemorrhagic fever were diagnosed between 1946 and 1958, followed by a temporary decrease in the number of human infections. After 1988, however, the disease reemerged and disease incidence in humans has increased in endemic areas, which remain within four Russian provinces.[6] The importation and release of 4000 North American muskrats into the region appears to have precipitated the initial disease outbreaks in Siberia. These economically valuable animals are highly susceptible to OHFV infection. People coming into close contact with muskrats or muskrat hides are at high risk of infection by the virus.[6]

THE DISEASE

Many OHFV infections are mild and may be unreported or misdiagnosed. These cases have no fever or hematological features. During a disease outbreak in 1988–1989, over 80% of the patients had a mild form of the disease. The highest incidence of reported disease is found in people between the ages of 20 and 40 years, although one-third of the infections are reported in children under the age of 15 years.[1]

Omsk hemorrhagic fever is biphasic, with patients being viremic during the first, but not the second, phase.[7] Symptoms include moderately severe hemorrhagic disease with a fever of 39–40°C and abundant bleeding from the nose, mouth, lungs, and uterus, as well as hemorrhagic rash and hemorrhaging of the skin. Other symptoms include dehydration, headache, nausea, severe pain in the calf muscles and regional joints, and cough. The fever usually is accompanied by chills that last for 8–15 days. Clinical signs early during the course of the disease include an enlarged liver; arterial hypotension and bradycardia; hyperemia of the face, neck, and breasts; a brightly colored mouth and throat; scleral injection; dryness of the tongue; a foul odor emanating from the mouth; and puffiness of the face.[1] These symptoms are then followed by increased amounts of bleeding, including gastrointestinal and pulmonary bleeding in serious cases.

After 1–2 weeks, 50%–70% of the patients completely recover. The remaining patients then enter into the second phase of illness, which lasts a further 5–14 days. This phase includes some of the initial symptoms, as well as spread of the disease to additional

Zika and Other Neglected and Emerging Flaviviruses. https://doi.org/10.1016/B978-0-323-82501-6.00017-7

179

anatomical sites.[1] Pathological changes involve several organ systems. Changes in the blood cells include high hemoglobin concentrations at disease onset, leukopenia and neutrophilia with left shifts, monocytosis, thrombocytopenia, and reduced complement levels. The cardiovascular system manifestations include diffuse or focal dystrophic degenerative changes of the myocardium, severe arterial hypotonia, hyperemia of the face and upper trunk, exanthema, a small degree of petechial rash, and hemorrhaging from the nasal, pulmonary, gastrointestinal, and uterine areas. The pulmonary manifestations include bronchitis and atypical pneumonia. Renal manifestations include moderate albuminuria and intermittent hematuria. Nervous system manifestations are also present, such as headache, muscle pain, Kernig's sign, occipital rigidity, Lasegne's sign, loss of taste, and decreased hearing, together with behavioral and psychological changes. One-third of the patients develop pneumonia, nephrosis, or meningitis.[1]

Despite the severity of illness, disease prognosis is typically favorable with most of the patients having a complete recovery after a long convalescent period. Infrequently, permanent complications are seen, including weakness, hearing and hair loss, and behavioral and psychological problems, including poor memory and difficulty concentrating or working. Mortality rates are low (0.4%–2.5%) and death occurs after a rapid onset of hemorrhagic symptoms or later, from septic complications.[1,8]

THE VIRUS

OHFV belongs to the TBE serocomplex of flaviviruses. Accordingly, comparison of the OHFV E protein to that of other tickborne flaviviruses reveals conserved N-glycosylation sites, cysteine residues, fusion peptides, and a group-specific hexapeptide. The E protein serves as the prominent immunogen. OHFV differs from the other members of the TBE serocomplex by possessing 20 unique amino acid substitutions scattered throughout the E protein, resulting in an amino acid identity of 93.0% with the other members of the serocomplex. One unique feature of OHFV is the presence of a sequence of amino acids (AQN) in other TBE viruses that is changed to MVG in OHFV. This change decreases its hydrophilicity in that potentially critical area of the E protein.[9] It is noteworthy that several amino acid residues in the E protein domain III differ between the neuropathological and hemorrhagic fever members of TBE serocomplex viruses.[10]

OHFV has been divided into two antigenic subtypes based on polyclonal antibody absorption and hemagglutination assays.[11] The genomes of the OHFV strains Kubrin (subtype I) and Bogoluvovska (subtype II) vary by six nucleosides that result in four amino acid changes, three of which are present in the E protein.[12] By contrast, OHFV and KFDV/AHFV differ by 35 amino acids even though both of these tickborne TBE serocomplex viruses cause hemorrhagic fever.[2] The nonstructural regions of both OHFV and ALKV, however, contain 15 amino acids that differ from other TBE complex viruses. The 5′ untranslated region of OHFV is unusual in which it contains a 5′-cap and a stretch of approximately 30 nucleosides that are not typical of tickborne flaviviruses. Its 3′ untranslated region is slightly shorter than that of other flaviviruses. Additionally, several amino acids in the E protein of OHFV and ALKV/KFDV, especially a $(T \rightarrow A)$ mutation at residue 76, differ from most TBE serocomplex viruses and may be important in membrane fusion and tissue tropism. Interestingly, this mutation is also present in a neuropathogenic, nonhemorrhagic strain of FE-TBEV.[2,13] Based on this and other genomic studies, both OHFV and ALKV/KFDV appear to be a part of separate clades within the TBE serocomplex and from each other.

OHFV antigen in infected mice is located in select regions of the brain.[14] At day 7 postinfection, more viral antigens are present in deep structures of the cerebrum, the thalami and basal ganglia, than in superficial regions, whereas in the cerebellum, both the cortex and deep cerebellar nucleus have high levels of the viral antigen. In focal areas of the brain, the antigen is also found in astrocytes. Later during the course of infection, the antigen is primarily restricted to the cerebellum, especially to Purkinje cells, although it is also still found in neurons of the deep cerebellar nucleus.[14] OHFV is also present in the enlarged spleens of experimentally infected mice, primarily in the red pulp and, to a lesser extent, in the white pulp. The viral antigen may also be present in the endothelial cells of the liver, but not the kidneys.

The two antigenically different strains of OHFV differ in plaque size, hemagglutination activity, and neurovirulence.[11,15] Although OHFV is closely related to the neurotropic TBEV, it causes less neurological and more hemorrhagic symptoms. Four amino acids located near the C terminal of the viral polymerase region of the NS5 protein are critical to neurological disease in TBEV, but not OHFV. These particular amino acids are linked to neuronal dysfunction, blocking neurite outgrowth, and neuron degeneration. They are not, however, linked to viral replication or histopathology, including inflammatory responses and viral antigen distribution. When the prM and E proteins of OHFV are replaced by those from TBEV, neuroinvasiveness is increased, but not neuropathology.[16]

Yoshii et al.[17] produced subgenomic OHFV with large deletions in the genes for the structural proteins. The resulting replicons can replicate in cell culture systems and secrete infectious virus-like particles that are unable to produce further infectious progeny viruses. Having such viral particles that are restricted to a single round of infectivity is useful since they can be studied using biosafety laboratory-2 (BSL-2) conditions, rather than in BSL-4 laboratories, which are used while studying the complete virus. This system also allows the particles to serve as delivery systems for genetically manipulated viral genes in order to better understand how changes in specific regions of the genome affect pathology, viral replication, and for inhibitor screening.[17] The particles may also be useful in developing self-replicating RNA vaccines that may produce long-lasting protective immunity that is similar to that already produced by replicons of several other flaviviruses, including TBEV, West Nile virus (WNV), and Japanese encephalitis virus (JEV).

Yoshii et al.[18] developed a full-length infectious cDNA clone from the Guriev strain of OHFV, which was originally isolated from human blood. Such infectious clones may also be used to study the molecular biology of virus replication, virus structure, and virulence determinants, as well as for vaccine development. In fact, during the production of this cDNA clone, several specific mutations in positions in the NS2A and NS5 proteins were found to decrease in OHFV RNA replication.

Several small animal models have been developed in order to better understand the underlying causes of disease pathology. It should be noted that infection in rodents differs in several key aspects from the disease in humans. In mice infected by the subcutaneous route, early localized viral replication is followed by viremia and invasion of internal organs. OHFV then crosses the blood–brain barrier and induces high levels of interferon production in the brains of juvenile mice.[1,19,20] Adult mice infected with high doses of OHFV, however, do not develop paralysis or have any significant infection of the cerebrum. They also do not develop encephalitis or meningitis, but rather have cerebellar involvement.[14] In these adult mice, clinical disease begins 7 days postinfection. Several aspects of antiviral innate and adaptive immune response peak at day 9. Unlike human infection, no viremia is present in these mice, but low levels of OHFV are found in most organs, with particularly high levels in murine spleens and livers.[21] It should be noted that this work was performed in BALB/c mice, and the results may differ in other mouse strains.

TRANSMISSION

OHFV is primarily transmitted by meadow ticks (*D. reticulatus*) in Siberian forest-steppe areas. Adult *D. reticulatus* also transmits to humans *Rickettsia* species that are linked to various types of spotted fever and the dog protozoan parasite *Babesia canis*, which is similar to the malaria parasite in addition to other medically important animal pathogens. These ticks reproduce and develop rapidly and can survive years of unfavorable conditions. They also can survive under water for months and are very cold-hardy. Adult ticks of this species additionally can survive for up to 4 years without taking a blood meal. These adaptive factors underlie the recent spread of *D. reticulatus* throughout western Russia and Europe.[6] The seasonal activity of this tick correlates with the numbers of human cases in Siberia.[22,23] While OHFV has been isolated from several species of mosquitoes (*Aedes excrucians*, *Aedes flavescens*, and *Mansonia richiardii*), mosquitoes do not appear to be important for viral transmission or maintenance.[3,24] *Dermacentor marginatus* ticks serve as the primary vector in the steppe areas of southern and western Siberia, while gamasid mites and the taiga tick (*Ixodes persulcatus*) may be important in maintaining the sylvatic cycle of the virus.[25,26] A study from the Republic of Korea found no OHFV in pools of six species of ticks: *Haemaphysalis longicornis* ($n=17{,}570$), *Haemaphysalis flava* ($n=3317$), *Ixodes nipponensis* ($n=249$), *Amblyomma testudinarium* ($n=11$), *Haemaphysalis phasiana* ($n=8$), and *Ixodes turdus* ($n=3$).[27] Agricultural workers and people who collect mushrooms or wild berries are among those at high risk of infection by these ticks, although dogs may also transmit ticks to people.[28]

D. reticulatus parasitizes more than 60 wild and domesticated hosts worldwide and at least 37 mammal and bird species in Siberia.[6] Their larvae feed on small mammals during June and July, and the adults feed on wild ungulates and humans in August and September. In forest-steppe regions, immature ticks preferentially feed on narrow-skulled voles, which serve as their major hosts. Water voles are also an important tick host.[1] The voles' cyclical population expansions correspond with those of virus-infected tick populations.[1,29] Since the 1960s, densities of both *D. reticulatus* and narrow-skulled voles have decreased.[1] It is unknown why Omsk hemorrhagic fever is confined to only certain parts of Russia since *D. reticulatus* and the virus' primary vertebrate hosts, water voles and muskrats, are distributed over much of northern Eurasia.[6]

OHFV has been isolated from other vertebrates found in the endemic area and many mammals, reptiles, and amphibians are seropositive.[3] Following experimental infection, other animals that develop symptoms include root voles, red-cheeked and spotted susliks, hedgehogs, and weasels.[1] Many other experimentally infected animals develop viremia, but remain asymptomatic.

D. marginatus frequently parasitizes humans in western Siberia.[29] In 1971–1989, the vole population and the area inhabited by ticks decreased in this region of Siberia as a result of a human activity, changing the forest-steppe landscapes. Before the emergence or reemergence of OHFV epidemic activity in 1999–2000, changes had occurred in the fauna of northern forest-steppe and the northern border of *D. marginatus* habitat moved southward. The population of *Ix. persulcatus* in forested regions overtook that of *D. reticulatus*, however, no change was seen in the population density of the latter.[1]

Muskrats are very susceptible to Omsk hemorrhagic fever, developing acute fatal neuroinfection with hemorrhagic symptoms, including high viremia and fever lasting at least 3 weeks. Viruses are released in the muskrats' urine, feces, and blood. OHFV may survive in lake water for over 2 weeks in June and July and for 3–5 months in the winter.[1] Disease outbreaks are linked to contact with infected muskrats, occurring most frequently in muskrat hunters and family members who remove and treat muskrat skins since OHFV may be contracted by contact with the animal's bodily fluids, including blood and urine, their feces, and their carcasses.[30,31]

The emergence of OHF is believed to have originated from the introduction of thousands of muskrats from Canada into Siberia during the late 1920s and 1930s for the harvesting of their valuable fur. This venture proved to be fruitless, however, due to many fatal epizootic outbreaks among the muskrats. The virus may have existed silently in Siberia prior to the muskrats' introduction, but large numbers of these highly susceptible hosts may have greatly increased infection rates in other animals, including humans.[1,32]

Omsk hemorrhagic fever has two seasonal peaks, correlating with tick activity. The initial outbreak begins in April and peaks during May and June, representing 73% of the total cases. The second yearly outbreak is seen in August and September, corresponding to the muskrat hunting season and affects people who are infected by contact with muskrats.[30]

Humans may also be infected by the respiratory route, but not by person-to-person contact.[28] OHFV is additionally transmitted through consumption of milk from infected goats or sheep.[3]

THE IMMUNE RESPONSE

During experimental infection of BALB/c mice, neutrophil numbers peak at day 9, while lymphocyte numbers are unchanged. Since activated neutrophils produce proinflammatory cytokines, chemokines, and reactive oxygen intermediates, increases in the numbers of these cells may be responsible for the rapid death found in this mouse strain, unlike the low mortality rate in humans.[21] C57BL/6 mice are much less susceptible to OHFV infection, perhaps due to their predominantly Th1 T helper cell response, instead of the Th2 response that occurs in infected BALB/c mice. No clinical disease is apparent in experimentally infected macaques, however, and, no virus can be isolated from tissues or blood, even though seroconversion occurs.[33]

OHFV infection stimulates an early production of the proinflammatory mediators IL-1α, TNF-α, IL-12p70, macrophage chemotactic protein-1 (MCP-1), macrophage inflammatory protein-1α (MIP-1α), and MIP-1β in the spleens, but not the brains, of infected BALB/c and C57BL/6 mice. The presence of antiinflammatory T regulatory cytokines is not detectable. Levels of proinflammatory cytokines and chemokines peak at day 3 postinfection. C57BL/6 mice have lower levels of these molecules, which may partially explain their decreased susceptibility to OHFV-induced disease.[34] Proinflammatory mediator levels appear earlier and at higher levels in mice spleens than in their serum, suggesting localized inflammation. The chemokines MCP-1, regulated upon activation, normal T cell expressed, and secreted (RANTES), and KC were also increased in the lungs and livers of OHFV-infected BALB/c mice.

Although both FE-TBEV and OHFV are members of the TBE viral serocomplex, they differ greatly in pathology. Mice infected by FE-TBEV develop neurological pathology, produce large levels of proinflammatory mediators in their brains, but not their spleens, after 7–9 days of infection. OHFV-infected mice, which primarily develop hemorrhagic fever, produce high levels of virus in their visceral organs, but not the brain, by day 3.[34] The differential localization of inflammatory agents in these two related flaviviruses may therefore contribute greatly to the differences in disease presentation.

TREATMENT

No anti-OHFV drug is currently approved for human use. Accordingly, the disease is treated by supportive care, including strict bed rest and administration of abundant levels of fluids and electrolytes. The disease is usually self-limiting, so aspirin and other nonsteroidal antiinflammatory drugs should not be used.[22] Several drugs have been tested in cell culture and animal models. High concentrations of Virazo or the interferon-inducers larifan and rifastin decrease viral reproduction moderately, while human interferon α-2b completely blocks viral reproduction in cell culture. Larifan had the greatest success against OHFV in animals. This drug protects 65% of infected mice and decreases disease severity in rabbits.[35]

In an attempt to rationally design drugs to block OHFV entry into host cells, a series of homology models of E proteins were produced with their β-OG pockets in the open state.[36] This type of virtual structure-based screening identified a group of compounds with highly specific activity against OHFV. These compounds did not protect cells against the closely related TBEV. Further studies are required to determine whether these, or other rationally designed flavivirus inhibitors, are active in vivo in animal models and in humans.

Another strategy to treat OHFV is to block viral polymerase activity using nucleoside analogs. One such analog is NITD008, an adenosine analog. It inhibits the levels of flavivirus antigen and viral titer in cell culture systems for both tickborne flaviviruses (OHFV, TBEV, KFDV, and Powassan virus) and mosquito-borne flaviviruses (WNV, DENV, and YFV).[37,38]

PROTECTION

No specific vaccine against OHFV is currently available. Vaccines against TBEV, however, are promising candidates for protection against OHFV infection since anti-TBEV antibodies cross-react with and neutralize OHFV in vitro. Sera from TBEV-infected mice have equal and high titers of neutralizing antibodies against TBEV and OHFV. More importantly, several immunizations with the TBEV vaccine yield 100% protection against OHFV challenge in mice.[39] Moreover, the dosage of OHFV used to challenge the immunized mice (30–1000 LD$_{50}$) and the timing of challenge after the final immunization do not significantly affect protection in vivo.[40] A hybrid vaccine vector that utilizes the prM/E proteins of the TBEV European subtype strain on a WNV background also induces neutralizing antibodies against OHFV.[41]

Four vaccines against TBEV are available, two of which are based on European subtypes of TBEV and two based on the Far-Eastern subtypes. In neutralization tests that utilize human sera after vaccination with the European TBEV subtypes, anti-TBEV and anti-OHFV neutralizing antibodies were found in 100% and 86% of the subjects, respectively.[39] Antibody titers ranged from 1:20 to 1:70, which is greater than the protective titer of 1:10.[40] Given the evidence of a protective effect, the TBEV vaccine was used in 1991 in an attempt to prevent an OHFV outbreak in Russia.[1]

SUMMARY OVERVIEW

Disease: severe hemorrhagic fever

Type of agent: tickborne encephalitis virus complex

Vectors: Dermacentor reticulatus and Dermacentor marginatus ticks

Common reservoirs: water voles and muskrats

Mode of transmission: tick bite, exposure to infected muskrats or their hides or bodily fluids, and consumption of raw, infected goat or sheep milk

Geographical distribution: in elevated northern lake-steppe, forest-steppe, and marsh regions of Western Siberia

Year of emergence: 1941 in humans

REFERENCES

1. Růžek D, Yakimenko VV, Karan LS, Tkachev SE. Omsk haemorrhagic fever. *Lancet.* 2010;376:2104–2113.
2. Lin D, Li L, Dick D, et al. Analysis of the complete genome of the tick-borne flavivirus Omsk hemorrhagic fever virus. *Virology.* 2003;313:81–90.
3. Kharitonova NN, Leonov YA. *Omsk Hemorrhagic Fever. Ecology of the Agent and Epizootology.* Oxonian Press; 1985:1–230.
4. Lebedev EP, Sizemova GA, Busygin FF. Clinical and epidemiological characteristics of Omsk hemorrhagic fever. *Zh Mikrobiol.* 1975;11:132–133.
5. Busygin F. Omsk hemorrhagic fever—current status of the problem. *Vopr Virusol.* 2000;45:4–9.
6. Földvári G, Široký P, Szekeres S, Majoros G, Sprong H. *Dermacentor reticulatus:* a vector on the rise. *Parasit Vectors.* 2016;9:314.
7. Novitskiy VS. Pathologic anatomy of spring-summer fever in Omsk region. *Proc OmGMI.* 1948;13:97–134.
8. Sizemova GA. Diagnostics of Omsk hemorrhagic fever. *Proc OmGMI.* 1957;21:256–260.
9. Gritsun TS, Lashkevich VA, Gould EA. Nucleotide and deduced amino acid sequence of the envelope glycoprotein of Omsk haemorrhagic fever virus: comparison with other flaviviruses. *J Gen Virol.* 1993;74:287–291.
10. Volk DE, Chavez L, Beasley DWC, Barrett ADT, Holbrook MR, Gorenstein DG. Structure of the envelope protein

domain III of Omsk hemorrhagic fever virus. *Virology.* 2006;351:188–195.

11. Clarke DH. Further studies on antigenic relationships among the viruses of the group B tick-borne complex. *Bull World Health Organ.* 1964;31:45–56.

12. Li L, Rollin PE, Nichol ST, Shope RE, Barrett ADT, Holbrook MR. Molecular determinants of antigenicity of two subtypes of the tick-borne flavivirus Omsk haemorrhagic fever virus. *J Gen Virol.* 2004;85:1619–1624.

13. Grard G, Moureau G, Charrel RN, et al. Genetic characterization of tick-borne flaviviruses: new insights into evolution, pathogenetic determinants and taxonomy. *Virology.* 2007;361:80–92.

14. Holbrook MR, Aronson JF, Campbell GA, Jones S, Feldmann H, Barrett ADT. An animal model for the tick-borne flavivirus—Omsk hemorrhagic fever virus. *J Infect Dis.* 2005;191:100–108.

15. Kornilova EA, Gagarina AV, Chumakov MP. Comparison of the strains of Omsk hemorrhagic fever virus isolated from different objects of a natural focus. *Vopr Virusol.* 1970;15:232–236.

16. Yoshii K, Sunden Y, Yokozawa K. A critical determinant of neurological disease associated with highly pathogenic tick-borne flavivirus in mice. *J Virol.* 2014;88(10):5406–5420.

17. Yoshii K, Holbrook MR. Sub-genomic replicon and virus-like particles of Omsk hemorrhagic fever virus. *Arch Virol.* 2009;154:573–580.

18. Yoshii K, Igarashi M, Ito M, Kariwa H, Holbrook M, Takashima I. Construction of an infectious cDNA clone for Omsk hemorrhagic fever virus, and characterization of mutations in NS2A and NS5. *Virus Res.* 2011;155:61–68.

19. Popov GV, Chumakov MP. Electron microscopic study of the central nervous system in mice infected by Omsk hemorrhagic fever (OHF) virus. *J Ultrastruct Res.* 1972;40:458–469.

20. Hofmann H, Radda A, Kunz C. Induction of interferon in the brain of baby mice by viruses of the tick-borne encephalitis (TBE) complex. *Arch Gesamte Virusforsch.* 1969;28:197–202.

21. Tigabu B, Juelich T, Bertrand J, Holbrook MR. Clinical evaluation of highly pathogenic tick-borne flavivirus infection in the mouse model. *J Med Virol.* 2009;81:1261–1269.

22. Mazbich IB, Netsky GI. Three years of study of Omsk hemorrhagic fever (1946–1948). *Trud Omsk Inst Epidemiol Microbiol Gigien.* 1952;1:51–67.

23. Chumakov MP. Results of a study made of Omsk hemorrhagic fever (OL) by an expedition of the Institute of Neurology. *Vestnik Acad Med Nauk SSSR.* 1948;2:19–26.

24. Netzki GI, Gagarina AV. Investigation of susceptibility of bloodsucking mosquitoes (Culicidae, Diptera) of OHF virus. *Med Parazitol.* 1950;19:545–546.

25. Gagarina AV. The spontaneous carriage of Omsk hemorrhagic fever virus by *Dermacentor marginatus* Sulz ticks. *Proc OmGMI.* 1957;4:15–21.

26. Kondrashova ZN. A study of the survival of the virus of Omsk hemorrhagic fever in Ixodes persulcatus in conditions of their massive infection. *Med Parasitol Parasit Dis.* 1970;39:274–277.

27. Yun S-M, Lee Y-J, Choi W-Y. Molecular detection of severe fever with thrombocytopenia syndrome and tick-borne encephalitis viruses in *Ixodid* ticks collected from vegetation, Republic of Korea, 2014. *Ticks Tick Borne Dis.* 2016;7:970–978.

28. World Health Organization. Viral hemorrhagic fevers. In: *Report of WHO Expert Committee*; 1985:128.

29. Estrada-Pena A, Jongejan F. Ticks feeding on humans: a review of records on human biting Ixodoidea with special reference to pathogen transmission. *Exp Appl Acarol.* 1999;23:685–715.

30. Fedorova TN, Sizemova GA. Omsk hemorrhagic fever incidence in man and muskrats in winter. *Zh Mikrobiol.* 1964;11:134–136.

31. Burke DS, Monath TP. Flaviviruses. In: Knipe DM, ed. *Fields Virology.* 4th ed. Lippincott Williams & Wilkins; 2001:1043–1126.

32. Avakyan AA, Lebedov AD, Ravdonikas OV, Chumakov MP. On the question of importance of mammals in forming natural reservoirs of Omsk hemorrhagic fever. *Zool Zhurnal.* 1955;34:605–609.

33. Kenyon RH, Rippy MK, McKee KT, Zack PM, Peters CJ. Infection of *Macaca radiata* with viruses of the tick-borne encephalitis group. *Microb Pathog.* 1992;13:399–409.

34. Tigabu B, Juelich T, Holbrook MR. Comparative analysis of immune responses to Russian spring-summer encephalitis and Omsk hemorrhagic fever viruses in mouse models. *Virology.* 2010;408(1):57–63.

35. la Loginova S, Efanova TN, Koval'chuk AV. Effectiveness of virazol, realdiron and interferon inductors in experimental Omsk hemorrhagic fever. *Vopr Virusol.* 2002;47:27–30.

36. Osolodkin DI, Kozlovskaya LI, Dueva EV. Inhibitors of tick-borne flavivirus reproduction from structure-based virtual screening. *ACS Med Chem Lett.* 2013;4:869–874.

37. Yin Z, Chen Y-L, Schul W, et al. An adenosine nucleoside inhibitor of dengue virus. *Proc Natl Acad Sci USA.* 2009;106(48):20435–20439.

38. Lo MK, Shi P-Y, Chen Y-L, Flint M, Spiropoulou CF. *In vitro* antiviral activity of adenosine analog against tick-borne flaviviruses. *Antiviral Res.* 2016;130:46–49.

39. Chidumayo NN, Yoshii K, Kariwa H. Evaluation of the European tick-borne encephalitis vaccine against Omsk hemorrhagic fever virus. *Microbiol Immunol.* 2016;58:112–118.

40. Chernokhaeva LL, Rogova YV, Vorovitch MF, et al. Protective immunity spectrum induced by immunization with a vaccine from the TBEV strain Sofjin. *Vaccine.* 2016;34:2354–2361.

41. Orlinger KK, Hofmeister Y, Fritz R. A tick-borne encephalitis virus vaccine based on the European prototype strain induces broadly reactive cross-neutralizing antibodies in humans. *J Infect Dis.* 2011;203:1556–1564.

CHAPTER 14

Conclusions

INTRODUCTION

We live in an age of constant change, due, to a large degree, to the continuing threat of infection by severe acute respiratory syndrome coronavirus-2 (SARS-CoV-2), the causative agent of COVID-19. This recently emerged pandemic coronavirus has spread throughout the world. Countries or parts of countries have responded by locking down segments of their areas, in some cases, literally preventing the population from leaving their homes. Some other places were less stringent and only locked down places where people may gather and spread the virus. Often, this led to only "essential" services remaining open, while small and large businesses, places of worship, and fitness facilities were closed. Much of life is a trade-off: The closure of business most likely was an important factor in slowing the spread of the disease and "flattening the curve" so as to prevent hospitals from being overwhelmed. Unfortunately, the closures will most likely lead to the permanent loss of jobs and income. The effects of these lockdowns have also triggered crises in mental health, increasing depression, and, in some cases, suicide incidence. Many of our elderly population, especially those living with comorbidities, are very vulnerable to developing fatal disease if they were to become infected. However, these people have been isolated from their families and many will die without having the chance to physically be with their loved ones. Our physical health is also threatened, not only for those sickened or killed by SARS-CoV-19, but also for people with other, noncritical, medical conditions, who may not have access to hospitals or testing facilities.

Many methods have been employed to slow the spread of this virus. We have either mandated or strongly encouraged people to wear various types of facial coverings whose effectiveness is controversial among those in the scientific and medical community. We have practiced social distancing. In many areas, we have closed parks and other recreational venues, replaced face-to-face schooling with online classes, and closed places of worship. We did succeed in flattening the curve in many places for months, yet some parts of the developed world are now seeing the numbers of reported cases spiraling out of control as the number of new cases breaks records daily. Some of the increase in the number of people testing seropositive may be due to the massive testing efforts detecting more cases. Some of the increase may result from the reopening of businesses and other venues, which led to the exposure and spread of disease among those previously isolated from contact with infected people. Fortunately, the mortality rate is decreasing.

A second round of COVID-19-related shutdowns has been advocated in some areas, but as time goes by, thoughts about implementing this drastic action continue to change. The economic and societal impacts of both our inactions and actions will likely be felt for many years. If another round of shutdowns is mandated, this action may save lives or damage the world's economic health even further or both. Shutdowns are particularly devastating to impoverished people in the developed world and, even more so, to those living in the developing world. As the numbers of COVID-19 cases and hospitalizations continue to increase in some parts of the world, our understanding of the disease and our responses to it must also change. However, the resulting uncertainty in what constitutes the best practice for different segments of the population has caused rifts among scientists, physicians, and public health workers, in addition to the general population. The world post-COVID-19 may in some respects not ever return to the world that we knew before the emergence of SARS-CoV-2. Our previous jobs and understanding of a work environment, manner and quality of education, societal and cultural norms, and personal liberties may be irreversibly altered.

These major changes in our lives and our world occurred rapidly from the time that the first cases of COVID-19 were reported in China in December 2019 to the time of this writing (late July 2020). The emergence, spread, and increased virulence of other neglected viruses and viral diseases have also occurred in the previous two to three decades, most notably the rapid emergence of Zika virus-induced microcephaly among newborns and infants and Guillain–Barré syndrome in some Zika virus-infected adults. While the recent, large, and deadly Ebola outbreak did not seriously threaten the lives of people living outside of

Zika and Other Neglected and Emerging Flaviviruses. https://doi.org/10.1016/B978-0-323-82501-6.00006-2

certain parts of Africa, it was devastating to the populations of the affected regions. Just as importantly, that Ebola outbreak occurred in an area of Africa that had previously been almost totally Ebola virus-free. Other large disease outbreaks in the previous decades include SARS, caused by a coronavirus that emerged in China and Hong Kong. It was quickly spread by air travel of infected people to other areas of the world and led to a major outbreak in Canada. The H5N1 avian influenza outbreak in 1997 was predicted to kill up to 100 million people, but instead killed less than 600 people over the course of two decades. The general public responded to the projected death rate with great fear that fortunately was unwarranted. Some leaders of the public health community are currently warning of a potential pandemic of a novel strain of H1N1 influenza during the next "flu" season, in addition to a second wave of COVID-19. Public health recommendations and mandates may again be implemented that threaten to rip apart the fabric of human society even further.

FLAVIVIRUSES AND THEIR VECTORS

This book dealt with the potential threats of novel or neglected flaviviruses or flaviviruses that have the potential to emerge or reemerge as they adapt to better survive and replicate in human hosts. Natural or man-made changes to the environment and ecosystems further disrupt long-standing viral transmission cycles as the behavior and range of the viruses' vector and reservoir species change. Since almost all flaviviruses are arboviruses, transmitted by mosquitoes and ticks, measures have been undertaken to decrease human exposure to the disease vectors, including extensive educational programs. The effectiveness of some of these measures is unknown. The vast campaign to contain West Nile virus in North America to New York City and the surrounding area appears to have been unsuccessful since the virus spread from coast to coast in the United States and southward and northward into Mexico and Canada in less than 5 years. We do not know, however, the extent to which this campaign mitigated the incidence of severe West Nile cases. Fortunately, while still a threat, the number of West Nile cases in much of North America peaked between 2003 and 2006. This is likely due to the decreased number of immunologically naïve human hosts resulting from herd immunity caused by large numbers of prior, asymptomatic cases.

Severe diseases caused by other flaviviruses, particularly dengue hemorrhagic fever and dengue shock syndrome, are continuing to spread as mosquitoes adapt to life in urban conditions (*Aedes aegypti*) and increase their range into more temperate zones (*Aedes albopictus*). Decreasing human exposure to mosquitoes and ticks should decrease disease incidence in humans. Large-scale, long-term elimination of these vector populations would, however, be extremely difficult. We have, however, had some significant successes in decreasing populations of disease-carrying mosquitoes. These successes include the dramatic reduction of yellow fever in Panama, which allowed the construction of the Panama Canal. Nevertheless, many areas that had substantially reduced mosquito populations are now seeing their return. Over a century ago, yellow fever was also virtually eliminated from the mainland of the United States, where it had previously occupied areas of the American South. These areas are still free of nontravel-related yellow fever.

FLAVIVIRUSES AND POTENTIAL ANIMAL RESERVOIR HOSTS
Flaviviruses in Bats

Bats have been suggested to be the original source of many viruses that are currently causing outbreaks in humans. Antibodies to several species of flaviviruses that are pathogenic to humans have been detected in bats, particularly in the Americas. A study conducted in Central and South America found that 20%–30% of the tested bats had neutralizing antibodies against dengue viruses 1–3 (DENV-1, DENV-2, and DENV-3).[1,2] All four DENV serotypes were present in Mexican bats. DENV has also been reported in Australian bats.[3]

In the northern United States, 1%–2% of big brown bats were seropositive for West Nile virus (WNV).[4] Several other North American bats are also seropositive for WNV. Antibodies to Saint Louis encephalitis (SLE) have also been found in about 9% of big and little brown bats.[5] SLE has also been isolated from Mexican free-tailed bats in Texas in the far south of the western United States. Neutralizing antibody was found in the sera of 20% of the tested bats.[6] In Trinidad, however, none of 14 tested species of bats ($n = 384$) were seropositive for WNV or SLE virus, another pathogenic flavivirus of humans found in North America.[7]

Flavivirus-seropositive bats have also been detected in Asia and Australia. Neutralizing antibodies against Japanese encephalitis virus (JEV) were found in the sera of 25% of the tested bats from southern China.[2,8] Viral RNA was not, however, detected in the brain of these animals. Five Australian flying foxes that were infected by exposure to JEV-infected *Culex annulirostris* mosquitoes remained asymptomatic and did not develop a detectable level of viremia.[9] Three species of Indian bats are also known to be seropositive for Kyasanur Forest disease virus.[2]

Flaviviruses and Rodents

In addition to bats, rodents have been implicated as major reservoir hosts for many microbes, including viruses. They have been, accordingly, the focus of a large amount of research in order to determine whether or not they are: (1) able to be infected with various types of viruses, (2) able to serve as competent hosts to pass the virus on to the virus' invertebrate vector, and (3) able to be used as sentinel animals to detect newly emerging human pathogens. Rodent species in most continents, to a greater or lesser degree, either have been reported to have flavivirus RNA in their tissues or are seropositive. Some of the tested rodents have close contact with humans in urban environments, while others have little contact with people. The former group is more likely to serve as important reservoirs of species of flavivirus that are or may become pathogenic to humans.

In North America, there is a paucity of pathogenic flaviviruses in rodent populations.

In Mexico, none of the rodent serum samples ($n = 708$) were positive for DENV-2, even though this virus is present in humans in the area.[10] While no Powassan flaviviruses have isolated from North American deer mice, they are seropositive for Powassan virus.[11]

In Europe, tickborne encephalitis virus (TBEV) was detected in six German rodent species: 13% of striped field mice, 8% of yellow-necked mice (8%), 29% of wood mice, 7% of field voles, 10% of common voles, and 13% of bank voles.[12] A study from Italy found that 4 of 90 yellow-necked mice from Italy were seropositive for WNV.[13] A study of 242 rodents and small mammals in Croatia, however, did not detect any flavivirus RNA.[14]

Several species of rodents are hosts to flaviviruses in Asia. In China, 46% of the tested brown and lesser ricefield rats ($n = 198$) were seropositive for anti-JEV IgG antibodies, but no viral RNA was found in the rodent brain samples.[15] In southern Vietnam, 5% of 275 tested rodents were seropositive for TBEV in an area in which 47% of 245 humans were positive.[16] TBEV RNA or E protein was present in 71% of the tested small mammals in Siberia, including northern red-backed voles, gray red-backed voles, northern bush mice, and striped field mice.[17]

In Africa, Usutu virus was isolated from two species of rodents in Senegal: the black rat and the multimammate mouse. Wesselsbron virus (WSLV) was isolated from a black rat in Senegal as well.[18,19]

Flaviviruses and Domestic Animals

In addition to adverse effects on humans throughout the world, some flaviviruses cause severe, life-threatening disease in animals, including birds, horses, and sheep. Some flaviviruses cause abortions in domestic animals, such as sheep and cattle. Other flaviviruses, however, use domestic animals as reservoirs or amplifying hosts. A meta-analysis found that only 4% of the tested bats were competent hosts for JEV, as opposed to 50% or more of the tested cattle, pigs, horses, donkeys, cats, and dogs.[20,21]

Due to our close interactions with our domestic animals, they may play a far greater role in zoonotic transmission of pathogenic flaviviruses than we realize. Agricultural animals, particularly cattle, as well as our companion animals, are known to be infected with several different flaviviruses. A study performed in Hungary found 27% of the tested cattle and 7% of the sheep, but no horses, were seropositive for TBEV.[22] TBEV is also excreted in the unpasteurized milk of goats, sheep, and cattle and is active for several days, even if refrigerated.[23] TBEV-FE has been isolated from dogs in Japan as well.[24] A high percentage of Australian cattle are seropositive for Murray Valley encephalitis virus.[25] Furthermore, serological evidence supports the presence of JEV antibody in 78% of the tested dogs, 52% of the cattle, 34% of the pigs, and 21% of the goats.[26] In a Malaysian survey, 80% of the dogs were seropositive for JEV, as well as 44% of the pigs, 32% of the cattle, and 16% of the cats.[27] In addition to causing disease in sheep and cattle, WSLV has been isolated from pigs, donkeys, camels, and horses in Africa.[28] A study of hunting dogs in southern Italy found serological evidence of Usutu virus in 13% of the tested animals as well.[29]

While some species of bats and rodents are infected with several flaviviruses that are pathogenic to humans, the number of flavivirus species and the incidence of infection in cattle and sheep are much greater than those found in bats or rodents. In light of the above information, perhaps more time and resources should be directed toward studying the risk of potentially pathogenic viruses using domestic animals as reservoir hosts.

PREPARATIONS FOR THE FUTURE

Once humans began to live in population centers that were large enough to allow sustained transmission of microbes from infected to immunologically naïve people, our species have been repeatedly hit by rounds of infectious disease outbreaks. Even the relatively slow methods of travel allowed the spread of infection to distant areas. However, with the discovery of compounds such as sulfa drugs and antibiotics and their increasing availability to the general population, humans began to curb the number of infections and deaths from infectious diseases in most of the developed world. Childhood diseases were disappearing due to the development of effective vaccines. During the late 1970s, a victory over infectious diseases, particularly over bacterial and parasitic illnesses, was proclaimed by many in the medical field as we began to increase our focus on preventing and treating other diseases, including those affecting the cardiovascular and respiratory systems, cancers, diabetes, and obesity.

Unfortunately, our proclamation of victory was premature as bacteria, including staphylococci and the *Mycobacterium* species responsible for tuberculosis, and parasites, such as the causative agents of malaria, became drug-resistant. Viruses, such as HIV, and influenza and Ebola viruses, are also not susceptible to antibiotics. The rapid rate of mutation of RNA viruses complicates the development of effective vaccines and drugs, making it very difficult to adequately prepare for large outbreaks of new strains of viruses as well as the emergence or reemergence of other viruses. The politicians and general population often fail to grasp the difficulty in the fight against viral infection. Many of the methods that had worked so successfully against bacterial infections for decades do not always work against viral infections. Other types of responses need to be developed to detect and mitigate outbreaks of viral diseases. This is especially important due to the rising number of our elderly population as well as the increased number of immunocompromised people, including those being treated for autoimmune conditions or cancer, those with respiratory or cardiovascular conditions, diabetics, and the obese.

To prepare more adequately for the next viral pandemic(s), we need to develop more broad-spectrum antiviral drugs in the same manner as we had previously developed different types of antibiotics. The process of producing antiviral compounds and vaccines will be much more difficult, however, given the rapid rate of mutation of some viruses and the tendency of antiviral drugs to produce serious side effects. We need to continue to repurpose older drugs as well. We also need to detect the emergence of new viral threats or the reemergence of older viruses to give ourselves the time in which to respond and curtail the spread of these diseases. Monitoring the potential for zoonotic transmission of newly emerging viruses or the spread or increased pathogenicity of neglected viruses could buy us this valuable time. While future viral pandemics are inevitable, we may then be better prepared to stop their spread and to treat them.

CANDIDATES FOR THE NEXT PANDEMIC?

Other mosquito-borne flaviviruses are also able to at least occasionally infect humans asymptomatically or may produce febrile disease that is usually self-resolving. The following flaviviruses are present in Australia or New Guinea: New Mapoon, Torres, Fitzroy, Edge Hill, Sepik, and Alfuy viruses. Infection with Edge Hill, Sepik, and Alfuy viruses may result in a mild, febrile illness. The following flaviviruses are from Africa: Bainyik, Koutango, Uganda S (including Banzi), Ntaya, and Spondweni viruses. Of these, Uganda S, Ntaya, and Spondweni viruses may cause a febrile illness. Ntaya virus may also cause headache, myalgia, and rigors. Spondweni virus is closely related to Zika virus, and infection may asymptomatic; mild and febrile; or cause headache, nausea, muscle and joint pain, conjunctivitis, and rash. It is also found in some Caribbean islands, including Puerto Rico and Haiti. In Asia, other neglected mosquito-borne flaviviruses include ThCAr virus.

Other tickborne flaviviruses may cause mild to severe illness as well. These include the nonpathogenic Gadgets Gulley virus from Australia and Kadam virus from Africa and the Middle East. Royal Farm (Karshi) virus from Afghanistan may cause a febrile illness, and Langat virus from Asia may cause Siberian fever and encephalitis. Two newly discovered members of the Flaviviridae family from China, the Alongshan and Jingmen tick viruses, while not from the flavivirus genus, cause mild, febrile disease in China.[30,31]

The above listed viruses are only some of the flaviviruses that may pose serious threats to humans if they increase their pathogenicity. Flaviviruses from other animals, especially our agricultural animals, also may at some point gain the ability to transition into new hosts, including humans. We need to remain vigilant in our monitoring of these and other microbes, but not panic. We need to carefully balance our safety and responsibility to our most vulnerable people against our economic and mental health needs as well as our personal liberties and the overall health of human societies. It is a difficult balancing act, but one that we have faced in the past and will continue to do in the future.

REFERENCES

1. Platt KB, Mangiafico JA, Rocha OJ, et al. Detection of dengue virus neutralizing antibodies in bats from Costa Rica and Ecuador. *J Med Entomol.* 2000;37(6):965–967.
2. Beltz LA. Other RNA viruses and bats. In: *Bats and Human Health: Ebola, SARS, Rabies, and Beyond.* Wiley-Blackwell; 2018:158–180.
3. O'Connor J, Rowan L, Lawrence J. Relationships between the flying fox (genus *Pteropus*) and arthropod-borne fevers of North Queensland. *Nature.* 1955;176:472.

4. Bunde JM, Heske EJ, Mateus-Pinilla NE, Hofmann JE, Novak RJ. A survey for West Nile virus in bats from Illinois. *J Wildlife Dis.* 2006;42(2):455–458.

5. Herbold JR, Heuschele WP, Berry RL, Parsons MA. Reservoir of St. Louis encephalitis virus in Ohio bats. *J Am Vet Res.* 1983;44:1889–1893.

6. Allen R, Taylor SK, Sulkin SE. Studies of arthropod-borne virus infections in Chiroptera. 8. Evidence of natural St. Louis encephalitis virus infection in bats. *Am J Trop Med Hyg.* 1970;19(5):851–859.

7. Thompson NN, Auguste AJ, da Rosa APAT, et al. Seroepidemiology of selected alphaviruses and flaviviruses in bats in Trinidad. *Zoonoses Public Health.* 2015;62(1):53–60.

8. Cui J, Counor D, Shen D, et al. Detection of Japanese encephalitis virus antibodies in bats in Southern China. *Am J Trop Med Hyg.* 2008;78(6):1007–1011.

9. van den Hurk AF, Smith CS, Field HE, et al. Transmission of Japanese encephalitis virus from the black flying fox, *Pteropus alecto*, to *Culex annulirostris* mosquitoes, despite the absence of detectable viremia. *Am J Trop Med Hyg.* 2009;81(3):457–462.

10. Sotomayor-Bonilla J, García-Suárez O, Cigarroa-Toledo N. Survey of mosquito-borne flaviviruses in the Cuitzmala River Basin, Mexico: do they circulate in rodents and bats? *Trop Med Health.* 2018;46:35.

11. Mlera L, Bloom ME. The role of mammalian reservoir hosts in tick-borne flavivirus biology. *Front Cell Infect Microbiol.* 2018;8:298.

12. Achazi K, Růžek D, Donoso-Mantke O. Rodents as sentinels for the prevalence of tick-borne encephalitis virus. *Vector Borne Zoonotic Dis.* 2011;11(6):641–647.

13. Cosseddu GM, Sozio G, Valleriani F. Serological survey of hantavirus and flavivirus among wild rodents in Central Italy. *Vector Borne Zoonotic Dis.* 2017;17(11):777–779.

14. Tadin A, Tokarz F, Markotić A, et al. Molecular survey of zoonotic agents in rodents and other small mammals in Croatia. *Am J Trop Med Hyg.* 2016;94(2):466–473.

15. Chen S-W, Jiang L-N, Zhong X-S, et al. Serological prevalence against Japanese encephalitis virus-serocomplex flaviviruses in commensal and field rodents in South China. *Vector Borne Zoonotic Dis.* 2016;16(12):777–780.

16. Van Cuong N, Carrique-Mas J, Be HV. Rodents and risk in the Mekong Delta of Vietnam: seroprevalence of selected zoonotic viruses in rodents and humans. *Vector Borne Zoonotic Dis.* 2015;15(1):65–72.

17. Bakhvalova VN, Chicherina GS. Tick-borne encephalitis virus diversity in Ixodid ticks and small mammals in South-Western Siberia, Russia. *Vector Borne Zoonotic Dis.* 2016;16(8):541–549.

18. Diagne MM, Faye M, Faye O, et al. Emergence of Wesselsbron virus among black rat and humans in Eastern Senegal in 2013. *One Health.* 2017;3:23–28.

19. Diagne MM, Ndione MHD, Di Paola N, et al. Usutu virus isolated from rodents in Senegal. *Viruses.* 2019;11(2):181.

20. Oliveira ARS, Strathe E, Etcheverry L, et al. Assessment of data on vector and host competence for Japanese encephalitis virus: a systematic review of the literature. *Prev Vet Med.* 2018;154:71–89.

21. Oliveira ARS, Cohnstaedt LW, Strathe E, et al. Meta-analyses of the proportion of Japanese encephalitis virus infection in vectors and vertebrate hosts. *Parasit Vectors.* 2017;10:418.

22. Sikutová S, Hornok S, Hubálek Z, Dolezálková I, Juricová Z, Rudolf I. Serological survey of domestic animals for tick-borne encephalitis and Bhanja viruses in northeastern Hungary. *Vet Microbiol.* 2009;135(3–4):267–271.

23. Wallenhammar A, Lindqvist R, Asghar N, et al. Revealing new tick-borne encephalitis virus foci by screening antibodies in sheep milk. *Parasit Vectors.* 2020;13(1):185.

24. Yoshii K. Epidemiology and pathological mechanisms of tick-borne encephalitis. *J Vet Med Sci.* 2019;81(3):343–347.

25. Liehne CG, Stanley NF, Alpers MP, Paul S, Liehne PF, Chan KH. Ord River arboviruses—serological epidemiology. *Aust J Exp Biol Med Sci.* 1976;54(5):505–512.

26. Angami K, Chakravarty SK, Das MS, Chakraborty MS, Mukherjee KK. Seroepidemiological study of Japanese encephalitis in Dimapur, Nagaland. *J Commun Dis.* 1989;21(2):87–95.

27. Kumar K, Arshad SS, Selvarajah GT, et al. Prevalence and risk factors of Japanese encephalitis virus (JEV) in livestock and companion animal in high-risk areas in Malaysia. *Trop Anim Health Prod.* 2018;50(4):741–752.

28. Wang Z-D, Wang W, Wang NN, et al. Prevalence of the emerging novel Alongshan virus infection in sheep and cattle in Inner Mongolia, northeastern China. *Parasit Vectors.* 2019;12:450.

29. Montagnaro S, Piantedosi D, Ciarcia R, et al. Serological evidence of mosquito-borne flaviviruses circulation in hunting dogs in Campania region, Italy. *Vector Borne Zoonotic Dis.* 2019;19(2):142–147.

30. Zhang X, Wang N, Wang Z, Liu Q. The discovery of segmented flaviviruses: implications for viral emergence. *Curr Opin Virol.* 2020;40:11–18.

31. Wang Z-D, Wang B, Wei F, et al. A new segmented virus associated with human febrile illness in China. *N Engl J Med.* 2019;380:2116–2125.

Abbreviations

25HC	25-hydroxycholesterol
ADE	antibody-dependent enhancement
AHF	Alkhurma hemorrhagic fever
AHFV	Alkhurma hemorrhagic fever virus
AKT	also known as protein kinase B
ALT	alanine transaminase
AMPK	adenosine monophosphate-activated protein kinase
ATF	activating transcription factor 4
ATK	autologous tumor killing
ATP	adenosine triphosphate
BANK1	B-cell adaptor protein with ankyrin repeats
BBB	blood–brain barrier
Bcl	B-cell lymphoma
BCR	B-cell receptor
BIK	BCL2-interacting killer
BMEC	brain microvascular endothelial cells
BMP	bis(monoacylglycero)phosphate
βPIX	PAK-interacting guanine nucleotide exchange factor
BST2	bone marrow stromal antigen 2
BTG2	B-cell translocation antigen 2
CARD	caspase activation and recruitment domain
CAV	caveolin
CCL	C–C motif ligand
CCR	CC-chemokine receptor
CD	complementary determinant
CDC	Centers for Disease Control and Prevention
CDK	cyclin-dependent kinase
CLU	clusterin
CNS	central nervous system
COL	colicinogenic
COX	cyclooxidase
C protein	capsid protein
CREB1	cAMP-responsive element binding protein 1
CSF	cerebral spinal fluid
CT scan	X-ray computed tomography
CTCF	CCCTC-binding factor
CXCL	C–X–C motif chemokine
CXCR	CXC receptors
DAA	direct-acting antiviral
DC	dendritic cells
DC-SIGN	dendritic cell-specific ICAM3-grabbing nonintegrin
DEET	N,N-diethyl-m-toluamide
DENV	dengue virus
DF	dengue fever
DHF	dengue hemorrhagic fever
DHODH	dihydroorotate dehydrogenase
DMP	dimethyl phthalate
dsRNA	double-stranded RNA
DSS	dengue shock syndrome
DTV	deer tick virus
ECOP	EGFR-coamplified and -overexpressed protein
EGCG	epigallocatechin gallate
eIF	elongation initiation factor
EMC	essential mixed cryoglobulinemia
Eomes	eomesodermin
E protein	envelope protein
ER	endoplasmic reticulum
FBP1	fructose-bisphosphatase 1
FcR	Fc receptor
G3PB	GAP SH3 domain-binding protein
GATA3	GATA-binding protein
GBS	Guillain–Barré syndrome
G-CSF	granulocyte colony-stimulating factor
GTP	guanosine triphosphate
GSK3β	glycogen synthase kinase 3β
HCV	hepatitis C virus
HLA	human leukocyte antigen
HI antibodies	hemagglutination-inhibiting antibodies
HMG-CoA	3-hydroxy-3-methyl-glutaryl-coenzyme A
HMGB-1	high-mobility group box-1
ICAM	intercellular adhesion molecule
IC_{50}	dose at which 50% of inhibition occurs
ID_{50}	dose at which 50% infection is obtained
IDO-1	indoleamine 2,3-dioxygenase 1
IFI44	interferon-induced protein 44
IFIT	IFN-induced proteins with tetratricopeptide repeats
IFITM	interferon-inducible transmembrane protein
IFN	interferon
IFNAR	interferon-alpha receptor

IFT	intraflagellar transport	NLRP3	NLR family pyrin domain containing 3
Ig	immunoglobulin		
IKK	inhibitor of κB kinase	NF-κB	nuclear factor κ of B cells
IL	interleukin	NK cell	natural killer cell
IL-1RA	IL-1 receptor antagonist	NPC1L1	Niemann–Pick C1-Like 1 cholesterol uptake receptor
ILHV	Ilhéus virus		
Imd	immune deficiency	OSM	osmotic avoidance abnormal
IMPDH	IMP dehydrogenase	NO	nitric oxide
IMP	inhibitors of metalloproteinase	NOD	nucleotide-binding oligomerization
iNOS	inducible nitric oxide synthase		
IP	interferon gamma-induced protein	NOX	NADPH oxidase
IPS-1	IFN-β promoter stimulator 1	NS proteins	nonstructural proteins
IRF	interferon regulatory factor	NTPase	nucleotide triphosphatase
ISG	interferon-stimulated gene	OAS	2′,5′-oligoadenylate synthase
ISGF3	interferon stimulating gene factor 3	OASIS	old astrocyte specifically induced substance
ITIM	immunoreceptor tyrosine-based inhibition motif		
		OSM	oncostatin M
JAM-A	junctional adhesion molecule A	PABPC1	polyadenylate-binding protein 1
JEV	Japanese encephalitis virus	PBMC	peripheral blood mononuclear cells
JNK	Janus kinase		
KFD	Kyasanur Forest disease	pDC	plasmacytoid dendritic cells
KFDV	Kyasanur Forest disease virus	PGE	prostaglandin
KOKV	Kokobera virus	PKC	protein kinase C
LARP1	La-related protein 1	PKG	protein kinase G
LD_{50}	dose at which 50% of the subjects die	PKR	protein kinase regulated by double-stranded RNA
LDL	low-density lipoprotein	PIK3CG	phosphatidylinositol-4,5-bisphosphate 3-kinase catalytic subunit gamma
LGP2	laboratory of genetics and physiology 2		
LIV	louping ill virus	PI3K	phosphatidylinositol 3 kinase
LMNA	laminin A/C	POWV	Powassan virus
MAIT	mucosal-associated invariant T	PPARα	peroxisome proliferator-activated receptor α
MAPK	mitogen-activated protein kinases		
MAVS	mitochondrial antiviral signaling protein	prM	precursor to membrane protein
		Rac1	Ras-related C3 botulinum toxin substrate 1
MBL	mannose-binding lectin		
MCP	macrophage chemotactic protein	RAG1	recombination-activating gene 1
MDA5	melanoma differentiation-associated gene 5	RANTES	regulated upon activation, normal T cell expressed, and secreted
mDC	monocyte-derived dendritic cells		
MHC	major histocompatibility complex	RdRp	RNA-dependent RNA-polymerase
MIF	migration inhibitory factor	RER	rough endoplasmic reticulum
MIP-1	macrophage inflammatory protein 1	RHOH	Ras homolog gene family, member H
miRNA	microRNA		
MLLT	myeloid/lymphoid or mixed-lineage	RIG-I	retinoic acid-inducible gene-I
MMP	matrix-degrading metalloproteinase	RLR	retinoic acid-inducible gene-I (RIG-I)-like receptor
M protein	membrane protein	RNA interference	EGFR-coamplified and -overexpressed protein
MRI	magnetic resonance imaging		
MTase	methyltransferase	ROCV	Rocio virus
mTOR	mechanistic target of rapamycin	ROS	reactive oxygen species
MVE	Murray Valley encephalitis	RSAD2	radical S-adenosyl methionine domains containing 2
MVEV	Murray Valley encephalitis virus		
MX1, MX2	MX Dynamin Like GTPase 1	RSSE	Russian spring–summer encephalitis
NCR	natural cytotoxicity receptor		
NDGA	nordihydroguaiaretic acid	RT-PCR	reverse transcription–polymerase chain reaction

RyDEN	Repressor of yield of DENV
SAMR	sterile alpha and HEAT/Armadillo motif; Myd88-5
SCID	severe combined immunodeficiency
SESTD	SEC14 and spectrin domain
sfRNA	subgenomic flavivirus RNA
SFV	Semliki Forest virus
SIAH	seven in absentia homolog
sIL-6R	soluble IL-6 receptor
siRNA	small interfering RNA
SLC	solute carrier
SLEV	Saint Louis encephalitis virus
SNP	single-nucleotide polymorphisms
SOCS3	suppressor of cytokine signaling 3
SREBP	sterol regulatory element binding protein
SSEV	Spanish sheep encephalitis virus
STAT1 and STAT2	signal transducer and activator of transcription
sTNFR	soluble TNF receptor
STING	stimulator of interferon genes
STRV	Stratford virus
SVR	sustained virologic response
TAB	TAK1-binding protein
TAK	transforming growth factor-β-activated kinase
TAM	Tyro3, Axl, and Mertk
TBE	tick-borne encephalitis
T-bet	T-box expressed in T cells
TBEV	tick-borne encephalitis virus
TBEV-Blk	TBEV-Bikalian
TBEV-Eur	tick-borne encephalitis virus—European
TBEV-FE	tick-borne encephalitis virus—Far East
TBEV-Sib	tick-borne encephalitis virus—Siberia

TBK1	TANK-binding kinase 1
$TCID_{50}$	dose at which 50% of the tissue culture cells are infected
TGF-β	transforming growth factor-β
Th	T-helper cells
TIAR	TIA-1-related protein
TIM-1	T cell/transmembrane, immunoglobin, and mucin gene family-1
TNF	tumor necrosis factor
TNF-R1	tumor necrosis factor receptor 1
TLR	Toll-like receptor
TRAIL	tumor necrosis factor-related apoptosis-inducing ligand
TRIF	Toll interleukin-1 receptor domain-containing adaptor inducing IFN-β
Treg	T regulatory cells
TRIM	tripartite motif
TSE	Turkish sheep encephalitis
UFR	unfolded protein response
uPA	urokinase plasminogen activator
UPR	unfolded protein response
USUV	Usutu virus
UTR	untranslated region
V-CAM	vascular cell adhesion molecule-1
VDLV	very low density lipoproteins
VEGF	vascular endothelial growth factor
Vipirin	virus inhibitory protein endoplasmic reticulum associated interferon inducible
viRNA	virus-derived small interfering RNA
WHO	World Health Organization
WNV	West Nile virus
YFV	yellow fever virus
ZIKV	Zika virus

Index

Note: Page numbers followed by *f* indicate figures and *t* indicate tables.

Printed and bound by CPI Group (UK) Ltd, Croydon, CR0 4YY

03/10/2024

01040300-0020